TREASURY
OF HOME REMEDIES

TREASURY OF HOME REMEDIES

Myra Cameron

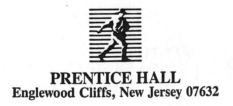

PRENTICE HALL
Englewood Cliffs, New Jersey 07632

Prentice-Hall International, Inc., *London*
Prentice-Hall of Australia, Pty. Ltd., *Sydney*
Prentice-Hall Canada, Inc., *Toronto*
Prentice-Hall of India Private Ltd., *New Delhi*
Prentice-Hall of Japan, Inc., *Tokyo*
Prentice-Hall of Southeast Asia Pte. Ltd., *Singapore*
Editora Prentice-Hall do Brasil Ltda., *Rio de Janeiro*
Prentice-Hall Hispanoamericana, S.A., *Mexico*

© 1987 *by*

PRENTICE-HALL, INC.
Englewood Cliffs, N.J.

10 9 8 7 6 5 4 3

Library of Congress Cataloging-in-Publication Data

Cameron, Myra.
  Treasury of home remedies.

  Bibliography: p.
  Includes index.
    1. Herbs—Therapeutic use.   2. Medicine—Formulae,
receipts, prescriptions. 3. Folk medicine—Formulae,
receipts, prescriptions. 4. Therapeutics, Physiological.
I. Title.
RM666.H33C36   1987   615.8′82   87-17553

ISBN 0-13-930637-4

ISBN 0-13-930645-5 {PBK}

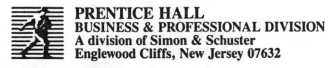

PRENTICE HALL
BUSINESS & PROFESSIONAL DIVISION
A division of Simon & Schuster
Englewood Cliffs, New Jersey 07632

Printed in the United States of America

Other books by Myra Cameron:

HOME-STYLE MICROWAVE COOKING

THE G.N.C. GOURMET VITAMIN COOKBOOK

PREFACE

Many of our mortal miseries can be prevented or successfully treated with natural remedies that may seem miraculous in our drug-oriented society. But this is not a collection of miracle cures to supplant or compete with necessary medical care. It is a "they say" book of options—an up-to-date distillation of the health wisdom of the ages.

There are nostrums from ancient Egyptian and Oriental physicians, medicine men and folk healers throughout the world, folklore from the Middle Ages, and common-sense cures from both Colonial and contemporary America. There is information shared by research scientists, biochemists, and nutritionists who have established the effectiveness of helping the body help itself through diet and supplements. Reputable orthomolecular physicians have expanded orthodox medicine by publicizing their successes in using vitamins and minerals to correct the cause of maladies and preserve or restore health without drugs or surgery. Holistic doctors and trained professionals have gone even further by including relaxation techniques, nerve massage, and nerve pressure in treating the whole person.

All of this material has been condensed into a comprehensive health manual with maladies and mishaps, and their remedies, arranged alphabetically. The efforts and accomplishments of those who provided the material from which this compendium was compiled are deeply appreciated. Crediting the sources for individual statements and remedies would create an impossibly bulky volume, so they are listed numerically in the Bibliography and referred to by number at the conclusion of each segment.

By definition, any treatment not generally accepted by the medical establishment qualifies as folk medicine and would, therefore, cover practically all natural remedies. For convenience, however, each type of natural remedy is explained in the Introduction and grouped accordingly as remedies for each ailment. Everything required is available in supermarkets or health food stores and can be self-applied with the explicit instructions.

Too much of anything—food, massage, vitamins, or even water—can be hazardous. Although all of the suggestions have been reported to be harmless when used as directed for temporary remedies, allergic reactions have been known to occur in response to any substance. The current practice of enriching numerous processed foods and beverages with a full day's requirement of the major vitamins and minerals should be taken into account before massive amounts of any of the fat-soluble vitamins are taken therapeutically.

Each remedy has proven effective in some instances and has been passed along with the goal of assisting others. Because of individual biological differences, not every remedy can be expected to be successful for every person, but there are many options for experimentation. In addition to after-the-fact remedies, there are countless tips for avoiding disease and discomfort as well as augmenting conventional medical treatment. It is hoped that this compendium will not only be of benefit but also be as fascinating to read as it was to compile.

Myra Cameron

CONTENTS

INTRODUCTION
TO NATURAL THERAPIES

DIET AND SUPPLEMENTS

For normally healthy people, governmental guidelines suggest less sugar, salt, meat, and fat; more fish and poultry; and more complex carbohydrates in the form of fruits, vegetables, and whole grains. Many nutritional experts stress the importance of eating a wide variety of natural foods while reducing or avoiding the intake of those that have been refined or processed. When maladies do attack, either from internal chemical imbalance or external sources, dietary alterations or restrictions may be necessary. Specific foods, vitamins, and minerals can act as medicines, often remedying the situation as effectively as drugs, and strengthen the body so that there is no recurrence. If medication or other treatment has been prescribed, no drastic change in either diet or supplements should be undertaken without medical approval.

Whenever feasible, obtaining vitamins and minerals from natural foodstuffs is preferred because of the as yet unidentified trace elements that may be included. In most cases, the large amounts needed for medicinal purposes make this impractical. For instance, acquiring enough vitamin C to squelch an incipient cold would require eating 15 oranges each hour for a day or two. Supplements, even in mega-doses, do not take the place of food. During any illness, a nourishing diet is essential to recovery. Some foods, such as acidophilus yogurt, serve a dual role. A wholesome food at any time, it is frequently advised as an accompaniment to antibiotics to counteract the destruction of helpful intestinal flora along with the harmful bacteria. For those who are not fond of yogurt, the beneficial acidophilus may be taken in capsules.

Precise amounts of vitamins and minerals for therapeutic use depend on existing deficiencies, body weight, and individual tolerance. Unless suggested as combinations, remedies should be experimented with one at a time and, when both minimum and maximum amounts are given, beginning with the lower dosage is recommended. If there is an adverse reaction to any supplement, a change of brands may solve the problem. (Milk sugar or other possibly allergenic substances are sometimes used in binding the nutrients into tablets.) Fat-soluble vitamins A, D, E, and K are stored in the body between doses but the remainder of the vitamins and minerals are water soluble. They are considered more effective when taken in two or more divided doses each day since any excess is flushed out of the body within a few hours.

1

Only a few of the 30-some essential minerals are used therapeutically. Chelated (chemically bonded to amino acids) minerals are advised as they are absorbed more efficiently and rapidly than other organic minerals or inorganic mineral compounds. Unless otherwise indicated, all the supplements are better assimilated when accompanied by food.

Vitamin A (Retinol, Carotene)

Although taking excessive amounts of vitamin A over long periods of time can cause unpleasant symptoms (which disappear in adults when the vitamin is discontinued), there have been fewer than 150 cases of chronic hypervitaminosis A in recorded medical history. Two-thirds of those were children given over 300,000 International Units daily. The others were adults who subsisted on polar bear liver, drank a gallon of carrot juice each day, or experimented with from 150,000 to 1 million units daily for many months.[4] According to Dr. Roger Williams[347], an adult would have to consume over 1,000 capsules a day to get a dangerous amount. Natural vitamin A (from fish liver) is less likely to cause disturbances than synthetic vitamin A. Carotene (a substance found in carrots, other vegetables and fruits, and now available as beta carotene capsules) is converted to vitamin A within the body. While an excess can cause temporary yellowing of the skin, it is not believed to create vitamin-A toxicity. To assure absorption, 1,000 IU of natural vitamin D plus 30 IU of vitamin E should be taken with each 10,000 units of vitamin A.[110,188] At least 15 milligrams of zinc per day are needed for mobilization of the vitamin A reserves in the liver.

Amino Acids

The body requires 22 of these organic compounds in order to synthesize the human protein vital to life. Eight of the amino acids must be supplied by diet but the remainder can be produced in the body. All the essential amino acids must be present simultaneously and in the proper proportions because they all are reduced to equal the one that is lowest or missing. Most meat and dairy products (termed "complete proteins") provide all of these amino acids, with eggs being the most perfectly balanced. Most vegetables, grains, and fruits are lacking in one or more and are considered "incomplete proteins." Judicious food combining can rectify these deficiencies for vegetarians. A number of the amino acids are available as individual supplements for therapeutic use.

Arginine
Asparic Acid
Cysteine
Cystine
Glutamine
Histidine
Isoleucine
Lysine
Methionine
Ornithine

Phenylalanine (should be taken as a supplement only under the supervision of a
   physician in cases of high blood pressure or pre-existing cancer)
Taurine
Threonine
Valine

Antioxidants (Antiradicals)

Supplements can help the body defend itself against self-produced oxidation or free radicals acquired from radiation or chemicals in the air, food, or water. When not controlled by antioxidants, the incomplete molecules of free radicals can cross-link in an involved chemical process to instigate practically any malady from arthritis to varicose veins, and are prime suspects in cancer and heart disease. The principal antioxidants are vitamins A, B-2, B-3 (niacin), B-5 (panthothenic acid), B-6, PABA, inositol, C and the bioflavonoids, E; the amino acids arginine, cysteine, and ornithine; the minerals selenium and zinc; and SOD (superoxide dismutase). Foods with antioxidant properties are bananas, grapes, and other fruits, celery, eggs, potatoes; and the seasonings, cloves, oregano, rosemary, sage, and vanilla.

B Complex

None of the B vitamins has been found toxic but they are so interrelated in function that large doses of any one of them may possibly cause a deficiency of the others. A daily tablet of the complete B complex is recommended whenever individual B vitamins are used therapeutically. Potencies range from 2 to 100 milligrams of each of the major B vitamins, with anything over 25 milligrams considered "high potency." Only recently available in the United States, B-15 is seldom included in the comprehensive supplements. The controversial Laetrile (B-17) is not present in either combination formulas or in brewer's yeast.

B-1   = Thiamine
B-2   = Riboflavin (once called vitamin G)
B-3   = Niacin—Nicotinic Acid (natural forms which often produce flushing),
        or Niacinamide—Nicotinamide (synthetic forms which have the vi-
        tamin effect of niacin without the flushing but are not effective for acne,
        cholesterol lowering, or migraine headaches). When taken in massive
        amounts, niacin may require "buffering" with milk, calcium tablets, or
        a bit of baking soda in order to prevent stomach irritation.
B-5   = Pantothenic Acid or Calcium Pantothenate
B-6   = Pyridoxine
B-9   = Folic Acid or Folacin (once called vitamin M)
B-12 = Cobalamin or Cyanocobalamin
B-13 = Orotic Acid or Calcium Orotate
B-15 = Pangamic Acid, Calcium Pangamate, or Dimethylglycine
Biotin = Co-enzyme R (once called vitamin H)
Choline

Inositol
PABA = Para-aminobenzoic Acid

Bioflavonoids (Citrus Bioflavonoids, Hesperidin, Quercetin, Rutin)

Found in apricots, black currants, blackberries, buckwheat, cherries, grapes, and the pulp and rind of citrus fruits, bioflavonoids are also available as supplements. Water-soluble and nontoxic, they were originally called vitamin P but are now regarded as part of the vitamin C complex. In addition to their own therapeutic properties, bioflavonoids increase the assimilation and effectiveness of vitamin C. Many authorities recommend that 100 milligrams of bioflavonids be taken with each 500 milligrams of vitamin C.

Brewer's Yeast (Nonleavening, Nutritional Yeast)

A composite of highly' concentrated nutrients, brewer's yeast once was a byproduct of beer making but now is "primary grown" (usually on molasses) for a food supplement. It provides complete protein containing 19 amino acids plus all the major B vitamins and 18 or more minerals. Available in flakes, powder, or tablets, the powdered form is the most potent. One or two tablespoons of brewer's yeast stirred into a glass of juice or milk may be used in place of, or to augment, a daily B-complex tablet. It is considered both an "energy food" and a remedy for certain ailments. Besides being the best natural source of chromium, it assists in the assimilation of chromium supplements. Beginning with no more than one teaspoonful per day and gradually increasing the dosage usually prevents any problems with intestinal gas.

Vitamin C (Ascorbic Acid)

According to Linus Pauling[251] and other vitamin-C experts, cost is the only difference between the natural and synthetic supplements. Both have the same beneficial effects. Vitamin C is nontoxic and water-soluble—as much as 20,000 milligrams has been taken daily for 25 years without adverse side effects. Early reports stating that vitamin C destroys vitamin B-12 and/or causes kidney stones have been proven incorrect.[7] Individual tolerance levels (usually indicated by intestinal gas or diarrhea) often can be extended by accompanying the vitamin C with bioflavonoids, B-6 and magnesium, calcium tablets, food, or milk. Those with digestive problems may need to take their vitamin C in the form of calcium ascorbate or sodium ascorbate, or accompany each dose with one-fourth teaspoon baking soda to neutralize the acid.

Smokers should allow 25 additional milligrams of vitamin C for each cigarette smoked. Aspirin also destroys vitamin C in the body. The level of vitamin C in the blood peaks two or three hours after ingestion, then decreases as this water-soluble vitamin is excreted. (The vitamin C "wasted" in the urine is believed to prevent intestinal polyps, kidney stones, and urinary infections.) Resistance to infection is determined by the lowest rather than the average concentration of vitamin C in the blood and tissues. It is estimated that 1,000 milligrams of vitamin C taken in four doses of 250 milligrams each throughout the day is as effective as 2,000 milligrams taken all at once.

When massive amounts of vitamin C are taken for a few days, body metabolism makes appropriate adjustments so it is wise to decrease the dosage gradually in order to avoid a "rebound effect" and susceptibility to disease.

Calcium

Calcium supplements are indicated for a variety of maladies. Clinical studies have shown that "average" adults absorb only 10 to 15 percent of the 400 milligrams of calcium they consume daily. Since the body requires at least 800 milligrams of calcium per day for nerve health as well as bone and teeth preservation, the negative balance can mount up to create an assortment of problems.[8]

In order to function, calcium must be accompanied by vitamins A, C, and D, and be balanced with approximately twice as much phosphorus and half as much magnesium. Some authorities feel the ratio of phosphorus should be as high as 5:2, others believe it should be lowered to 1,100 milligrams of phosphorus for each 1,000 milligrams of calcium.[194] (One cup of milk supplies 291 milligrams of calcium, 228 milligrams of phosphorus, and 33 milligrams of magnesium.)

Calcium gluconate, Calcium lactate, and Calcium orotate are easily absorbed, natural derivatives of calcium. Oyster shell calcium, which has been filtered through the oyster's body, is considered exceptionally pure. Bone meal contains calcium carbonate (also derived from limestone) plus phosphorus and other minerals. (Beef has 22 times as much phosphorus as calcium—bone meal has only half as much phosphorus as calcium, so helps serve as a balance.[261]) Bone Ash is not recommended as a food supplement. It is manufactured by burning the bones, which destroys organic matter.[78] For convenience, calcium supplements prebalanced with the necessary vitamins and minerals are available.

Taking some form of acid (vitamin C or a teaspoon of apple cider vinegar in a glass of water) with the calcium increases its absorption, but taking calcium with an alcoholic beverage reduces its assimilation. Physical inactivity leads to calcium loss; mild but consistent exercise helps maintain calcium-nutrient balance.

Chromium

Only about 3 percent of dietary chromium is converted into the biologically active form of GTF (Glucose Tolerance Factor) and the percentage decreases with age. Accompanying chromium supplements with brewer's yeast increases the chromium absorption.

Vitamin D (Ergosterol, Calciferol, Viosterol)

Natural vitamin D from fish liver oils is preferred and is best utilized when taken with vitamin A. The official RDA of 400 IU resulted from cases of infantile hypervitaminosis D in Great Britain following the supplementation of babies' milk with 2,000 IU of synthetic vitamin D daily. These synthetic forms, calciferol or ergosterol [D-2 and D-3] differ structurally from natural vitamin D and are considerably more toxic.[183,260] Excess amounts of this fat-soluble vitamin are stored in the liver. Continued use of large amounts of vitamin D can produce toxicity—1,000 IU daily is considered the upper limit of safety for infants—but over 5,000 IU of natural vitamin D have been taken daily by adults over long periods of time with no symptoms of overdosage.[89,189]

Vitamin E (Tocopherol)

Caution: Those with diabetes, heart disease, high blood pressure, or an overactive thyroid should take no more than 30 to 100 IU daily for six weeks, then gradually increase the amounts as body tolerance rises. Those who have had rheumatic heart disease should never take more than 50 to 100 IU daily.

Natural vitamin E (indicated by "d" rather than "dl") should be taken with meals containing fat. "Dry" vitamin E is suggested for those allergic to wheat since the oil-based vitamin usually has a wheat-germ-oil base. The vitamin E in many multivitamin formulas is "used up" by the synthetic vitamins A and D they contain. Inorganic iron taken within eight or ten hours of a vitamin E supplements inhibits its absorption.

Alpha tocopherol is the most potent form of this vitamin but many authorities believe there are advantages in including the other seven tocopherols. For instance, if 600 IUs of vitamin E are indicated, 400 IUs of alpha tocopherol could be taken in the morning and 200 IUs of mixed tocopherols in the evening. Taking 25 micrograms of selenium with each 200 IUs of vitamin E increases its effectiveness.

Vitamin F (Unsaturated Fatty Acids)—Arachidonic, Linoleic, and Linolenic

Vitamin F cannot be manufactured within the body but is necessary for many bodily functions. The best sources of these "essential fatty acids" are cold-pressed vegetable oils such as corn, peanut, safflower, soybean, sunflower, and wheat germ. (Olive oil contains little linoleic acid; neither coconut nor palm oil have any.) These oils may be eaten on salads, in foods, or taken in capsules. They should be kept refrigerated to prevent rancidity, which nullifies their beneficial effects, as does high heat and exposure to air. According to many nutritionists, at least 10 IU of vitamin E should be taken for each tablespoon of unsaturated oil ingested to prevent its oxidation within the body. Vitamin F is best absorbed when taken with vitamin E at mealtimes.

Iron

Very little of the iron used to enrich or fortify processed foods is absorbed by the body—less than 1 percent according to a study reported in *The American Journal of Clinical Nutrition* [February, 1977]. But the need for supplemental iron is better determined by a physician on the basis of a blood test. When overdoses are chronic, the extra iron can build up to toxic levels, since, other than through bleeding, the body has no way to dispose of significant amounts of excess iron.

Iron supplements should be taken only as directed and should be combined with an organic compound as in ferrous citrate, ferrous fumarate, ferrous gluconate, or ferrous peptonate. The iron in these forms, or in foods, does not interfere with the absorption of vitamin E as does the inorganic ferric phosphate or ferric sulfate, but most authorities suggest that supplements of iron and vitamin E be taken eight to 10 hours apart. Drinking large amounts of coffee or tea inhibits iron absorption. Taking 500 to 1,000 milligrams of vitamin C with each meal or iron supplement has been shown to increase iron absorption by as much as 50 percent.[282]

Lecithin

A combination of unsaturated fatty acids, choline, inositol, and phosphorus, lecithin is a component of all body cells and tissues. It is made by the body, is present in foods such as corn, egg yolks, or unsaturated vegetable oils, but is most concentrated in soybeans. Soy lecithin is available in capsules, granules, liquid, or powder. (One tablespoon of liquid or granules equals 10 1,200-milligram capsules.) When using large amounts of lecithin, calcium and magnesium should be increased to balance its phosphorus content.

Magnesium

An overbalance of calcium can crowd out the magnesium since they share a single system of bodily transportation and assimilation. The ideal proportions are a two-to-one ratio of calcium to magnesium. Dolomite supplies this combination, or separate tablets of magnesium may be used with calcium supplements. Principal food sources of magnesium are nuts, seeds, and uncooked green vegetables. Magnesium is more effective when taken with adequate protein plus vitamins B-6, C, and D. Some authorities suggest that magnesium supplements be taken between rather than with or after meals since this mineral tends to neutralize stomach acids.[228]

Selenium

Once considered a possibly harmful supplement, selenium has been shown to have antioxidant properties, increases the effectiveness of vitamin E, and to be of value in correcting many maladies. Minute amounts—not more than 250 micrograms per day—are the most that are required. The best natural sources of selenium are bran, broccoli, onions, tomatoes, tuna, and wheat germ.

Tissue Salts (Biochemical Cell Salts)

These 12 inorganic mineral components of the body's tissues were isolated by a German doctor, Wilhelm H. Schuessler, in the 1870s and have been used with success in both Europe and America. The natural minerals are finely ground and mixed with milk sugar by a process called "trituration," then molded into tiny tablets that can be dissolved under the tongue for instant assimilation. [Only microscopic amounts of the cell salts are contained in the tablets so they should be taken as directed for specific maladies and not as a substitute for mineral supplements.] Therapeutic effectiveness is believed to be increased by the tremendous reduction. The most generally useful potency is 6X, a dilution of 1 to 1 million. The 3X potency indicates a dilution of 1 to 1,000. Dosages range from one to five tablets taken at frequent intervals.

The 12 tissue salts are available in health food stores or through mail-order homeopathic or vitamin suppliers. They are nontoxic, nonhabit-forming, and may be taken alone or with each other without side effects.[165]

Calc. Fluor. = Calcarea Flurica = Calcium Fluoride = Fluoride of Lime
Calc. Phos. = Calcarea Phosphorica = Calcium Phosphate = Phosphate of Lime.
Calc. Sulph. = Calcarea Sulphurica = Calcium Sulphate = Sulphate of Lime
Ferr. Phos. = Ferrum Phosphoricum = Iron Phosphate
Kali. Mur. = Kali Muriaticum = Potassium Chloride = Chloride of Potash
Kali. Phos. = Kali Phosphoricum = Potassium Phosphate = Phosphate of Potash
Kali. Sulph. = Kali Sulphuricum = Potassium Sulphate = Sulphate of Potash
Mag. Phos. = Magnesia Phosphorica = Magnesium Phosphate
Nat. Mur. = Natrum Muriaticum = Sodium Chloride = Chloride of Soda
Nat. Phos. = Natrum Phosphoricum = Sodium Phosphate = Phosphate of Soda
Nat. Sulph. = Natrum Sulphuricum = Sodium Sulphate = Sulphate of Soda
Silicea = Silicon Oxide or Dioxide = Silicic Acid

Zinc

Not established as an essential nutrient until 1934, zinc's therapeutic importance seems to have been acknowledged in direct proportion to the soil depletion and general deficiency of this mineral. In order to be efficiently absorbed, zinc should be taken with vitamins B-6 and E.

FOLK REMEDIES

A number of ancient folk remedies have received medical sanction. Others have been found to have a scientific basis. Some have been handed down through the generations simply because they work. The remedies listed require only easily available ingredients. The herbs and spices can be purchased as teas, pulled from the spice rack, or found in supermarkets along with the foodstuffs called for. Possibly harmful or illegal substances such as Indian hemp (marijuana) or laudanum (opium) have been bypassed, along with exotic plants and ground unicorn horns. Quantities and instructions have been adapted for modern usage, and contemporary folk-medicine suggestions included.

NERVE MASSAGE (Reflexology, Reflex Balance, or Zone Therapy)

Believed to have originated in China, nerve massage was used by African natives as well as some American Indian tribes. Utilized by natural healers in the United States during the 1930s, its popularity has increased since the 1960s. Related in theory to acupuncture, nerve massage is based on the premise that invisible nerve currents run throughout the body in longitudinal lines or zones, with their nerve endings easily accessible in the feet and hands. Every malady is thought to indicate maladjustment of the intricate balance within the body. Massage of a specific area is used to release nervous energy to the respective organ, balance the body's electromagnetic field, and restore normalcy.

Unless otherwise indicated, the designated area should be rubbed once each day until a tender button of concentrated crystals is felt, then massaged for a minute or two. Trained reflexologists have recorded amazing curative results. As suggested in this book, self-applied nerve massage is merely for symptomatic relief but may help the body's self-healing mechanism do its job more efficiently. Only moderate pressure is required and, when applied to others, a very gentle touch should be used with the very young or the very old.

NERVE PRESSURE (Acupressure, Finger Pressure, or Shiatsu)

An ancient Oriental therapy now becoming better known in the United States, "shiatsu" means "finger pressure" in Japanese. It is similar to both acupuncture and nerve massage in that it is thought that there are various points on the body (possibly far removed from the part that sustains the malady) which, when stimulated, bring about beneficial results. Called "meridian paths," most of the points are the same as those used in acupuncture, but a few seconds of firm pressure replaces the use of needles. Recent studies theorize that pressure on specific points may trigger the release of a type of endorphin that blocks pain. (Endorphin, "the morphine within," is a natural painkiller released by the brain.) Impressive cures have been reported by advanced practitioners but, as used in this compendium, self-applied nerve pressure is for symptomatic relief only. Experts suggest finger pressure of from 5 to 15 pounds and recommend practicing on a bathroom scale to judge the amount of finger force required. Less pressure should be used for infants and the elderly.

RELAXATION TECHNIQUES AND POSITIVE THINKING

The interrelationship of mind and body has been recognized for thousands of years. Many methods of "mind over matter" therapy have been used to aid the healthy in staying well or contribute to recovery from illness. As the Stoic philosophers stated, "Man is troubled not by things, but by the view he takes of them."

Studies show that a stressed, nervous person is more susceptible to pain. Psychological stress and tension are such all-pervasive threats that scientists have assigned values to vast numbers of stressful events. They believe that the more "points" amassed, the greater the likelihood of physical illness. Both catastrophic and joyful events, as well as daily aggravations, contribute to the ever-accumulating total. Brief daily periods of relaxation have been shown to reduce this accumulation and activate the endorphin-releasing mechanisms of the brain. (Endorphins are natural painkillers that block pain in the same manner as morphine.) According to some experts, even two minutes of slow, deep breathing will discharge the effects of immediate stress.

From 5,000-year-old yoga to progressive relaxation, transcendental meditation and biofeedback clinics; from autogenic training and mind control to psychocybernetics—all operate on the theory that physical relaxation is the state in which the body can best begin to heal itself, and that the human brain can transmit the idea of wellness into the cell tissues of the body so that disease can give way to healthy tissue. Tests have indicated that there is no one "best" method. It is a matter of individual compatibility. All are equally effective when performed with patience and persistence. Detailed instructions for each technique of self-induced relaxation and positive thinking are available in books and on tapes, but the basic patterns are quite similar and remarkably simple.

Sit comfortably or recline in a quiet room with eyes closed. Tense, then consciously relax all the muscles. Begin with the feet and move up through the legs, torso, arms, neck, and face. Concentrate on breathing deeply while either repeating one number or word (called a "mantra") or counting down from 10 to one, with one number for each exhalation. Imagining descending a staircase deeper and deeper into an area of relaxation may increase the effect.

The object is to relax the mind as well as the body. Absence of thought, not profound ruminations about the nature of the universe, is the goal of this type of meditation. Random thoughts should be dismissed rather than pursued. Outside distractions can be minimized by thinking, "External sounds do not matter." Visualizing a peaceful scene and/or thinking, "I am calm and serene" may enhance the effectiveness.

After continuing this for two to 20 minutes, reverse the procedure by slowly counting up from one to five. Open the eyes, then yawn and stretch. Daily practice makes it possible to accomplish complete relaxation merely by closing the eyes and concentrating on deep breathing for a few seconds while in an office or on public transportation.

Making positive self-suggestions while in this relaxed state can be beneficial, particularly when reinforced by visual imagery. For instance, thinking, "My sinuses are cool," and visualizing the nasal passages returning to normal may help reduce congestion in that region. Painful muscles or joints may be relieved by imagining lying on a beach, covering the painful areas with warm sand, listening to the sound of the ocean, smelling the fresh breeze, feeling the warmth of the sun, and thinking how wonderful it is to be comfortable and pain-free. Any malady may be treated in a similar manner to augment natural or orthodox remedies.

Auto-suggestion or self-hypnosis is quite different from the antics of stage hypnotists and their subjects. There is no loss of consciousness and no technical knowledge of anatomical details or biochemical functions is required. Simply visualizing the area of discomfort and then mentally painting it with white light has been effective in many instances.

Daily practice combined with pleasant imagery and brief, positive statements are the key to this form of relaxation and internal communication. Even generalizations such as: "The pain is fading," or "When I open my eyes I will feel refreshed and alert," have been found to be helpful.

ACNE (Acne Vulgaris and Acne Rosacea or Spider Veins)—See Also Eczema and Psoriasis

Acne vulgaris, the scourge of teenagers, usually appears during adolescence as a result of temporary hormonal imbalances complicated by dietary deficiencies and/or indiscretions. A waxy substance secreted by the sebaceous gland plugs up channels leading to the skin surface, creating visible little lumps called "comedones." If the lump remains closed, it is a "whitehead." If it opens and is oxidized to a dark color, it is a "blackhead." If it ruptures and spreads into the surrounding skin, pimples or abscesses may form and there may be permanent scarring—particularly if the pustules are squeezed. Medical attention may be required for severe acne, but natural remedies have proven successful in many cases.

Acne rosacea, called "grog blossoms" in colonial times, is a malady of the middle-aged. Also instigated by nutritional deficiencies and hormone changes, a red flush or visible veins (spider veins) radiating out from a central point appear in the outer layers of the skin around the nose and cheeks. Tiny pimples may develop on the flushed areas, but there are few blackheads and no danger of scarring. Occasionally, an overgrowth of nose tissue may create the bulbous, red appearance associated with chronic alcoholism.

The standard treatment calls for a bland diet and the elimination of alcoholic or caffeine-containing beverages. Orthomolecular physicians and nutritionally oriented dermatologists attribute these conspicuous veins to a deficiency of B vitamins (especially B-2), and have reported consistent success when a B-complex tablet plus one or two tablespoons of brewer's yeast and 25 milligrams of B-2 were taken daily. Improvement has been noticeable within one month and may be speeded by taking 1,000 milligrams of vitamin C with 400 to 800 milligrams of bioflavonoids, plus a multivitamin-mineral tablet containing at least 15 milligrams of zinc each day.

All types of acne benefit from gentle but thorough cleansing, an adequate diet, mild exercise without excessive perspiration, and sufficient relaxation and sleep. Acne that does not respond to natural remedies may be due to allergies. If avoiding commercial cosmetic preparations and processed foods containing chemical additives does not correct the problem, allergy tests may be necessary.

Diet and Supplements

Although there is considerable disagreement about the significance of diet as a causative factor in acne, the "half rations" prescription of the 1800s has borne the test of time. A calorically reduced natural diet accentuating fresh fruits, vegetables, and whole grains while avoiding refined sugar, saturated fats and fried foods, chocolate, alcohol, and anything containing caffeine or artificial coloring and flavoring has eliminated acne problems in many cases. Raw or juice-packed canned fruits plus small amounts of honey or molasses can be used to allay the craving for sweets. Carob powder can serve as a substitute for chocolate or cocoa. Low-fat or skim milk can replace whole milk. Two daily glasses of vegetable juices (carrot, cucumber, lettuce, or spinach—in any combination but with carrot juice predominating) have been reported to improve acne within a few weeks.[152,243] Herbal teas specified for acne by folk healers are: comfrey root, dandelion, red clover, strawberry leaf.

Dietary supplements have long been used for prevention and/or treatment of acne.

Vitamin A—10,000 to 25,000 units once or twice each day (under medical supervision, up to 100,000 units daily). The dry form of vitamin A should be used if fats are eliminated from the diet.

Acidophilus—One or two capsules or a serving of acidophilus yogurt with each meal. Helpful for all types of acne, acidophilus is of particular importance if antibiotics have been prescribed as part of the treatment.

B Complex—One comprehensive tablet daily plus up to 300 milligrams each of B-6, niacin, and/or pantothenic acid in divided doses each day. Vitamin B-6 is especially effective for acne that flares up during menstrual periods.

Brewer's Yeast—One to two tablespoons (or the equivalent in tablets) daily have cleared many cases of acne. Combining the yeast therapy with dessicated liver and B-complex tablets has been more effective for others.

Vitamin C—1,000 to 3,000 milligrams (preferably with 200 to 1,000 milligrams of bioflavonoids) in two or three divided doses each day.

Calcium—When milk and dairy products are restricted in order to avoid fats, calcium supplements of one or two dolomite and/or bone meal tablets are recommended to avoid calcium deficiency and the nervous tension that may help instigate acne.

Charcoal—Taking two tablets (not bits of charcoal briquettes) after each meal for two weeks, then two tablets daily have accomplished astounding results in clinical tests.[151]

Vitamin E (see Caution, page 6)—100 to 800 IU daily. (The dry form should be used when fats are severely restricted.) Vitamin E protects vitamin A from destruction within the body and helps prevent vitamin-A toxicity. When the two are taken in combination, dramatic improvement in teenage acne has been reported.

Vitamin F—One to two tablespoons (or the equivalent in capsules) of cold-pressed vegetable oil. Animal fats may make acne worse but small amounts of polyunsaturated oils are believed to help the skin combat acne.

Tissue Salts—Three tablets of 6X Calc. Phos. three or four times daily is the suggested remedy for adolescent acne. If the skin is red and blotchy: alternate doses of Calc. Sulph., Kali. Sulph., and Silicea may be added. If accompanied by inflammation of the skin: Ferr. Phos. and Nat. Phos. should be included. When acne is slow to heal, Nat. Sulph. may be of benefit.

Zinc—50 milligrams, one to three times daily. Considered the best modern remedy for acne, tests reported in the *British Journal of Dermatology* in 1977 showed that 135 milligrams of zinc per day were more effective than tetracycline (the then-favored prescription for acne). Other tests have shown spectacular results when zinc therapy was combined with vitamin A and E supplementation.

Facial Cleansing and Masques

Scrupulous cleansing is a vital constituent of acne treatment. Gently washing the face with mild soap and warm water two to four times daily is the most generally accepted method. For those who would rather not use soap, optional washing liquids are milk, diluted lemon juice, or a solution of one part alcohol to 10 parts warm water. The face should be thoroughly rinsed with warm water and patted dry, not vigorously toweled. Washing with buttermilk and blotting the face without rinsing was an old folk remedy, as was rubbing the affected area with lemon juice or fresh garlic several times a day to speed the healing of existing pimples. Warm, double-strength papaya-mint tea has been used as an emergency treatment for acne eruptions. Other foods to apply to the cleansed skin as facial masques for 30 minutes before rinsing off with lukewarm water are:

Carrots—Cook in as little water as possible, then mash and apply when comfortably cool.
Cucumber—Peel if coated with wax. Slice very thin and soak in rum, or simply grate before applying.
Egg Yolk—Whisk and pat over the skin.
Oatmeal—Cook in milk until thickened, then cool and apply.

Another option is to apply a paste of baking soda mixed with water, rinse immediately with water, then follow with a rinse or spray of apple cider vinegar and water. Add a final clear-water rinse.

Modern folk medicine suggests covering the freshly washed and dried skin with the oil from a vitamin E capsule. After 30 minutes, a coating of lightly whisked egg white should be applied and allowed to remain for another 30 minutes before being rinsed off with plain water. An overnight masque said to dry the skin without irritation can be made by diluting liquid hand soap or shampoo with water and patting it onto the face after washing and rinsing.

Case History

Gordy W. was a straight-A student who had been looking forward to his first week in high school. His schedule was in his new notebook, his books were in his assigned locker, and the first "zit" on his previously unblemished face did not deter his enthusiasm. The second and third "zits," however, destroyed his self-confidence. With "Best Looking" printed beneath his picture in the junior-high-school annual, Gordy was not about to put up with a "Hey, Pimples" designation. He knew his mother could not afford an expensive dermatologist; so Gordy arranged for a job as a carry-out boy, and told his mother that he wanted to quit school and go to work. She countered with a suggestion for clearing his incipient acne with the natural remedies she had read about —they should be worth a try if they would allow him to continue his studies and attain his goal of becoming a lawyer. Gordy agreed to give it a shot. He washed his face with pure white soap, and rinsed it thoroughly, each morning and again when he came home from school. Following the nighttime washing and rinsing, he patted a bit of the soft white soap on each eruption and allowed it to remain overnight. Gordy also took the multiple-vitamins and the 30-milligram zinc tablet his mother proffered with his morning juice—and he swore off his favorite chocolate bars in exchange for the carob treats she concocted. Their combined efforts were successful. Gordy, smooth-faced and handsome as ever, went on to college to acquire his degree and later became a trial lawyer.

Light

Sunlight, or a sunlamp, can aid self-help acne treatment. Exposure to ultraviolet or infrared light should be carefully monitored to prevent deep burns or a leathery, wrinkled skin. An alternative is to use a plain 60-watt light bulb in an unshielded lamp base to help dry up pimples and oozing skin.

Nerve Pressure

Stimulating any or all of the following points once each day is believed to bring relief from acne. Each point should be pressed and released three times for 10 seconds each.

- On each shoulder, press the outer edge of the hollow just beneath the collarbone.
- Bend the left arm at a 45-degree angle. Use the right thumb to press the point where the elbow crease ends on the outer arm. Repeat with the right arm.
- Clench the left fist, leaving the thumb extended against the index finger. With the right thumb, press the highest point of the mound formed between the thumb and index finger. Repeat with the other hand.
- On both legs, press a point on the inner thigh 2 inches above and 2 inches to the inside of the center of the knee.

Sources (See Bibliography in Back of Book)

6, 13, 22, 52, 53, 61, 62, 68, 81, 82, 83, 84, 88, 89, 92, 119, 128, 152, 165, 168, 169, 174, 211, 213, 228, 243, 254, 260, 261, 291, 312, 315, 318, 335, 353.

ALLERGY (See Also Hay Fever)

The word allergy means "altered reaction"—an unusual sensitivity to a substance or circumstance that is harmless for most people. While occasionally present in primitive areas, allergy is steadily becoming more prevalent in "civilized" societies as more and more potentially allergenic substances are introduced into the environment. Sometimes referred to as a backfiring of the body's protective system, allergy may manifest itself as an obvious mishap such as breaking out with a rash after eating strawberries (see Eczema—Hives), or becoming sneezy and itchy-eyed when in the same room with a bouquet of roses (see Hay Fever). Delayed or cyclical allergic reactions may masquerade as practically any malady: arthritis, asthma, bronchitis, canker sores, diarrhea, heart irregularity, migraine headache, etc.

The offending factor, called an allergen, may be anything from animal dander, chemicals, cosmetics, drugs, foods, or house dust to emotional stress or temperature fluctuations. After a medical examination has ruled out the possibility of physical causes, identifying combinations of subtle allergens requires considerable self-detective work—especially since the symptoms usually appear only after a second exposure.

Inhaled substances are considered the most frequent cause of allergy but food allergies have beset mortals since earliest recorded times. The much-used expression, "One man's meat is another man's poison," is paraphrased from the statement made by Lucretius in the first century B.C., "What is food for some may be fierce poison for others." The same method used today for building up a tolerance for food allergens was described in the Babylonian Talmud.

Chief offenders among foodstuffs are artificial colorings and preservatives, chocolate, citrus fruits, corn, cow's milk, peanuts, peas, tomatoes, and wheat. The first step in self-testing is to avoid all these foods for two or three weeks. If the allergic symptoms disappear, the foods may be reintroduced, one at a time at two-day intervals, until the culprit is identified. Any food can cause allergic reactions for certain individuals. If this first test does not bring relief, other favorite, frequently eaten foods should be eliminated on a trial basis. (A compulsion for a specific food can be similar to drug addiction. The craving is not only for the "high" but also for protection from withdrawal symptoms.) If the isolated allergens cannot conveniently be avoided, it may be possible to build up a tolerance by eating a miniscule amount of the food each day and gradually increasing the amount over a period of weeks or months (i.e., two grains of wheat or one-eighth teaspoon cooked egg per day).

Temperature extremes, indoors or out, may be unsuspected allergens. Statistics indicate that cold allergy is more common in children, heat allergy in adults. To test for a reaction to cold: place an ice cube on the skin for a minute or two—if a red, inflamed area or hives develop, a cold allergy is indicated. Heat allergy is confirmed if definite hives develop after the hand is soaked in 100-degree water for a few minutes. If either heat or cold are recognizable allergens, the treatment consists of desensitization by careful exposure. Tub baths are the most convenient home method. Begin with body-temperature water and increase or decrease the water temperature a degree weekly (using a thermometer) until relatively hot or cold baths can be tolerated without a reaction.

There are a number of other natural remedies for all types of allergies.

Acidophilus—Two capsules or a serving of acidophilus yogurt with each meal have often alleviated both mouth sores and intestinal tract disturbances instigated by allergies.

Case History

When Thelma R. moved to Arizona from Oklahoma she was so thrilled about having orange and grapefruit trees in her own backyard that she juiced oranges for breakfast and ate grapefruit as a before-dinner appetizer every day. She noticed a burning sensation in her mouth but hoped it would go away as her system adapted to the fresh fruit. However, after a week of this regimen her mouth and tongue became so sore and inflamed she had to stop using any of the citrus. Thelma offered the grapefruit and oranges to a neighbor, and explained why she could not use them herself. The neighbor was appreciative but suggested that Thelma try taking acidophilus capsules or eating yogurt with each meal before she gave away the fruit she enjoyed so much. This simple remedy worked like a charm. Thelma took two acidophilus capsules with her morning juice, ate yogurt with her lunch, took two more acidophilis capsules at dinner time—and indulged in as much citrus as she wanted without any mouth irritation.

Apple Cider Vinegar and Honey—One or two teaspoons of each stirred into a glass of water and sipped with each meal has relieved allergic reactions for many people.

Bee Pollen—One teaspoon of granules or the equivalent in tablets daily. Bee pollen is a respiratory-strengthening food believed to prevent and correct allergic disturbances by elevating the gamma globulins and immune responses of the body.

Vitamin B-6—450 to 1,000 milligrams daily in divided doses. Clinical studies have shown this vitamin to be a vital factor in relieving maladaptive reactions to food and chemicals.[350] Chest congestion and wheezing due to allergy have shown improvement within a week and been cleared in less than a month when B-6 was taken in massive amounts. It is particularly effective in combination with vitamin C and pantothenic acid.

Vitamin C—300 to 10,000 milligrams daily in divided doses. Mild allergies have responded to the lesser amount of vitamin C but up to 1,000 milligrams per hour have been given for one or two days in severe cases.[89] It is most effective when taken before exposure to known or suspected allergens. The vitamin C acts as a detoxifying agent and antihistamine as well as improving the immune system's regulatory mechanism. Accompanying vitamin C with bioflavonoids increases its beneficial action. Taking at least 50 milligrams of B-6 with each massive dose of vitamin C is recommended both for allergy control and to avoid any possibility of kidney-stone development.

Vitamin E (see Caution, page 6)—100 to 800 IU daily. Research has shown that vitamin E has anti-allergenic properties and acts as an antihihistamine.[261] Vitamin E is more effective when taken before the irritation than after the allergic reaction has begun.

Garlic—One or two cloves of garlic, or the equivalent in capsules, each day are believed to destroy bacteria causing the absorption of histamines resulting in intestinal disturbances.

Pantothenic Acid—40 to 800 milligrams in divided doses daily. (Up to 6,000 milligrams under medical supervision.) Pantothenic acid stimulates both adrenal gland function and the production of cortisone within the body. The amount required to alleviate allergies varies with individual requirements. It is more efficient for allergy control when accompanied by vitamins B-6, C, and/ or brewer's yeast.

Sources (See Bibliography)

9, 13, 19, 39, 52, 66, 76, 89, 92, 128, 153, 156, 168, 171, 181, 205, 216, 229, 258, 261, 270, 288, 297, 312, 315, 327, 330, 350, 353.

ANEMIA

Anemia occurs when there is an insufficient number of able-bodied red blood cells to carry the oxygen required by the body. It can be caused by anything from loss of blood or poor nutrition to the location of the ancestral homeland or reactions to medications. An insufficiency of any of the amino acids can produce anemia as may deficiencies of vitamins B-3, B-6, B-12, C, E, folic acid, pantothenic acid, or the minerals copper and zinc. Iron-deficiency anemia (tired blood), the most well-known form, is common among menstruating women. It is becoming more prevalent in all those who subsist on a modern diet of highly refined foods. An adequate amount of iron is necessary in order for red blood cells to be produced and to function, but, because of the many forms of anemia, it can appear or continue even when ample iron is supplied. Anemia can be treated most efficiently when the particular type is determined by a blood test.

Hemolytic Anemia (Vitamin-E Deficiency Anemia)—A lack of vitamin E can cause the premature breakdown of red blood cells. Some premature babies have this type of anemia. They usually respond to 75 to 100 IU of vitamin E given daily in their formula. Adults may require 200 to 400 IU daily. (See Caution, page 6)

Megoblastic Anemia (Folic-Acid Deficiency Anemia)—A "large cell" anemia, it is common among children, pregnant women, and persons who have a high intake of refined foods, aspirin, or alcohol. Daily doses of from 250 micrograms to 5 milligrams of folic acid plus at least 500 milligrams of vitamin C have often corrected this form of anemia.

Pernicious Anemia (Vitamin B-12 Deficiency Anemia)—The absorption of B-12 through the stomach depends on an "intrinsic factor." Persons lacking this factor develop pernicious anemia. For most victims of this form of anemia, professional care and regular injections of B-12 are absolutely mandatory. If the anemia does not respond to the B-12 injections, the addition of oral folic-acid supplements may bring improvement. The book, *Life Extension*[252], states that the sugar-substitute, Sorbitol, taken with oral supplements of B-12 restores proper assimilation of the vitamin. (Ruth Winter's *Consumer's Dictionary of Food Additives* (Crown, 1978), however, warns that Sorbitol may alter the effect of other drugs and can cause gastrointestinal disturbances if used to excess.)

Sideroblastic Anemia (Vitamin B-6 Deficiency Anemia)—This type of anemia develops when both the number of red blood cells and the amount of hemoglobin are decreased. In many such cases, taking 100 milligrams of B-6 daily has proved more effective than any amount of supplemental iron. Adding a magnesium supplement is sometimes helpful as it tends to reduce the body's requirement for B-6.

Hereditary and Rare Anemias—These require specialized medical care. They include the hereditary sickle-cell, Mediterranean, and sperocytosis anemias as well as the rare aplastic, and G6PD—which is a discriminatory anemia that attacks only the males of a few nationalities.

As optional additions to professional diagnosis and prescribed medical treatment, the following natural remedies have been found beneficial.

Diet and Supplements

The body's production and maintenance of healthy red blood cells depends on adequate protein, vitamins, and minerals—including iron. Incorporating iron-rich foods in the diet is both prevention and treatment for anemia. Tests have shown that liver, kidneys, apricots, and eggs produce the most hemoglobin, but all meats, dried legumes, wheat germ, and whole grains are excellent sources of natural iron. Bananas contain folic acid and B-12 besides easily assimilable iron. Other iron-rich fruits are apples, dark grapes, raisins, and strawberries. Sunflower seeds contain almost as much iron as liver. Sesame seeds are another good source if used in sufficient amounts. Nutritionists recommend one or two daily glasses of any combination of the following fresh fruit and vegetable juices: apricot, beet, blueberry, carrot, celery, cucumber, parsley, prune, red grape, spinach. Parsley, beet greens, and spinach contain a lot of iron but much of it is held in insoluble compounds that cannot be absorbed. If excess amounts of spinach are eaten, the oxalic acid it contains can rob the body of calcium.

Phosphate additives used in baked goods, beer, candy, ice cream, soft drinks, and other foods reduce the absorption of iron. The inorganic iron used to enrich white flour and other processed foods is not absorbed as well as the organic iron present in natural foods. Coffee, tea, chocolate, and caffeine-containing soft drinks should be limited or avoided because caffeine interferes with iron absorption in the body. (Taking lemon or vitamin C with tea nullifies the action of its tannic acid, but the caffeine-effect remains.)

Vegetables contain a "nonheme" iron that is only one-sixth as absorbable as the "heme" iron in meats. Vitamin C and meat are the only two substances with the ability of increasing iron absorption. According to *Federation Proceedings* (June, 1977), studies showed the amount of iron absorbed from corn to be doubled when eaten with meat or fish. Adding 60 milligrams of vitamin C to the meal boosted iron absorption 500 percent. Cooking in cast-iron utensils increases the iron content of foods three or four times—with new iron pots contributing more than old ones. For use as sweeteners, both honey and blackstrap molasses are useful. Honey is rich in copper, which assists iron assimilation. One-third cup of blackstrap molasses contains more iron than a 3-ounce serving of liver, plus many of the minerals that help prevent and control anemia.

Case History

Judy S. was so tired all the time that she dragged through each work day and could no longer participate in the outdoor activities she had enjoyed. A medical examination had revealed that Judy was anemic, but the liver and iron pills prescribed by the doctor upset her stomach to such an extent that she took them only on weekends. A sympathetic friend suggested a home remedy that had been successful for her mother: Eat liver every day, and cook everything in a cast-iron skillet. Judy began the regimen enthusiastically. She liked liver and onions. After one week of nightly liver and onions, however, the dish had lost its appeal. Rather than give up, Judy delved into her cookbooks and resorted to ingenuity. Besides experimenting with the gourmet recipes, she simmered a whole liver in her iron skillet, thinly sliced part of it for sandwiches, and made "liver sausage" from the remainder by pureeing it in her food processor with boiled eggs and mayonnaise. On the days she could not "face" any more liver, Judy mixed a jar of baby-food liver with ground beef for patties or meatloaf. She even spread some of the baby food in a thin layer, froze it, and broke off tiny pieces to swallow like capsules. Several months later, Judy bumped into her sympathetic friend. In response to a query about how she was feeling, Judy responded, "Miserable." The friend was in the midst of regretful comments about her suggested remedy for anemia being ineffective when Judy interrupted. "My blood is fine," she said, "the anemia is gone—it's my shoulder that's bothering me. I twisted it while I was skiing last weekend."

B Complex—One comprehensive tablet daily, plus other B vitamins as indicated. Researchers in London found that 50 to 100 milligrams of B-2 per day increased the effectiveness of iron in raising low red-cell counts (*Proceedings of the Nutrition Society,* February, 1980). Injections of B-12 are required by those with pernicious anemia but others, particularly vegetarians, may benefit from daily oral doses of from 50 to 750 micrograms of B-12.

Bee Pollen—One teaspoon of pollen granules (or the equivalent in tablets) daily. Tests by French scientists showed that bee pollen serves as a biological stimulant to increase the content of hemoglobin and the red blood cells occurring in bone marrow.[328]

Vitamin C—500 to 1,500 milligrams daily to increase the absorption of iron.

Desiccated Liver—Available in either tablets or a powder to be stirred into foods or liquids by those who do not enjoy eating liver but want its benefits.

Iron—The treatment of iron-deficiency anemia usually requires therapeutic doses of iron in addition to a nutritious diet. Ferrous gluconate appears less likely to cause distress than ferrous sulfate, but either should be taken with vitamin C to increase absorption, and only as medically advised.

Tissue Salts—Three 6X-potency tablets three times a day of any or all of these three tissue salts are recommended:

- Calc. Phos.—believed to increase the number of red blood cells by nourishing the bone marrow.
- Calc. Sulph.—considered a blood purifier, it may help correct the gray, pasty-appearing skin sometimes associated with anemia.
- Ferr. Phos.—helps increase hemoglobin and is a constituent of red blood corpuscles.

Zinc—15 to 30 milligrams daily. Studies indicate that zinc is necessary for the utilization of B-12, and that its lack may contribute to anemia.

Folk Remedies

In ancient times, "physicians" would dip a sword in water or wine, then have the anemic patient drink the liquid to absorb the strength of the sword. Later, the folk-practitioner's treatment was to stick rusty nails into a sour apple, allow them to remain overnight, then remove the nails and have the anemic person eat the apple. Neither of these is recommended as a modern remedy because of the possibly harmful alloys included in present-day metals. Currently practical folk remedies include:

Apple Cider Vinegar—One teaspoonful stirred into a glass of water and sipped with each meal is believed to increase the amount of hemoglobin in the blood. Adding another teaspoon of vinegar plus two teaspoons of blackstrap molasses is said to cause iron to be assimilated when other forms are rejected by the body.[293]

Beet Juice—Thought to regenerate and reactivate red blood cells, the juice from fresh red beets has been a remedy for anemia since the Middle Ages.

Brandy Tonic—Steep 1 ounce each camomile tea leaves and ground orange peel with ½ teaspoon ground ginger in two cups boiling water. When cool, add ½ cup brandy. Take half a cupful several times each day.

Herbal Teas—Comfrey tea is suggested as a substitute for regular tea or coffee. It contains the anti-anemia vitamin, B-12, as well as four of the essential amino acids—including methionine, which most vegetables lack. Dandelion and fenugreek teas are other folk-medicine favorites for anemia.

Watercress—Eating a generous portion of watercress every day was believed to strengthen the blood. Modern analysis has shown watercress to contain easily assimilable enzymes, minerals, and vitamins.

Nerve Massage

A daily massage of the outer edge of the left hand between the base of the little finger and the wrist, and/or the outer edge of the underside of the left foot between the center of the arch and the little toe, is believed to help produce new red blood cells by stimulating the spleen and liver.

Nerve Pressure

Pressing each of these two points for 10 seconds, releasing for 10 seconds, and repeating for a total of 30-seconds pressure once each day is thought to increase the manufacture of red blood cells within the body.

- Press just under the base of the skull on each side of the spinal column.
- Hook the left index finger as far up as possible under the inside margin of the left rib cage, then press inward and upward.

Sources (See Bibliography)

3, 13, 23, 34, 44, 48, 51, 63, 76, 78, 82, 83, 88, 89, 98, 114, 133, 146, 151, 156, 165, 171, 172, 180, 184, 189, 190, 228, 243, 250, 252, 254, 255, 261, 281, 293, 315, 330, 349.

ARTHRITIS AND RHEUMATISM

One of the oldest of all maladies, arthritis has been found in the skeletons of dinosaurs and Neanderthal Man. Hieroglyphics depict Egyptians using hippopotamus fat to treat arthritic joints in 3000 B.C. In ancient Rome, those crippled with arthritis were exempt from paying taxes—an impractical system for the United States where it is estimated that at least one person out of seven suffers from arthritis.

The symptoms of arthritis and rheumatism are so similar that the terms have long been used interchangeably. Technically, "rheumatism" applies to disorders of the muscles, ligaments, and tendons with joint stiffness and soreness. "Arthritis" refers to actual inflammation of the joints resulting from destruction or wearing away of the cartilage which covers the ends of the bones at the joints. There are over 100 different types of arthritis. The two most common forms are osteoarthritis and rheumatoid arthritis. Known as degenerative or wear-and-tear arthritis, osteoarthritis usually develops in middle age and attacks the much-used joints of fingers, hips, knees, etc. Rheumatoid arthritis is a crippling type of joint disease that strikes at any age, may flit from one spot to another, and can affect the entire body.

Excess body weight aggravates joint distress, as does stair-climbing and slumping in overstuffed furniture. To take advantage of the healing value of rest, eight or nine hours in bed each night plus several daily rest periods of 15 to 30 minutes each are recommended. While not the cause of arthritis, emotional stress can trigger or aggravate the established disease. Utilizing some form of deliberate positive thinking or auto-suggestion (see pages 9-10) often serves to counteract the physical effects of mental upheaval. Daily exercise, stopped when the first sense of fatigue is felt, may arrest or improve arthritic problems. When a joint is not used for a period of time, it tends to "freeze" and the surrounding muscles may atrophy to make movement even more difficult. Exercising for 20 minutes a day while soaking in a tub of warm water reduces the pain of moving elbows and knees. Rolling an empty bottle back and forth across the floor with the feet whenever sitting and relaxing provides exercise for painful knees. An elastic bandage applied in a figure-eight may ease the pain of an arthritic knee. During cold weather, wearing 8-inch knitted cylinders over knees and elbows avoids aggravating the condition by chilling.

The confusion over terminology extends to the treatment—one person's "arthritic condition" may be another's "rheumatiz." Remedies recommended specifically for osteoarthritis, rheumatoid arthritis, or rheumatism are listed separately after the general suggestions, but all might bear investigation. If medications have been prescribed, the physician's approval should be obtained before making extensive alterations in food or vitamin intake.

Even though there is no one, simple cure, arthritis is not hopeless. Many different regimens have been used to alleviate or even reverse it. Nutritionally oriented physicians and biochemists agree that individual experimentation with various healthful diets and natural remedies, both old and new, is the key to its control. Most feel that arthritis causes sufficient body stress to justify a daily multiple-vitamin-mineral tablet in addition to any other supplements.

Diet and Supplements

Allergy may be the inciting factor for some cases of arthritis and may account for individual successes achieved with arthritis diets such as Dr. Dong's.[100] Avoiding all members of the Nightshade Family (eggplant, peppers, tomatoes, tobacco, white potatoes) has been the solution for many, particularly those with degenerative arthritis. More than just creating an allergic reaction, a substance called "solanine" contained in those plants can invade body cells to cause arthritic symptoms which may require from one month to one year of abstinence to correct. For quick relief, there is the much-publicized diet evolved by Ruth Stout (sister of author, Rex Stout) who cured her arthritic pains in 10 days by eating a healthful diet with the addition of one avocado, one banana, 12 pecan halves, one heaping teaspoon each of wheat germ and brewer's yeast, and taking several alfalfa tablets each day. Others have found surcease from painful joints simply by including generous servings of cabbage and onions with their daily menu.

Eating two or three cups of acidophilus yogurt every day has reportedly cleared arthritis resulting from low-grade infections of the intestines. The daily use of sprouted soybeans has relieved other cases of painful arthritis and rheumatism. Gouty arthritis usually necessitates limiting the purine-rich foods (see Gout) and, for some, eating at least one cup of cherries each day has brought relief. Celery, either raw or cooked, has been found to act as a neutralizing agent against uric acid, so is recommended for those with gouty arthritis.

For over 60 years, clinics in Switzerland have been treating arthritis with the Bircher-Bennet diet consisting of raw foods and fresh juices. Even with a normal diet, drinking one or two glasses of any combination of the raw juices from alfalfa, beets, carrots, celery, cucumbers, parsley, or potatoes has been found beneficial. Fresh pineapple juice contains an enzyme, bromelain, which is thought to reduce swelling and inflammation in arthritic joints when used regularly. According to several nutritionists, only small amounts of citrus juices should be used by those with arthritis, but other authorities recommend fresh grapefruit juice daily to help dissolve calcium deposits in the joints.

For most people, however, merely avoiding concentrated sweets and white sugar, coffee, tea, and alcohol (all of which can aggravate arthritis) and up-grading the diet with more whole grains, fresh fruits and vegetables, plus at least some of the optional supplements, produces beneficial results.

> **Vitamin A**—10,000 to 50,000 units daily. Vitamin A is particularly important for those who are taking cortisone, aspirin, or other anti-inflammatory drugs that increase the risk of infection and retard the healing of wounds. Painful heel

spurs have been relieved by taking 30,000 units of vitamin A plus several bone meal and/or dolomite tablets daily for one month.

Alfalfa—6 to 20 tablets daily. Besides Ms. Stout's astounding results with alfalfa tablets, others have reported that including alfalfa sprouts on the menu, eating three tablespoons of ground alfalfa seeds daily, or drinking four or five cups each day of a tea made from alfalfa seeds (with or without the contents of a ginseng capsule) has brought relief within two weeks.

Apple Cider Vinegar and Honey—A standard folk-remedy for arthritis is to sip with each meal a mixture of one or two teaspoons each apple cider vinegar and raw honey stirred into a glass of water.

B Complex—One comprehensive tablet daily plus optional, individual B vitamins. 50 to 100 milligrams of B-2 daily (up to 1,000 milligrams under medical supervision) have been found to accelerate the body's production of cortisone to combat arthritis. 300 to 4,000 milligrams of niacinamide (not the flush-producing niacin) have decreased pain and improved mobility with both degenerative and rheumatoid arthritis in less than two months. Beginning with 100 milligrams three times daily and gradually increasing the niacinamide to 1,000 milligrams per dose is suggested. (More massive supplementation should not be attempted without a doctor's approval.) Dr. Wright[353] suggests accompanying the niacinamide with 1,000 milligrams of vitamin C three times daily, and 2,000 IU of natural vitamin D taken twice each day. Some individuals require additional amounts of the complete B complex, especially B-1, B-6, folic acid, and B-12. After the condition is corrected, the niacinamide should be continued to prevent recurrence.

- 50 to 2,000 milligrams of PABA daily has produced good results in combatting stiffness. 150 to 1,000 milligrams of pantothenic acid each day stimulates the body's production of cortisone to alleviate all arthritic problems and is of particular benefit with the rheumatoid form. In *Let's Get Well*[89], Adelle Davis recommended a daily intake of 600 milligrams of pantothenic acid divided into six doses. She suggested taking it with milk and accompanying each dose with 500 milligrams of vitamin C. In addition to a high-protein diet and a calcium supplement, Ms. Davis also advised that 25,000 units of vitamin A, two B-complex tablets, 2,500 IU of natural vitamin D, and 100 IU of vitamin E be taken daily until definite improvement was noticed, then the amounts reduced by one-half for maintenance.

- Arthritic bone spurs have been corrected by injections of 1,000 micrograms of B-12 each day until the pain has been abolished. *Dr. Mandell's Lifetime Arthritis Relief System* (Coward-McCann, Inc., 1983) states that many cases of carpal-tunnel syndrome have shown improvement after taking 500 milligrams of B-6 three times a day for 12 weeks.

Barley Water—An old-fashioned cure for arthritis was to drink several cups of barley tea each day. It can be prepared in quantity (one cup of unhulled barley steeped for one hour in two quarts of boiling water) and refrigerated in a glass container.

Bee Pollen—One teaspoon of pollen granules (or the equivalent in tablets) daily for three to four months has brought improvement for many of those suffering from arthritis or rheumatism.[205]

Brandy and Rosemary—Steep two parts dried rosemary in three parts brandy in a closed container for five hours. Strain, then use the liquid to sponge the painful joints each morning. Once each week, take two tablespoons of the liquid internally.[201]

Brewer's Yeast—Stir two tablespoons Primary Grown brewer's yeast into a glass of juice or milk and drink with breakfast each morning.

Case History

Nora J. was so proud of her long fingernails that she protected them (and the surfaces they encountered) by utilizing the knuckles of her first two fingers for opening file cabinets at work and operating controls on kitchen appliances at home. By the time she was in her late forties these knuckles were becoming painfully stiff—justifiably so, said her physician as he explained the process of degenerative arthritis on overworked joints. Nora "accepted the inevitable" as the aching in her fingers spread to wrists, elbows, and shoulders; but she decided to try to prevent further "ravages of age" by following a friend's advice and stirring two tablespoons of brewer's yeast into her glass of juice at breakfast to avoid thinning hair and loss of stamina. After two weeks of this regimen, Nora could discern no perceptible improvement in either her hair or her energy level (both of which had always been excellent). She had, however, discovered the true meaning of "serendipity"—all the pain and stiffness in her joints had disappeared! It took several weeks of off-and-on experimentation to convince Nora that such a small amount of such a simple food supplement could perform such wonders, but Nora is now a confirmed brewer's yeast addict—an addict with flexible pain-free fingers.

Vitamin C—3,000 to 8,000 milligrams, plus 300 to 4,000 milligrams of bioflavonoids taken in divided doses daily. This combination, especially when taken with supplements of vitamin B-6, has relieved arthritic pain and improved joint mobility in many cases.

Calcium—500 to 2,250 milligrams daily. It has been found that calcium deficiency rather than excess calcium can be responsible for arthritic enlargement of joints and that the body's attempt to repair itself by withdrawing calcium from the skeleton can create the additional problem of osteoporosis. A survey conducted by *Prevention Magazine* several years ago revealed that over 46 percent of the almost 3,000 arthritic-pain sufferers participating had their pain either relieved or completely abolished by taking calcium. Providing the body with adequate calcium (plus good nutrition) has been shown to halt calcifying of the joints, prevent degeneration of the joint tissues, reduce or reverse the collection of fluid at these joints, and allay pain.

Cod Liver Oil—One capsule to two tablespoons three times daily. Another old-fashioned remedy that has borne the test of time, an experiment reported in the *Journal of the American Medical Association* (July, 1959), showed that taking one tablespoon of cod liver oil in a glass of warm milk twice a day before meals reduced arthritic tissue inflammation. A vitamin source as well as a joint lubricant, cod liver oil has relieved many forms of arthritic pain, particularly that of arthritic bone spurs.

Vitamin D—800 to 1,200 IU daily. Necessary to prevent the fragile, easily broken bones which can accompany arthritic conditions, the amount of vitamin D should be in proportion to the calcium intake—at least 400 IU of natural vitamin D for each 800 milligrams of calcium.

Vitamin E (See Caution, page 6)—100 to 1,000 IU daily. Vitamin E protects the essential fatty acids and vitamin A from destruction by oxygen within the body, helps stimulate cortisone production, and often reduces pain. When taken in combination with steroid therapy, it may be possible to reduce the amount of the drug by as much as one-third.

Herbal Teas—Teas made by steeping one teaspoonful of any of the following substances in one cup of boiling water have been used to soothe the pain of arthritis and contribute to the healing process: alfalfa leaf, buckthorn, camomile, celery seed, comfrey, corn silk, juniper berry, parsley, peppermint, rosemary, sage, sassafras, slippery elm, wintergreen.

Kelp—One to 10 tablets daily. This natural product of seaweed offers a mineral supplement believed especially beneficial for arthritis sufferers. Dr. Airola[12] recommends that an equal amount of bone meal tablets be taken with the kelp. Both are available in powdered form to incorporate with foods, and the kelp can serve as a salt replacement.

Sea Water—One teaspoon to three tablespoons daily of the bottled sea water available in health food stores. Its natural minerals have proven helpful to many arthritics.

Selenium—150 to 250 micrograms daily. Selenium's ability as a scavenger of free radicals (molecular fragments considered a contributory factor in arthritis) may account for its success in reducing inflammation and pain with both rheumatoid and osteoarthritis.

Tissue Salts—Taking one tablet of 3X Calc. Fluor. each morning and evening plus one tablet of 6X Silicea three times daily is believed to restore elasticity and strength to joints. If the condition has not improved within a few weeks, one 6X tablet of Nat. Phos. can be taken with each dose of the Silicea.

Yucca—One to three tablets, three times daily. This is a new-old remedy that has been successful for some arthritics.

Zinc—15 to 80 milligrams daily. Persons on cortisone therapy may require larger amounts (up to 650 milligrams daily) in order for wounds to heal. Zinc has been effective in relieving calcium deposits and spurs, but massive doses of zinc require a compensating increase in the calcium intake as the two minerals are antagonistic—and should be taken only under medical supervision.

Case History

Dorothy W., an enthusiastically energetic little woman of almost 70, became listless and depressed after a hospital stay for treatment of her bleeding ulcers.

She "rested" most of the time, could not walk more than a few steps because of her painful arthritis, and wept because she could not care for her ailing husband. Her physician offered to prescribe an antidepressant but Dorothy hesitated to add more drugs to those she was already taking for her arthritis. Instead, she made an appointment with a local nutritionist. The long list of suggested supplements appeared forbidding until the nutritionist explained that one mega-vitamin-mineral tablet contained most of the essentials, including 50 milligrams each of the B vitamins. The brewer's yeast could be stirred into her breakfast tomato juice; the calcium taken with her bedtime glass of milk; leaving only the lecithin capsule and 500-milligram vitamin C tablet to take with each meal, plus 200 IUs of vitamin E with her dinner. Dorothy faithfully followed instructions, began to feel like her old self within a few weeks, and, with her doctor's approval, gradually tapered off the arthritis medication. Her arthritic stiffness disappeared so completely that now she not only takes care of her husband, but does her own yardwork and actually dug the trenches and installed her own sprinkler system. Truly a new lease on life through natural remedies.

External Remedies
Applications

- **Cold**—A 20-minute application of ice three times a day may temporarily abolish arthritic pain and increase joint mobility, but it is important that the ice pack be removed as soon as the area has become numb. A flexible, reusable ice pack may be made by filling a sturdy plastic bag with a mixture of two-thirds water and one-third alcohol. When frozen, it will be slushy enough to conform to the joint and may be held in place with a turkish towel.
- **Liniments**

- For an old-fashioned remedy that can be made with bottled horseradish: liquefy one-half cup prepared horseradish in an electric blender, then mix with an equal amount of melted paraffin. Store in a covered jar at room temperature. Rub into the affected joint, bandage with a soft cloth, and leave on overnight. Rinse off with warm water. Repeat each night until the pain and swelling have subsided.
- Combine one-third cup dry mustard with an equal amount of table salt. Stir in enough melted paraffin to make a thick cream, then store in a covered glass container at room temperature. Rub a small amount into the swollen joints and do not rinse off for 24 hours. Repeat each day whenever needed.
- Combine the lightly beaten whites of three eggs with one-half cup each turpentine and vinegar. Or, mix equal parts of turpentine, vinegar, and olive oil. Either liniment may be rubbed into the affected joint each night.

- **Poultices** made from comfrey tea leaves moistened with warm water and bound over aching joints each night are said to have brought relief within two weeks.

Baths

- **Bran**—Add one pound of unprocessed bran to a tub of comfortably hot water and soak for 30 minutes nightly.

- **Epsom Salts**—Dissolve one cup of epsom salts in a tub of warm water and soak for 20 minutes every night. Rinse off with a warm shower. For chronic arthritic pain: dissolve 5 pounds of epsom salts in 6 inches of water in the bathtub. Fill the tub with water as hot as can be borne. Start with 10 minutes of soaking daily and gradually increase the time to 20 minutes. Applying an ice pack to the back of the neck and/or the forehead makes the heat more bearable. Those with high blood pressure should check with their physicians before taking these hot baths and should have someone nearby to call in case of dizziness.

  Hand or foot baths may be made by dissolving 1 pound of epsom salts in a large pan of hot water. Soak the afflicted hands or feet for five minutes. Massage thoroughly, rotating the joints, then soak again for five to 10 minutes. After rinsing with warm water, massage peanut oil into the affected areas.
- **Sea Salt**—Dissolve one cup of sea salt (available in health food stores) in a tub of hot water and soak for 30 minutes each day. Rinse off with a warm shower. For those near a seashore, swimming in the ocean for 20 minutes twice each day may be of benefit.
- **Seaweed**—Soften a clump of dried seaweed (available from health food stores) in a tub partially filled with very hot water. Add enough cool water for comfort and soak for 30 minutes.

Nerve massage (Afflicted areas should be massaged for one or two minutes each day)

- For relief from arthritis of the arms: massage the tip of each elbow and completely across the inside of each wrist with a slow, kneading motion.
- To improve flexibility and reduce the aching of arthritic fingers: hold the last joint of each finger and slowly pull until the knuckle is about to crack, then reverse and push while gently squeezing the finger.
- For arthritis of the legs: massage a circle around the outside of each kneecap.

Nerve pressure (Press for 10 seconds, release for 10 seconds, and repeat for total of 30-seconds pressure once each day)

- For arthritis of the arms: press a point at the tip of each shoulder where the bone ends.
- For arthritis of the legs: press a point in the hollow behind and slightly below each anklebone.

Remedies for Osteoarthritis

For stiffness and pain—Take one B-complex tablet plus 50 to 200 milligrams of B-6 daily. This has been found especially beneficial for stiffness of the hands.[24,52] A type of degenerative arthritis identified by swollen, hard nodules (called Heberden's Nodes) on the fingertip joints often responds to treatment with large amounts of the B vitamins. In his *Book of Nutritional Therapy*,[353] Dr. Wright recommends taking 200 milligrams of B-6, a B-complex tablet containing 50 milligrams of each of the Bs, and three dolomite tablets three times each day plus adding one tablespoon of unsaturated oil to the daily diet. This regimen has reduced pain in the fingers (and other joints as well) within one month and brought complete relief to some cases in less than three months. A control rather than a cure, the nodes on the fingers did not disappear but the joints usually remained pain free on a daily maintenance dose of 300 to 400 milligrams of B-6.

To relieve aching hands—Twice each day soak them in warm water for four minutes, then in cold water for one minute. Repeat three or four times.

To retain finger flexibility—At least once each day, squeeze a rubber ball for a count of five, release for a count of five, and repeat 12 times.

Remedies for Rheumatoid Arthritis

Alfalfa Seed Tea—Combine two tablespoons alfalfa seeds and two and one-half cups water. Bring to a full boil, cover and let stand for 30 minutes. Strain, then add cold water to make five cups. Refrigerate in a glass jar and drink during the day, adding honey if desired. Fresh tea should be made each day. In some cases, improvement has been noticeable within two weeks.

Vitamin B-15—50 to 100 milligrams daily. European studies have shown this vitamin to restore normal blood sedimentation rates in rheumatoid arthritis patients.

Citrus Bioflavonoids—200 milligrams three times daily. Studies reported in the *Journal of the American Geriatrics Society* (March, 1957), recommended bioflavonoids as a supplement to other methods of treatment.

Vitamin E Ointment or Oil—Gently rub into the affected joint for 10 minutes each night, then cover with a heat pack for 10 minutes.

Fat-Free Diet—As reported in *Clinical Research* (vol. 29, no. 4, 1981), experimentation with fat-free diets produced complete remissions in some patients with rheumatoid arthritis. Eating plenty of fresh fruits and vegetables, plus bran if necessary to avoid constipation, is advised.

Pantothenic Acid—50 to 100 milligrams daily. Pantothenic acid has been found especially beneficial for rheumatoid arthritis when coupled with capsules of Royal Jelly.[128]

Paraffin Treatment for Hands—Once each day, dip the hands in melted paraffin and allow the coating to remain for half an hour before peeling off into the container for remelting. It is wise to use a candy thermometer to make sure the paraffin is never heated above 125 degrees. If desired, one-half cup of mineral oil may be added to each two cups of paraffin.

SOD (Superoxide Dismutase)—200 to 800 milligrams daily in divided doses. A natural antioxidant, SOD inactivates the peroxide radicals which are believed prime suspects for initiating the rheumatoid process.

Zinc—150 to 660 milligrams in three divided doses daily. Beginning with 50 milligrams three times a day and gradually increasing the dosage is recommended. Many studies have shown positive results with zinc therapy. As reported in *Lancet* (September 11, 1976), zinc reduced the joint swelling and morning stiffness of rheumatoid arthritis. Accompanying the zinc with vitamin B-6 often accelerates its effectiveness.

Folk Remedies for Rheumatism

Oliver Wendell Holmes was said to have carried a horse chestnut in one pocket of his greatcoat and a potato in the other to protect himself from rheumatism. Those for whom this preventive measure was unsuccessful found relief with remedies such as:

Apple Cider Vinegar—Drink one to 10 teaspoons of apple cider vinegar in a glass of water four times a day.

Cayenne Pepper Liniment—Boil one tablespoon cayenne pepper in two cups of apple cider vinegar for 10 minutes. For an even more potent version: combine one-fourth cup cayenne pepper with four teaspoons of bruised mustard seed. Stir into one pint of whiskey and simmer for a few minutes. Saturate cloths in either hot liquid and apply to the afflicted joints.

Garlic—Eat minced raw garlic, take garlic perles, and/or rub the afflicted parts with garlic or garlic oil to relieve rheumatic pain.

Herbal Teas—Drink one cup at bedtime and another before breakfast of any of these teas: buckthorn, cayenne, celery seed, peppermint, rosemary, sarsaparilla, skullcap, slippery elm, uva ursi. For parsley tea: place a handful of fresh parsley in a glass jar. Add two cups boiling water, cover, and let cool. Strain, then drink one glassful an hour before meals. For watermelon seed tea: steep one tablespoon dried, ground watermelon seeds in one cup boiling water. Drink a cup two or three times a day.

Lemon or Lime Juice—In the 1870s, the liberal use of these juices was said to relieve rheumatism in three days when all stimulating liquids were avoided.

Mint—Rub fresh mint leaves on the affected areas to help relieve pain.

Potatoes—Grate raw potato and spread over the sore spots. Or, boil chopped potatoes until very well done, then bathe the affected parts in the hot cooking liquid just before going to bed.

Pyridoxine and Antioxidants—Massive amounts of B-6 and the other antioxidants (see page 3) are a modern folk remedy for relieving rheumatism.

Tissue Salts for Rheumatism (3X-potency tablets dissolved under the tongue)

For chronic rheumatism—Take three tablets of Silicea twice each day. If the condition is worse in damp weather, add three tablets of Nat. Sulph. on rainy days.

When the pain is worse with movement—Alternate one tablet of Ferr. Phos. with one tablet of Kali. Mur. each day.

When the pain lessens after continued movement—Alternate Mag. Phos. and Nat. Phos. three times a day between meals.

When the pain is worse with warmth—Alternate Mag. Phos. with Kali. Sulph. morning and evening, increasing the dosage if the condition is acute.

Sources (See Bibliography)

3, 12, 13, 17, 22, 24, 35, 37, 47, 52, 53, 62, 66, 68, 76, 82, 84, 88, 89, 92, 98, 100, 110, 118, 121, 124, 128, 142, 152, 153, 160, 165, 168, 171, 180, 181, 189, 190, 201, 205, 211, 215, 226, 228, 229, 243, 249, 250, 252, 253, 256, 260, 272, 276, 280, 282, 289, 293, 297, 299, 300, 311, 316, 318, 328, 333, 334, 335, 345, 348, 353.

ASTHMA AND EMPHYSEMA

Asthma has beset mortals since they first began reacting to their environment. Residents of India and China suffered through its choking spasms 2,000 years ago. Ephedrine, as well as several other modern medications were developed from the plants used in Chinese and Indian folk medicine and an ancient Egyptian papyrus contains 10 prescriptions for asthma. Physical treatments have changed little from those advised by the Roman physician, Aurelianus, in the fifth century: breathing exercises, change of climate, cold baths, sunbathing, walking.

Although breathing difficulties are symptomatic of both, asthma and emphysema are direct opposites. Asthma is characterized by intermittent attacks of shortness of breath due to interference with the free flow of air through the small bronchial tubes. Instead of expanding, the little air sacs (alveoli) contract so that it is hard to get air *in*. Emphysema creates constant difficulty in breathing because the tiny air sacs are permanently inflated, retain carbon dioxide, and do not empty as they should—making it difficult to get air *out*. Inhaling pure oxygen may benefit an asthmatic but could be harmful for a person with advanced emphysema.

The causative factors vary with each individual: allergies, disorders of the adrenal glands, emotional or physical stress, environmental pollution, infections, low blood sugar. Asthma may appear with a sudden attack but emphysema, which today is almost a national epidemic, develops gradually from years of respiratory irritation. Repeated bouts of coughing can break the walls of the alveoli, leaving larger, less efficient, flabby air sacs. Many bronchial irritants can be removed with a home air filter. Smoke-filled rooms should be avoided and tobacco use eliminated or limited to no more than five cigarettes per day. Asthma and emphysema frequently co-exist, most remedies apply to both, and relief depends largely on factors under individual control.

Diet and Supplements

Documented tests[2,48] showing that most asthmatics have low blood sugar have led many orthomolecular physicians to recommend a functional hypoglycemia diet (see Low Blood Sugar) for those with asthma. Even when allergies are involved, the level of blood sugar may be the deciding factor in an asthmatic attack.

Most diets for asthmatics prohibit dairy products because of their mucus-producing qualities but milk, buttermilk, and yogurt have been found helpful in some cases. Horseradish is an excellent solvent of excess mucus in the system. It may be mixed with honey or lemon juice and taken by the spoonful, combined with butter for sandwiches, or used in sauces or salad dressings. Apples, apricots, cabbage, carrots, celery, cherries, citrus fruits, green beans, onions, peaches, peppers, turnips, and turnip greens are also recommended for those with asthma or emphysema. Sweets and caffeine-containing beverages should be severely limited because they raise the blood-sugar level for a short time, then cause it to fall lower than it had been. However, in the 1880s, black mocha coffee was a European treatment for bronchial asthma. Cold beverages can shock the sensitive airways into spasms, and drinks that contain food dyes can trigger some forms of asthma. Room-temperature or hot liquids act as natural expectorants, keeping mucus thin and coughable. Drinking one-half to one cup of fluid every waking hour is recommended. When taken at the onset of an asthmatic attack, a cup of hot apple cider, herb tea, hot lemonade, or soup may serve to abort it.

Supplements also play a role in the treatment of respiratory conditions. Without relating asthma to low blood sugar, Adelle Davis[89] obtained definite improvement for youthful asthmatics within one month by putting them on a·high-protein diet with no refined carbohydrates. The supplements given daily were: 20,000 units of vitamin A, a B-complex tablet, 600 milligrams of vitamin C, 800 IU of natural vitamin D, 32 IU of vitamin E.

A rule generally accepted by nutritionally oriented asthma authorities is that if cortisone will help the condition, strengthening the adrenals with vitamins will be equally effective without producing unwanted side effects. Vitamins A, B-6, C, and pantothenic acid seem to be the most important, but additional B vitamins and vitamin E may be needed. As cited in *Orthomolecular Nutrition*[171], 5,000 asthma patients responded favorably to daily doses of 28,000 to 75,000 units of vitamin A and 5,000 to 14,000 IU of natural vitamin D plus bone meal supplements. All the antioxidants (see page 3) are recommended for those with asthma or emphysema. They help control the free radicals which may be at least partially responsible for emphysema, and several of them have an antihistamine action. Some emphysema sufferers have reportedly benefited from taking four tablespoons brewer's yeast, one tablespoon lecithin granules, 50 milligrams B-15, and 400 micrograms folic acid every day. Other options for individual experimentation:

Vitamin A—10,000 to 50,000 units daily to protect the mucous membranes from air pollution and infection.

B Complex—One comprehensive tablet daily plus individual B vitamins as indicated. Vitamin B-6 acts as a natural antihistamine and has produced improvement in bronchial asthma within two weeks when 100 milligrams were taken two or three times each day. (The effect is enhanced when each dose of B-6 is accompanied by 500 milligrams of vitamin C and 100 milligrams of pantothenic acid.) At least 30 micrograms of B-12 are needed for proper functioning of pantothenic acid and vitamin C—larger amounts of B-12 have helped some asthmatics. Taking 200 milligrams of PABA on a regular daily basis has brought relief to others. Vitamin B-15 is believed to be an anti-allergy vitamin that promotes cell oxidation—50 milligrams daily has relieved asthma symptoms in some cases.

Bee Pollen—Two teaspoons of pollen granules, or the equivalent in tablets, daily. Even though pollens are a common irritant for asthmatics, taking pollen in this form has proven beneficial for many.

Bioflavonoids—200 to 1,000 milligrams daily to strengthen the fragile walls of the air sacs and capillaries and to insulate the bronchial tubes against the irritating effects of inhaled allergens. A high concentration of bioflavonoids is found in the white underskin and segment parts of citrus fruits. Berries, cherries, grapes, plums, and sun-dried apricots are also good sources. Eating some of these fruits each day is believed to increase the effectiveness of the bioflavonoid supplements and has improved or cleared some asthmatics in less than 10 days.

Vitamin C—600 to 5,000 milligrams daily. Since this vitamin has both a detoxifying and antihistamine action, it is especially beneficial for those whose asthma is of allergic origin. Taking 300 milligrams every 15 minutes during attacks has brought immediate relief in some instances. Vitamin C also helps widen air passages during exercise or exertion. In a study reported in the *Journal of the American Medical Association* (February 13, 1981), asthma sufferers given 500 milligrams of vitamin C before an exercise test doubled their tolerance.

Calcium—1,000 to 3,000 milligrams daily. Calcium relaxes the muscles surrounding the bronchial tubes to ease breathing, and its lack is considered a contributory factor in allergy responses. Taking one or two calcium tablets containing vitamin D each hour during an asthma attack often decreases its severity.

Vitamin D—800 to 2,000 IU daily to assure calcium absorption. When correlated with supplements of vitamin A, 10,000 IU natural vitamin D daily for a few weeks has proven helpful for some asthmatics.

Vitamin E (see Caution, page 6)—100 to 1,600 IU daily. Vitamin E is an antioxidant that also decreases the body's need for oxygen.

Manganese—5 milligrams taken twice each week for 10 weeks. [European doctors have had good results with this treatment for asthma.[62]]

Case History

Kevin J. had always struggled for breath. Playing tag with fellow Cub Scouts had made his face turn blue, and one of his more embarrassing memories had to do with having to help his Den Mother prepare refreshments instead of participating in their games. By the time he was a seventh-grade science teacher, however, Kevin had been through the medical mill and learned to live with his limitations. He compensated for time lost through his seasonal asthmatic absences by offering extracurricular projects to his students. Then he read an article about the value of vitamin supplements for asthmatics. He discovered that vitamin C plus bioflavonoids did not create the diarrhea caused by plain vitamin C, so he took a 500-milligram combination three times a day. Kevin also switched to a more potent daily multiple-vitamin-mineral supplement, and added a B-complex tablet. The spring term ended without Kevin having to use the remainder of his sick-leave; the fall term left him with accumulated sick-leave credit; and by the following summer he began to wonder if he had ever had asthma—there were no more attacks.

Tissue Salts—One 6X tablet of Kali. Mur. and/or one 6X tablet of Kali. Phos. dissolved under the tongue each 20 minutes during an attack, then once every three hours for the remainder of the day.

Exercise and Relaxation

Walking or swimming are ideal for asthmatics, provided rest is taken at frequent intervals. Activities that involve brief spurts of action, separated by periods of relaxation, are much less apt to trigger asthma than sports that call for continuous exertion. Deep breathing is vital for warding off wheezing, chest tightness and shortness of breath, and is especially important for those with emphysema. The *American Lung Association Newsletter* (May, 1981) suggests thinking of the chest and stomach as a container for air. Slowly breathe in through the nose to fill the bottom of the container first. Then exhale slowly through the mouth until all the air is expelled. Repeat 12 times at intervals during the day.

When the air is cold, either indoors or out, breathing through the nose helps warm the air before it reaches the lungs. Wearing a gauze face mask or a scarf pulled up over the mouth and nose before going out in the winter is helpful in extreme cases.

Simple exercises such as bending over and attempting to touch the toes while exhaling helps to get rid of trapped air, as does blowing up balloons for five minutes three times a day. A passive exercise that allows gravity to help clear mucus from the lungs is to lie over the edge of a bed with the elbows on the floor and the head dependent, then give several good coughs while turning from side to side.

Deliberate relaxation (see pages 9-10) is such a useful shield against asthma that many doctors recommend variations of the technique taught by Dr. Rapp.[268] First tense all the muscles, then relax until limp. Imagine floating on a cloud or down a river on a soft raft while breathing softly and easily. By practicing this and recalling the "wet-noodle" feeling, relaxation can be accomplished whenever needed. Concentrating on and repeating the phrase, "My breathing tubes are expanding," can relieve tightness or stop an impending attack for many people.

Folk Remedies

Keeping a chihuahua dog in the house is believed to cure the asthma of its owners, but there are many other suggestions for pet-less sufferers of either asthma or emphysema.

Anise Oil (available from pharmacies)—Five drops mixed with a teaspoon of honey and taken before each meal has helped some persons with emphysema.

Apple Cider Vinegar—To relieve wheezing, add one tablespoon of the vinegar to a glass of water and sip for half an hour. Wait 30 minutes, then repeat.

Apple Water—Pour boiling water over sliced apples, let stand until cool, then strain and drink to relieve shortness of breath.

Cherry Stems—Steep a handful of cherry stems in a pint of boiling water until cool. Strain and make into a syrup with honey, then take one tablespoonful every hour as needed.

Cranberries—Store cooked, mashed cranberries in a glass jar in the refrigerator. When an asthmatic attack occurs, mix two teaspoons of the pulp in a cup of hot water and sip. (Cranberries are believed to contain an ingredient that dilates bronchial tubes to help restore normal breathing.)

Garlic—Long used as a remedy for asthma, one or more minced raw garlic cloves were the prescription for adults. A bowl of garlic soup taken before retiring was believed soothing. A concoction of garlic cloves boiled with vinegar and sugar, then taken by the spoonful each morning was a favorite cure during the 1800s.

Heat—Allowing any part of the body to become chilled can trigger an asthmatic spasm. During an attack there should be adequate fresh air but the body must be kept warm. Hot packs placed over the stomach, chest, back, and soles of the feet, or a 45-minute tub bath in water held at 100 degrees, has been found helpful.

Herbal Teas—Folk healers suggested several daily cups of any of these teas: anise seed, camomile, cayenne, comfrey, eucalyptus, garlic, ginger, ginseng, horehound, marjoram, thyme.

Honey and Bee Pollen—Apply a poultice of honey and bee pollen granules around the throat to ease breathing.

Honey, Lemon Juice, and Whiskey—Combine one tablespoon of each and take during asthma attacks.

Lemon Juice—Take half a tablespoon of lemon juice before each meal and before bedtime. Do not eat anything for at least four hours before retiring.

Mustard Seed—Mix one tablespoon of bruised mustard seed with molasses or water and take each morning and evening.

Oil—To relieve nighttime wheezing, take one tablespoon corn oil or sunflower oil just before going to bed.

Onion—Place thin slices of raw onion on a plate. Spread with honey, cover, and let stand overnight. Take one teaspoonful of the resulting liquid four times each day.

Potatoes—Inhaling the steam from boiling potatoes is a Russian folk remedy for asthma.

Rosemary—To relieve difficult breathing, smoke crumbled, dried rosemary in a clean tobacco pipe.

Salt and Soda—If neither ACTH nor cortisone have been prescribed, increasing the blood sodium by taking one-half teaspoon each salt and baking soda dissolved in a little water, then drinking a glass of orange juice or milk has been beneficial during asthmatic attacks.

Nerve Massage

To relieve shortness of breath: bend the head forward, then use the thumbs and index fingers to massage toward the spine 2 inches below the shoulders, 1 inch on each side of the spinal column. Or, use the index finger to press inward, then massage downward in the depression at the hollow of the throat between the collarbones.

Nerve Pressure

- Using a tongue depressor or the handle of a tablespoon, press down on the floor of the mouth at the root of the tongue, then on top of the tongue as far back as possible without causing gagging. Even biting the tongue (firmly but without inflicting injury) for several minutes at a time may help in an emergency.
- Press the center of the sternum between the second ribs. (About 2 inches below the hollow of the throat, just beneath the bony prominence across the breastbone.) Once each day, maintain pressure for 10 seconds, release for 10 seconds, then repeat for a total of 30 seconds of pressure.

- Place moderately tight rubber bands on the thumbs and first two fingers of both hands for 10 to 15 minutes—less if the fingers start to turn blue—as often as needed for relief.

Sources (See Bibliography)

2, 3, 6, 12, 13, 24, 34, 37, 40, 48, 52, 53, 62, 63, 64, 67, 76, 78, 82, 89, 92, 129, 152, 153, 165, 168, 171, 173, 174, 176, 180, 184, 189, 190, 215, 226, 227, 229, 252, 253, 254, 261, 268, 289, 293, 297, 305, 315, 327, 328, 330, 333, 334, 345, 350.

ATHLETE'S FOOT

Scientifically termed "dermatophytosis" or "tina pedis," athlete's foot is not limited to either athletes or feet. It is an infection caused by a fungus commonly found in public showers or swimming-pool walkways and usually begins on the skin between the toes. Wearing sandals or well-ventilated shoes avoids the excessive perspiration that can help instigate or aggravate athlete's foot. It is highly contagious and can spread from the toes to the fingernails, scalp, or moist skin folds such as armpits or groin. Showers rather than tub baths are recommended and the hands should be scrubbed with soap after touching the infected areas.

While no one natural remedy is effective for everyone, each of the following treatments has proven successful for some individuals.

Alcohol—Apply a mild solution of alcohol and water to the affected area. Allow to dry, then sprinkle with cornstarch or talcum powder before dressing.

Aloe Vera Gel—Apply the gel (either bottled or fresh) every morning and evening.

Apple Cider Vinegar—Pour apple cider vinegar over the infected area each morning and night and/or saturate cotton with the vinegar and place between the toes—taping in place if necessary. Cover with a sock in the evening and leave on overnight.

Garlic—Spread crushed raw garlic over the infected area. A feeling of warmth can be expected for about five minutes, but, if the skin burns, rinse off immediately with clear water. The next day, experiment with garlic diluted with water. The garlic should remain on the skin for 30 minutes daily before being washed off.

Honey—Saturate cotton with raw honey. Each night for one week, place small pieces of the saturated cotton between the affected toes and cover with a sock.

Mutton Tallow and Garlic Powder—Cook the fat from lamb kidneys over low heat and strain to prepare the tallow. Store in a covered jar and apply to the infected area each night before bed. Sprinkle with garlic powder and cover with a sock.

Nerve Pressure—Use the eraser on a pencil to press the top of the foot at the base of the little toe where it joins the fourth toe. Press for 10 seconds, release for 10 seconds. Repeat for a total of 30 seconds pressure each morning and night.

Red Clover Tea—Stir dry red clover tea with hot water to make a paste. Spread on the affected area, cover with a sock, and leave on overnight.

Salt Water—Add one or two tablespoons of salt to a basin of water and bathe the feet several times each day.

Sunlight—Mild cases of athlete's foot have been cured by being exposed to sunlight for one hour each day.

Vitamins and Minerals

- Vitamin A is well-known as an infection fighter. In his book *Feed Your Kids Right*[305], Lendon Smith recommends 25,000 units A and 1,000 IU of D from cod liver oil, plus 500 to 2,000 milligrams vitamin C, 100 milligrams zinc, and one tablespoon vegetable oil daily for six weeks.
- B vitamins are especially important in treating fungus infections. In addition to taking a daily B-complex tablet orally, a B-vitamin salve may be prepared by crushing 10 high-potency B-complex tablets, adding one tablespoon brewer's yeast, then stirring in sesame oil to make a paste. Store tightly covered, thinning with more oil if the mixture becomes too dry. Apply to the affected skin before bed and cover with a sock.
- Nutritionist Adelle Davis[89] reported permanent cures of athlete's foot following one week of eating liver, wheat germ, and yogurt plus three tablespoons of brewer's yeast daily.
- Vitamin C powder or crystals applied directly to the fungus infection has effected a cure in some instances.
- Covering the infected skin twice each day with vitamin E squeezed from a capsule has been reported to bring improvement within one week. After the athlete's foot has cleared, continuing to rub on vitamin E once each week has prevented recurrence.

Sources (See Bibliography)

3, 13, 19, 52, 53, 62, 89, 156, 174, 226, 228, 254, 261, 272, 276, 288, 305, 312, 315, 335, 345.

BACKACHE, LUMBAGO, AND SCIATICA

Among mankind's most common complaints, an aching back can result from a variety of causes. Poor posture, inadequate nutrition, or lack of exercise can weaken the spine and its supporting muscles so that sitting for a prolonged period, strenuous exertion, or even bending over to tie a shoelace may cause the back to "go out." A too-soft mattress or improper footwear, especially heels that are too high, may be partly responsible for a nagging backache. Back pain can be partially or wholly psychological in origin or may be a symptom of disorders in the ligaments, bones, or underlying organs. Any backache that is accompanied by fever or headache, or a severe one that does not improve within a week, should receive medical diagnosis.

Lumbago was once considered "rheumatism in the small of the back" but now is used as a general term to describe pain in the middle or lower back—the lumbar region. Sciatica (sometimes labeled as disc trouble, a slipped disc, or lumbago) may occur independently or in conjunction with other back pain. A damaged spinal disc or osteoarthritis of the spine may cause inflammation of the sciatic nerve which extends from the base of the spine down the leg to the ankle.

Sciatica, or the sudden pain brought on by strain, normally responds to bed rest on a firm mattress (with a pillow under the knees), and local applications of moist or dry heat for an hour four times a day. When heat is not being used, rubbing the painful area with ice cubes wrapped in a towel helps combat muscle spasms. Alternating hot and cold packs or using a spray hose in the bathtub to apply hot water for five minutes, then cold water for two minutes and repeating several times may help decrease the pain. Sprinkling turpentine on a towel over the painful area, then ironing with a medium-hot iron was a folk method for providing deep heat. Improving posture, avoiding overly soft beds or chairs, performing a few spine-straightening exercises, and upgrading nutrition usually alleviates chronic back discomfort.

Diet and Supplements

Proper nutrition not only prevents but corrects many back problems. Protein and vitamin C are essential for firm supporting tissue. B vitamins are needed for healthy nerve tissue. Calcium and other minerals are necessary to avoid or relieve backaches caused by the gradual demineralization of the bones. A daily multi-vitamin-mineral tablet containing manganese; 500 to 3,000 milligrams vitamin C; a B-complex tablet; and 1,000 to 2,000 milligrams of calcium help maintain a healthy back and often bring relief from an ailing one.

Case History

Mike H. was a truck driver with a "bad back." When the occasional bouts of back discomfort became more frequent, sometimes seeming to "freeze" his back in one position, Mike went to his physician. The doctor found nothing medically wrong but agreed that Mike did have a "bad back," probably due to weak back muscles that could not keep his spine aligned, and referred him to an osteopath. Even with these manipulative treatments Mike's painful back caused him to miss several days' work each month and he worried about losing his job. Mike's mother-in-law came to visit during one of his stay-in-bed-with-a-heating-pad periods. She told Mike about a friend who had had a similar problem with his back and had "cured" it with vitamins. Mike was skeptical but dutifully swallowed the 400 IUs of E and 1,000 milligrams of C with bioflavonoids she insisted he take in addition to his daily multiple vitamin-mineral supplement. Nothing happened. Mike drove his 18-wheeler for a month, then for another month, and still nothing happened—his back did not "go out" or "freeze." Mike has almost forgotten that he ever had a "bad back" but he does not forget to take his vitamins.

Sciatic pain has responded to a month of therapy with those vitamins and minerals plus 1,000 micrograms of oral or injected B-12, 50 milligrams each B-1 and B-15, and 50 IU of vitamin E each day. Drinking a daily glass of fresh, raw potato juice (mixed with beet, carrot, or celery juice for palatability) has brought relief to some sciatica sufferers.

The tissue salt, Mag. Phos., is recommended for acute back pain that comes in spasms. One teaspoonful of the tablets may be taken each three hours for 12 hours, then three tablets dissolved under the tongue three times each day. Folk remedies for back problems were uva ursi tea, bed rest, and one or two alcoholic drinks as a mild sedative—especially if the back pain was triggered by an emotional crisis.

Exercise and Posture

Correct sitting and standing habits can do much to prevent and relieve chronic backache. Slumping should be avoided, as should sitting without any back support. Constantly changing position or using a footstool to elevate one foot while standing is helpful. When sitting in an upholstered chair, elevate the feet on a hassock (or use a reclining chair) so that the knees are higher than the hips. Rocking chairs help reduce the spinal strain of prolonged sitting.

Once an acute attack is over, any of the well-documented back-strengthening exercises may be of benefit. Weakness of the abdominal muscles increases strain on back muscles, making them more readily subject to injury. Two unobtrusive exercises that can be practiced regularly to strengthen all these muscles are:

- Stand with the back to a wall, the feet 12 inches away from the wall. Tip head and shoulders forward and press the beltline against the wall.
- Sit on a straight chair with both feet on the floor. Gradually allow the body to drop forward until the head is between the knees. Then tighten the abdominal muscles and pull back up to a sitting position.

Nerve Massage

Every other day, completely massage the bottom of each foot for a minute or two. On the alternate days, massage both hands—especially the pad at the base of the thumb, the center of the palm, and the pad between the thumb and first finger.

For pain in the upper back and shoulders—Massage the bottom of the foot just below the big toe and/or the palm of the hand near the base of the thumb.

For pain in the center of the back—Massage the center of the arch at the rim and/or the top surface of the hand between the wrist and web of the thumb.

For low back pain—Massage the inside of the foot from the arch to the heel and/or massage the top surface of the hand at the base of the thumb.

Nerve Pressure

Press inward and upward with the thumbs under the arch of each eyebrow, about 1 inch from the bridge of the nose. Maintain pressure for 10 seconds, release for 10 seconds, and repeat for a total of 30 seconds of pressure each day.

Sources (See Bibliography)

3, 4, 13, 34, 46, 52, 62, 63, 64, 76, 84, 88, 89, 118, 142, 156, 168, 174, 186, 189, 190, 229, 241, 243, 254, 260, 261, 282, 288, 289, 297, 304, 315, 316, 350, 353.

BALDNESS AND THINNING HAIR

The loss of scalp hair (alopecia) has been a persistent problem throughout the ages. An Egyptian papyrus written in 1550 B.C. gives instructions for growing hair on bald pates by annointing them with a mixture of crocodile, elephant, lion, and hippopotamus fat.

The human scalp holds approximately 100,000 hairs, all of which are in different stages of growth, and normally sheds 50 to 100 hairs daily. Scientific evidence indicates that excessive hair loss is due to a combination of heredity, hormones, emotional factors, inadequate nutrition, and mistreatment by harsh brushing, pulling the hair too tightly in braids or around curlers, the use of hair dyes, etc. Stress and tension constrict the blood vessels of the scalp, prevent the hair from receiving nourishment, and can cause it to fall out. This may account for the ever-increasing rate which "male pattern baldness" (center baldspot with receding hairline) is affecting today's females.

Patchy hair loss (alopecia areata) may be a symptom of an underlying disease and should be examined by a physician even though emotional upheaval plays a role in many cases. The loss of hair caused by diabetes or other illness (or the medications prescribed as treatment) usually self-corrects once health is regained. If all else fails, there is this "simple and effectual cure" recorded in *Dick's Encyclopedia of Practical Receipts and Processes*,[98] "Moisten the part affected with saliva and rub it over thoroughly three times a day with the ashes of a good Havana 'segar'."

Diet and Supplements

Hair is composed almost entirely of protein. Many American and European doctors recommend a high-protein diet including meats, fish, eggs, cheese, and milk to help control excessive hair loss. Brewer's yeast, liver, and green vegetables are well supplied anti-stress factors that may help overcome the problem of falling hair. Other foods believed beneficial are: asparagus, barley, cabbage, celery, figs, lettuce, oats, onion, rutabaga, spinach, strawberries, tomatoes, turnips, wheat germ. A daily glass of mixed vegetable juices (carrot, cucumber, lettuce, and spinach) is thought to promote hair growth, as is a mixture of alfalfa and beet juice with a bit of onion juice added. In his book, *Helping Yourself with New Enzyme Catalyst Health Secrets*[334], Carlson Wade suggests drinking several glasses each day of a blenderized mixture of grapefruit juice, unprocessed bran, and wheat germ.

An excessive amount of carbohydrates and animal fats in the diet may adversely affect the sebaceous glands to inhibit new hair growth. Some Scandinavian doctors[154] believe that ingesting too much salt is a cause of baldness. The use of tobacco in any form constricts small blood vessels. This may deprive the hair of nutrients and possibly contribute to its loss.

Vitamins and minerals are so essential for a healthy head of hair that hair-nourishing combination-supplements are now on the market. According to *Earl Mindell's Vitamin Bible*[228], taking a high-potency B-complex tablet each night and morning plus 1,000 milligrams each calcium, choline, and inositol, and a multi-mineral tablet with 500 milligrams of magnesium daily will help combat hair loss. Other authorities suggest individual experimentation with these optional supplements.

Vitamin A—10,000 to 30,000 units daily. Vitamin A is essential for a healthy scalp and prevents the destruction of hair follicles from infection.

B Complex—One or two comprehensive, high-potency tablets daily. Early baldness or a receding hairline may indicate an unusually high hereditary requirement for B vitamins. Taking large amounts in the form of tablets and/or brewer's yeast has stimulated hair growth for many men and women. An additional 50 to 100 milligrams of B-2, B-6, PABA, and pantothenic acid plus 50 micrograms of biotin, 800 micrograms of folic acid, and the 1,000 milligrams of choline and inositol recommended by Dr. Mindell has been helpful in some instances. Niacin, in two or three daily doses of 100 milligrams each, dilates the capillaries to furnish increased nutrition to the hair follicles. Excessive amounts of any liquid—alcohol, coffee, soft drinks, tea, or even water, can wash the needed vitamins out of the system and contribute to hair loss.

Vitamin C and Bioflavonoids—500 to 1,000 milligrams of vitamin C plus 50 to 100 milligrams of bioflavonoids. The vitamin C complex strengthens capillaries to provide adequate nourishment to the hair.

Cysteine—500 to 2,000 milligrams daily. Hair is approximately 8 percent cysteine. Supplements of 1,000 milligrams of this amino acid each day have been found to make hair grow faster but should be accompanied by at least three times that amount of vitamin C to prevent the possibility of bladder or kidney stones.[252]

Vitamin E (see Caution, page 6)—100 to 1,200 IU daily. When taken orally, vitamin E stimulates blood flow to promote hair growth. Rubbing the scalp before each shampoo with vitamin E squeezed from a capsule has halted some cases of hair loss.

Vitamin F—One to two tablespoons of cold-pressed vegetable oil, or the equivalent in capsules daily, to encourage healthy hair growth.

Kelp—1 to 15 tablets or up to one teaspoon of kelp granules daily. A natural source of minerals, kelp is high in the iodine that may correct hair loss due to an underactive thyroid gland but large amounts should be taken only with a physician's approval.

Lecithin—One teaspoon to two tablespoons of granules, or the equivalent in capsules, daily. Lecithin contains the hair-growth-stimulators biotin, choline, and inositol.

Minerals—One high-potency multi-mineral tablet daily. All the minerals are required for hair growth. A deficiency of iron is often a contributory factor in hair loss but medical diagnosis is wise before taking more iron than is contained in the combination supplement. Taking an additional 15 to 50

milligrams of zinc daily has halted hair loss and encouraged growth in a
number of cases.

Tissue Salts—Hair loss may be caused by a deficiency of Calc. Phos., Calc.
Sulph., Kali. Sulph., Nat. Mur., and/or Silicea. Suggested dosage is three 6X-
potency tablets dissolved under the tongue twice daily.

Case History

Connie V. had fine hair that would not hold the back-combing required for the
bouffant hair styles then in vogue. With an executive position that required an
attractive appearance at work, and a family that required too much attention at
home to allow for daily hair styling, Connie wore a wig to work. Her perfectly
coiffeured hair was greatly admired—no one even suspected her secret. After a
few years, however, Connie noticed that her hairline was beginning to recede,
and that an excessive amount of hair was accumulating in her hairbrush. When
she overheard a colleague mention that he had forestalled his incipient baldness
with brewer's yeast and B vitamins, Connie decided to experiment for herself.
She began taking a daily multiple-vitamin-mineral containing 25 milligrams of
each of the major B vitamins, and gradually increased her intake of brewer's
yeast from one teaspoon to one-fourth cup each day. Within a month, Connie
could tell the difference in her hair. It still won't hold back-combing, but she no
longer wears a wig; and Connie's co-workers insist that her luxuriant short-and-
curly hair is far more flattering and youthful than her previous hair style.

External Remedies

Exercise

- To help stop a receding hairline: without using the hands, wrinkle up the
  forehead then pull it down as forcefully as possible. Repeat 10 times at least
  twice each day.
- To stimulate hair growth: twice each day, lie on the back with the legs lifted
  high and the body supported by elbows and hands (as for the bicycling
  exercise). Or, relax on a slantboard for 15 minutes with the head 18 inches lower
  than the feet to bring blood to the scalp.

Nerve Massage—Briskly rub the fingernails of one hand directly across the nails
of the other hand for a total of five minutes, three times a day.

Scalp Stimulation

- Brush with a hairbrush with natural bristles for three to five minutes each day.
- Twice each day, massage the scalp and temples in a circular motion with the
  fingertips or an electric vibrator. *Margo*[218] recommends rubbing both the bare
  scalp and areas of existing hair with a turkish towel each day, preferably
  following shampooing. Enough friction should be generated to turn the skin
  pink without irritating it and gradually resupply the capillary network of the
  scalp. The time can vary from 30 seconds to two minutes a day. Remarkable
  successes have been recorded when this was continued for three or four months.

Shampooing—Whether the hair is washed daily or once a week, authorities agree that commercial shampoos should be diluted half-and-half with water before being applied to the hair.

Folk Remedies

Aloe Vera Gel—Rub into the scalp and allow to remain overnight. Rinse with plain water or shampoo each morning. (If fresh aloe vera is not available, the gel may be purchased in health food stores.)

Apple Cider Vinegar—Sipping a glass of water containing one teaspoon of the vinegar three times a day is believed to restore hair, especially when reinforced by eating one teaspoon of horseradish with each of two meals daily. When hair falls out in patches, brushing the naked scalp twice each day with a soft toothbrush dipped in the vinegar has been known to stimulate regrowth. To counteract the alkaline effect of shampoos, add one tablespoon of apple cider vinegar to each two cups of water for the final rinse.

Cayenne Pepper—Rub the balding spots with the ground red pepper to stimulate new hair growth.

Cold Water—Immerse the head in plain cold water, or a mild salt-water solution, each morning and night. Dry the hair thoroughly, then brush to produce a warm glow.

Eggs—Eating at least one egg each day is an old suggestion substantiated by modern science. (As part of its complete protein, each egg contains 250 milligrams of the amino acid, cysteine.) For a "protein pack" to thicken hair: a whole egg, or an egg yolk, may be blended with water or one tablespoon vegetable oil, rubbed onto the scalp and hair, then covered with a towel or shower cap for 20 minutes before shampooing. For added benefits, an egg yolk may be whisked with the shampoo just before using.

Garlic—rub sliced garlic cloves over thin or balding spots each night. (New hair growth has occurred within weeks when the garlic was applied three times daily and allowed to dry before being rinsed off.[3])

Herbal Teas—Drinking several cups daily of alfalfa, camomile, fenugreek, parsley, rosemary or sage tea, singly or in combination, is suggested. Double-strength teas may be used as a hair rinse or sponged onto the scalp once a day as a tonic.

Honey—Eating four tablespoons of raw honey with each meal is a folk-remedy for falling hair. This is not recommended for those with diabetes or low blood sugar, however.

Jojoba Oil—Now available in various hair preparations, jojoba oil rubbed onto the scalp before shampooing has long been considered a stimulant for hair growth.

Olive Oil or Lard—To check falling hair: massage the scalp with olive oil or lard each night, cover with a protective cap, then shampoo out in the morning.

Onion—An old favorite for curing baldness, fresh onion juice may be rubbed onto the scalp, or the onion may be combined with other ingredients for more complex remedies.

- Steep slices of a large onion in a pint of brandy for two weeks. Strain and add two cups of water, then rub on the scalp each day.
- Each morning and evening, rub the head with fresh onion until red, then massage it with honey, rinse off with rosemary tea, and towel dry.

Peaches—Both the fruit and the kernels were used by folk practitioners to restore hair.

- Combine one-half cup chopped ripe peaches with two cups apple cider vinegar. Wash the bare spots on the scalp with the mixture three times a day.
- Grind or pound peach kernels, then simmer in vinegar to make a thick paste. Rub on the naked scalp or receding hairline.

Vodka—Mix three tablespoons vodka with two tablespoons honey. Rub onto the scalp and allow to remain for two hours before rinsing or shampooing.

- An even more stimulating tonic may be made by mixing one-fourth cup cayenne pepper with one and one-fourth cups vodka. Cover and steep for two weeks, shaking the bottle once each day. Strain and store in a tightly closed glass container. Rub a small amount on the scalp twice daily. (Keep away from the eyes and wash the hands after using!)

Sources (See Bibliography)

3, 11, 12, 13, 15, 24, 40, 53, 63, 68, 78, 84, 88, 89, 92, 98, 110, 150, 152, 154, 160, 174, 184, 189, 190, 211, 215, 218, 227, 228, 229, 238, 247, 252, 254, 261, 270, 272, 276, 282, 293, 315, 318, 333, 334.

BEDSORES

An added misfortune of the bedridden, bedsores are caused by unrelieved pressure on bony areas such as the hips, and aggravated by improper care or a poor nutritional state which weakens the skin and slows healing. These sores are easier to prevent than cure. When the physical condition allows, the position should be changed from back to side and back again each two hours. Bathing and gentle friction should be performed daily and clean, wrinkle-free sheets kept on the bed.

Other preventives that also speed healing are: placing a thick section of textured foam rubber under the sheet, placing a sheep skin (or man-made fur fleece) with the fleece side up between the sheet and the body, or lying on a warmed water bed. A large rubber ring under the hips helps protect tender areas from too much pressure. A small doughnut-shaped pad (made of rolled nylon stockings) can be arranged under the feet to relieve pressure on the heels. If moist sores have developed, they may be dried with the cautious use of a heat lamp or an ordinary light bulb in an unshielded lamp base.

Diet and Supplements

Illness creates a stress situation within the body, uses up nutritional elements rapidly, and requires a super-nutritious diet. Even with proper physical care, the development, severity, and healing time of bedsores can depend on nutritional factors. From two to seven times the normal maintenance level of protein is recommended. (A lack of certain amino acids can lead to bedsores. Up to 400 grams of protein daily may be required for their healing.[7,89]) Reinforcing other remedies with vitamin and mineral supplements has achieved amazing results in many cases.

Vitamin A—10,000 to 25,000 units daily. This "healing" vitamin is partially responsible for the strength of new tissue formed at the site of the sore.

B Complex—one or two comprehensive, high-potency tablets daily. All the B vitamins are needed to combat the stress of illness. Additional supplements of 25 milligrams B-2, 50 milligrams B-6, and 400 to 800 milligrams of folic acid may be beneficial—a deficiency of any of these vitamins can delay the healing of bedsores.

Vitamin C—1,000 to 4,000 milligrams in divided doses daily. Vitamin C prevents the capillary fragility which allows bedsores to form. Once they are present, it reduces healing time from months to weeks. Taking 500 to 1,000 milligrams of bioflavonoids each day enhances the effectiveness of vitamin C. Spraying the sores with a mild solution (3 percent) of vitamin C powder and water has been shown to further speed healing.

Vitamin E (see Caution, page 6)—100 to 1,200 IU daily. When taken orally, vitamin E works through the blood supply to help avoid bedsores or heal them more rapidly. Applying vitamin E ointment, or the oil from a punctured capsule, directly over the sore minimizes the pain and speeds healing even more. If the sores are draining, cornstarch may be sprinkled over the coating of vitamin E.

Minerals—One multi-mineral tablet plus a zinc supplement daily. A number of minerals are necessary for the synthesization of new proteins for wound healing but the key mineral is zinc. Bedsores have healed up to three times faster when 30 to 150 milligrams of zinc were taken daily. (Under medical supervision, 660 milligrams of zinc sulfate per day has cleared bedsores without any serious side effects.[282])

Folk Remedies

Alcohol—As a preventive, rubbing alcohol may be sponged over the back and hips three or four times a day. If sores have formed, bathing them several times daily with a mixture of one tablespoon powdered alum (available in pharmacies) combined with three-fourths cup whiskey was a standard folk-medicine curative.

Cornstarch—Dust the sores with cornstarch whenever they appear moist or reddened. (Mixing the cornstarch half-and-half with unscented talcum powder helps prevent the formation of a pasty mass.)

Cucumber—European folk-practitioners have achieved good results by applying the juice of fresh, ripe cucumbers to bedsores.

Egg White—Beat an egg white with two tablespoons of wine and apply to the sores.

Flour—Bake wheat flour in a moderate oven until golden brown, then dust over the bedsores several times each day.

Garlic—Combine freshly grated garlic with vegetable oil to make a poultice for the sore. Reduce in strength if a burning sensation is felt.

Honey—Raw honey spread on a gauze pad and placed over the bedsore each night has produced healing within two weeks.[53] Physicians in British hospitals have found that this ancient remedy promotes healing better than any other local application. Neither the honey nor the dressing seems to stick to the sore.

Lecithin—Coating bedsores with liquid lecithin (available in health food stores) and covering them with a dry bandage is a modern folk remedy. Some practitioners suggest cleansing the sores with hydrogen peroxide before applying the lecithin.

Sugar—Packing an open bedsore with sugar and covering it with an airtight dressing was believed to close up bedsores by instigating healing from the inside. Several doctors have adopted this method and achieved excellent results with either granulated or powdered sugar.

Case History

Uncle Josh insisted he was doing just fine, a few more weeks in bed and he would be up-and-at-'em. Ellen was his favorite niece, he appreciated her taking time from her lecture tour to stop and see him, and did not intend to waste their visit on his complaints. She admired his new remote-control TV, and agreed that the neighbor lady who came over twice each day was wonderful—there was a thermos of hot soup for his lunch, and the house was spotless. Ellen also noticed the wince of pain each time Uncle Josh changed position. Her doctorate was in archeology, not medicine, but Ellen had acquired a lot of practical health experience, and was accustomed to taking charge. One look convinced her that what Uncle Josh referred to as an irritated hip was a bedsore. While she packed the raw sore with granulated sugar and covered it with an airtight bandage, Ellen elicited the fact that he hadn't bothered with any vitamins since he came home from the hospital. She found a bottle of multiple vitamins in the bathroom, had him take one with his lunch, and drove off on a foraging expedition. The neighbor lady arrived just as Ellen returned with her parcels. Together they unrolled the fleecy pad she had purchased at the hospital, and smoothed it between the sheet and Uncle Josh. He was pleased with the assortment of fruit and cheese Ellen had brought for his snacks, promised to continue taking his multiple vitamins plus the zinc tablets and vitamin C with bioflavonoids she placed on his bedside table, but almost rebelled at the directions for replacing the sugar dressing on his hip each morning and evening. However, Uncle Josh followed Ellen's instructions, and when she stopped for another whirlwind visit two weeks later, the bedsore was healing beautifully.

Sources (See Bibliography)

3, 7, 19, 52, 53, 86, 89, 98, 128, 142, 152, 168, 227, 260, 282, 288, 301, 316, 349.

BED-WETTING (ENURESIS)

All infants have enuresis but if bed-wetting persists past the sixth birthday it calls for investigation rather than punishment. A physician should be consulted if natural remedies are not effective. Disorders of the urinary tract, infections, or spinal nerve pressure may be responsible for bed-wetting, especially in older children and adults. Allergic reactions can create bladder hypersensitivity which in turn causes bed-wetting. Low blood sugar (which see) may leave the nervous system without enough energy to transmit a message from a full bladder up to the area of social concern in the brain. Anxiety, excitement, and emotional stress are contributory factors as they cause blood sugar to fall just as low as if sugar had been ingested.

Clinical studies have shown that enuretic children sleep more deeply than others, have a smaller bladder capacity, and that the disturbance tends to run in families.[292] In many cases, the underlying cause stems from too-frequent visits to the bathroom. When the bladder has constantly been emptied before it is fully filled, the controlling muscles become weakened and the natural warning system no longer functions properly. Gradually lengthening the time between daytime trips to the lavatory and increasing muscular control by voluntarily starting and stopping the flow two or three times during each act of urination may remedy the situation.

Diet and Supplements

The kidneys become active for only a short period after a drink is taken, so there need be no restriction of liquids except for an hour before bedtime. The every-night bed-wetter is usually prone to deep sleep caused by food allergy or low blood sugar. The most likely allergens are chocolate, citrus fruits, components of processed foods, corn, eggs, milk, sugar, tomatoes, and wheat; but an allergy to anything can trigger enuresis. Nutritional deficiencies, or a hereditary need for exceptionally high amounts of certain vitamins and minerals, may be responsible for bed-wetting at any age. Including cabbage, cantaloupe, fish, green leafy vegetables, and organ meats provides a supply of the nutrients needed to prevent bed-wetting, but additional supplements may be required. Taking a multi-vitamin-mineral table that included 10 to 25 milligrams of iron has benefited some of those with enuresis.

> **B-6 and Magnesium**—25 to 100 milligrams of B-6 and 200 to 600 milligrams of magnesium, depending on body weight, daily. Vitamin B-6 helps correct muscle weakness and improves bladder control, but increases the need for magnesium—which is one of the nutritional keys to the problem. Taking magnesium in the form of dolomite is advantageous when dairy products are being restricted.

> **Vitamin C and Niacin**—500 to 1,000 milligrams of vitamin C plus up to 150 milligrams of niacin have proven beneficial when taken in divided doses each day.

> **Vitamin E** [see Caution, page 6]—100 to 800 IU of alpha tocopherol each day has been reported helpful in some cases of bed-wetting.

Tissue Salts—One tablet each of 3X-potency Ferr. Phos., Kali. Phos., and Nat. Phos. dissolved under the tongue three times each day has corrected the condition in some instances.

External Remedies

Exercise—Walking, running, and bicycle riding are beneficial for strengthening the muscles of the urinary apparatus.

Nerve Pressure—Press each point for 10 seconds, release for 10 seconds, and repeat for a total of 30 seconds pressure each day.

- The hollow on each side of the back of the neck between the spine and the bottom of the ears.
- The joint-crease closest to the tip of the little finger and/or the second crease closer to the hand. Apply pressure on both hands.
- The center of the abdomen, approximately 1½ inches below the navel.
- Three inches below the bottom of the kneecap, 1½ inches toward the outside of the leg.
- The hollow behind and slightly below each anklebone.
- The web of skin where the big toe and the next toe meet.

Relaxation—Lying quietly while reading or listening to music releases tension and encourages kidney secretion which should be voided after half an hour. Massaging the abdominal region with a firm, circular motion, then rubbing the back and buttocks with long, even strokes for a total of five minutes just before bed has been found beneficial. Parental tenderness and positive suggestions about remaining dry can be helpful, but scolding or threats can create anxiety which upsets all the reflex mechanisms of the body (See also, Relaxation, pages 9-10).

Love in Action

"Twas once upon a midnight blur,
   my jammies wet and cold,
I staggered through the hall to her,
   not feeling very bold.

Of all the children she had borne
   I was the last in line—
My feelings mixed, my thoughts were torn,
   clean jammies I should find.

Somehow, she knew that I was there
   dejected and forlorn.
Reached out to me, and held me near.
   Do all Moms feel that warm?

Lois Currie

Sleeping Coverings—Bedcovers should be light in weight but an incontinent individual should keep warm at night, possibly with the aid of a hot water bottle or heating pad next to the abdomen.

Sleeping Patterns—Bed-wetters often are such heavy sleepers that messages from the bladder do not register. Various mechanical alarm systems are available for after-the-fact rousing, but older children and adults can use an alarm clock for prevention by setting the alarm for two hours after bedtime, getting up to empty the bladder, and resetting the alarm for another two hours. Progressively lengthening the intervals frequently results in being able to stay dry with no more than one noctural awakening.

Folk Remedies

Cinnamon—Chewing stick cinnamon just before retiring is thought to have an astringent effect on the urinary system.

Cranberry Juice—Four ounces of cranberry juice for a child, twice that amount for an adult, has reportedly stopped enuresis on the first night.

Epsom Salts—One-half teaspoon stirred in liquid and taken after supper was an old-fashioned remedy that has been scientifically justified—epsom salts equals magnesium sulfate.

Herbal Teas—One cup of corn-silk or fennel-seed tea, sweetened with honey if desired, and taken during the day (not at bedtime) was recommended to control bed-wetting.

Honey—One teaspoon to one tablespoon raw honey taken just before retiring. (Honey acts as a mild sedative for the nervous system and is believed to attract and hold body fluid to spare the kidneys.)

Sources (See Bibliography)

19, 52, 53, 62, 67, 68, 81, 88, 89, 126, 152, 153, 168, 171, 181, 227, 254, 261, 288, 292, 305, 306, 315, 318, 328, 353.

BLOOD PRESSURE, HIGH (HYPERTENSION)

The pressure produced when the heart muscle contracts to push blood through the body's 60,000 miles of blood vessels is the systolic, or higher number. The lower figure (diastolic) represents the pressure when the heart muscle relaxes between beats. The diastolic reading is considered the more important since the more rigid an artery when relaxed, the greater the chance of its causing coronaries or strokes. Called "essential hypertension" when the high blood pressure is without known cause, and "secondary hypertension" when it stems from kidney or other disease, these sphygmomanometer readings should be taken by a physician at least once each year as high blood pressure may be present without producing any symptoms.

Blood pressure rises and falls during any 24-hour period and is stimulated by excitement, whether conscious or during dreams while asleep. It was formerly believed that a gradual elevation of blood pressure was a natural part of the aging process, with a systolic rate of 100 plus the person's age being the body's method of adapting to hardening or narrowing of the arteries. Most doctors now consider blood pressures greater than 140/90 potentially dangerous, regardless of age. Studies have shown a much higher risk of heart attacks, strokes, kidney problems, and premature deaths among those with even small elevations over the 140 systolic figure.

Causes of high blood pressure are varied and complex, with less than 10 percent being related to physical abnormalities. Atherosclerosis, environment, genetic inheritance, high salt and sugar consumption, lack of exercise, nutrient-poor diets, obesity, oral contraceptives, reactions to medications, smoking, and all forms of stress are contributory factors. Stress may be either mental or physical (see Relaxation, pages 9-10)—a result of high-pressure lifestyles or physical abnormalities such as Low Blood Sugar (which see).

The first line of attack against high blood pressure is weight control. For each extra pound of body weight the heart must pump blood through an added mile of capillaries. Studies have shown that up to two-thirds of overweight hypertensives can substantially lower their blood pressure by losing their excess weight.[84,134]

Smoking is especially detrimental for those with high blood pressure. Pipes and cigars are considered less harmful than cigarette smoking which constricts the blood vessels, raises blood pressure, and increases the amount of potentially harmful fats in the blood. *The Harvard Medical School Health Letter* (August, 1983) reported that the systolic blood pressure of hypertensives rose ten points after they smoked two cigarettes, and that their diastolic pressure went up eight points. In addition, when the carbon monoxide from the smoke is inhaled, it reduces the amount of oxygen available to the heart. For those who must smoke, choosing cigarettes with low tar and nicotine and then avoiding smoking them all the way down is suggested—the last third of a cigarette produces twice as much tar and nicotine as the first third.

Even though the following remedies have been proven effective in lowering blood pressure for some people, each case is individual. Medically prescribed medications should be continued as directed until improvement is sufficient for the attending physician to reduce or eliminate the drugs.

Diet and Supplements

Hypertension is considered the greatest threat to our health. It affects one out of every four average Americans and over half the population over 65. It is a good example, however, of a malady that can be controlled by natural methods. The typical American diet with its one or two large daily meals, high proportion of meat, heavy use of salt and refined sugar, and extensive consumption of processed foods in which natural mineral and vitamin balances have been disrupted seems to have been designed to create high blood pressure.

A diet for preventing or controlling high blood pressure should be low in sugar and salt; high in protein, B vitamins, calcium, potassium, and all the elements helpful in lowering the cholesterol level (see Hardening of the Arteries). Dr. Berenson, of the Louisiana State School of Medicine, maintains that sugar is an important factor in the development of hypertension.[24] Another doctor at the University of Maryland has induced rises in blood pressure by feeding sugar to his patients. Adding sugar to a high-salt diet increases blood pressure much more rapidly than the high-salt diet alone.[52,282]

A current research project on a nondrug approach to hypertension has shown that the simple mechanisms of potassium and calcium produce better clinical results than the use of diuretics.[22] The widely accepted belief that reducing the amount of salt in the diet will help prevent or reduce high blood pressure for everyone is now being questioned. As reported in *American Health* (July/August 1982), hospital studies of hypertensive patients showed that an extremely low-sodium diet lowered blood pressure to normal within a few days in about half the cases tested. Other tests have shown only one-third of hypertensives to be affected by the amount of salt used.[134,262] The blood pressure of the remaining patients was not affected by either further sodium reduction or by increasing dietary salt to 3,000 milligrams daily. (The average American consumes over 5,000 milligrams of salt each day.) For the one-third to one-half of hypertensives who are salt-sensitive, limiting sodium intake to between 250 and 500 milligrams per day usually brings quick results, but adding even one-fourth teaspoon of salt can raise their blood pressure, so the restriction must be continued on a permanent basis.

Many investigators believe that concentrating on foods high in potassium can be just as important as salt reduction. Sodium and potassium must be in balance for proper body chemistry. An imbalance with too little potassium can cause the body to retain so much sodium that high blood pressure develops. According to a report in *Medical World News* (December 11, 1978), a study of 2,500 volunteers showed that a high potassium intake negates the harmful effects of excess sodium consumption. Good food sources of potassium are blackstrap molasses; fresh fruits (especially bananas and watermelon); fruit juices such as apple, citrus, cranberry, grape, and pear; raisins; sunflower seeds; unsalted nuts; vegetables; and wheat germ. Granulated kelp is high in potassium with relatively little sodium and has a slightly salty flavor when sprinkled on foods. Commercial salt substitutes with a high potassium content may be helpful for those with high blood pressure.

One teaspoon of table salt contains approximately 2,300 milligrams of sodium. If many canned or processed foods are included in the diet, a potassium supplement may be needed to maintain an equal balance with the sodium. But, it is possible to upset the balance in the other direction, so dietary adjustments are believed preferable.

A diet high in complete proteins has been successful in lowering blood pressure but a definite correlation has been established between the amount of animal foods in the diet and elevations of blood pressure. Whole grains, seeds, nuts, and legumes are suggested replacements for at least part of the protein customarily derived from meats. Eating four to six small meals daily allows better nutrient absorption with less heart effort than one to three larger ones, and is less likely to cause weight gain. Both the Pritikin Program.[266] and Paavo Airola's vegetarian diet[13] have been successful in decreasing hypertension. The Kempner Rice Diet usually lowers blood pressure but should not be continued for longer than one or two weeks as nutritional deficiencies might result. The Kempner diet consists of one and one-half cups dry rice (approximately 1,000 calories) cooked without salt, and 1,000 calories of cooked or raw fruit (with sugar, if desired) each day.

POTASSIUM-SODIUM COMPARISON CHART*

	Potassium	Sodium
1 cup chicken-noodle soup	55	979
3-ounce serving roast turkey	315	111
11-ounce "TV dinner" of turkey, potato, and peas	549	1,247
3-ounce serving lean, broiled sirloin steak	320	50
8-ounce frozen beef potpie	211	830
1 medium potato, baked in its skin	407	3
1/2 cup green peas, cooked without salt	157	1
1/2 cup canned green peas, drained	81	200
1 medium apple, raw	182	2
1 serving apple pie [1/6 of 9-inch pie]	128	482

*From *The Dieter's Companion,* Nikki & David Goldbeck, Signet, 1977, and *Nutrition Almanac,* McGraw-Hill, 1979, revised edition

Most naturopaths and some physicians recommend "juice fasts" of from two to four days out of alternate weeks for six months. The daily pattern for juice-fasting usually includes three or four cups of herb tea and/or unsalted vegetable broth plus one quart of water interspersed with two 8-ounce glasses of raw vegetable juices and one glass of fresh fruit juice. Dr. Airola suggests one week of eating nothing but watermelon to lower blood pressure. Either of these treatments should be undertaken only with medical supervision.

Coffee, tea, colas, and other caffeine-containing beverages should be avoided as they can raise blood pressure from 10 to 14 points and encourage fluid retention. Five cups of a caffeine drink doubles the intake of cadmium, which contributes to hypertension. Alcohol should be limited as it causes a rapid rise of fatty substances in the blood, but small amounts taken before or with meals open the blood vessels and seem helpful to both circulation and digestion.

Tests have shown that the nitrates or nitrites usually added to bacon, cold cuts, ham, hot dogs, etc. can elevate blood pressure, so these foods should be avoided or at least restricted. Commercial or home water softeners increase both the sodium and cadmium content, so "softened" water should not be used for drinking or cooking. Current findings indicate that the harder the water, the lower the death rate from hypertensive heart disease.

When taken in addition to a daily multi-vitamin-mineral tablet, the following optional supplements have shown excellent results in reducing high blood pressure for many individuals.

Vitamin A—Up to 150,000 units daily for two weeks only has lowered blood pressure when taken in conjunction with vitamin E.

B **Complex**—One comprehensive, high-potency tablet and/or one or two tablespoons brewer's yeast daily, plus optional, individual B vitamins.

- **B-6**—50 to 200 milligrams. Hypertension has been found to require extra amounts of this vitamin, but magnesium should be increased at the same time.
- **B-15**—50 milligrams daily to increase the supply of oxygen reaching the heart.
- **Niacin**—100 to 500 milligrams daily to increase blood circulation.
- **Pantothenic Acid**—100 to 1,500 milligrams daily as a natural tranquilizer to lower blood pressure.
- **Choline**—500 to 3,000 milligrams daily helps strengthen weak capillary walls and dilates the blood vessels to decrease the blood pressure required.
- **Inositol**—500 to 3,000 milligrams in divided doses to act as a tranquilizer and help prevent fatty deposits in the arteries.

Vitamin C and Bioflavonoids—1,000 to 5,000 milligrams C plus 500 to 2,000 milligrams bioflavonoids. Large amounts of vitamin C have been known to lower blood pressure. The complete C-complex works with vitamin E to strengthen the blood vessels and help prevent cerebral hemorrhage or stroke.

Calcium—1,000 to 3,000 milligrams daily. Calcium calms nerves and increases the excretion of salt through the urine to lower blood pressure. The *Journal of the American Medical Association* (March 4, 1983) reported an average reduction of 7.3 percent in the diastolic pressure of those taking calcium supplements.

Vitamin E (see Caution, page 6)—Starting with 100 IU of alpha tocopherol and increasing gradually to 400 to 800 IU daily is suggested. Vitamin E not only decreases the need for oxygen and lowers blood pressure, it seems to enhance the action of most antihypertensive drugs. It also provides insurance against cerebral hemorrhage or stroke by working with vitamin C to strengthen the blood vessels.

Lecithin—Suggested dosages vary from three 1,200-milligram capsules to three tablespoons of lecithin granules daily. (One tablespoon granules is the equivalent of 10 1,200-milligram capsules.) Lecithin is a good source of both choline and inositol.

Magnesium—500 milligrams daily. Magnesium has been a mainstay in treating hypertension for the past half century. It induces muscle relaxation and is necessary for potassium function. Dolomite tablets offer magnesium plus calcium.

MaxEPA—Eicosapentaenoid Acid is a substance isolated from fatty salt-water fish. When taken as directed on the container, it has proven successful in helping reduce high blood pressure. According to *Health News and Reviews* (May/June 1983), researchers believe the Eskimos and Japanese are so free of high blood pressure because of their abundant consumption of cod, herring, mackerel, and other cold-salt-water fish.

Selenium—50 to 200 micrograms daily to intensify the action of vitamin E and to prevent sticky accumulations in the blood which can cause hypertension.

Tissue Salts—Two or three 3X-potency tablets, two or three times daily, of Ferr. Phos. (to increase the amount of oxygen reaching the cells) and Silicea (to improve circulation).

Zinc—10 to 50 milligrams daily. Zinc increases blood circulation, helps compensate for stress, and is of value in reducing high cadmium levels.

Exercise

Any strenuous exercise program should be attempted only under the direction of a physician but mild exercise, such as walking or swimming for 20 minutes each day, offers threefold benefits for hypertensives.

- Gentle exercise helps blood vessels become more elastic and regulates the body's output and response to certain hormones thought to influence high blood pressure.
- Literally walking away from mental pressures and irritants for a few minutes can be more effective than tranquilizers.
- The calories expended in exercise help burn up excess pounds which contribute to hypertension.

Folk Remedies

Apple Cider Vinegar—Stir one or two teaspoons apple cider vinegar into a glass of water and sip with each meal. An equal amount of raw honey may be mixed in, if desired, but the vinegar alone has brought a 20- to 40-point drop in blood pressure in half an hour after a high-protein meal.[180] (Protein eaten without acid is believed to thicken the blood and raise blood pressure.)

Garlic—One or two cloves of fresh garlic (or several garlic perles) taken with two meals each day is a time-honored remedy for dilating constricted blood vessels and reducing blood pressure. Recent scientific tests showing that 40 percent of hypertensives respond to the garlic treatment reinforce this belief.[228]

Case History

Calvin D. was discouraged about his continued high blood pressure. He had followed his doctor's orders; had eliminated caffeine, cut down on salt, even lost his 10 pounds of excess weight—but his blood pressure remained higher than it should. When a friend asked if he had tried adding garlic to his diet, Calvin laughingly replied that he was already using garlic in cooked dishes and rubbing it on the salad bowl. The friend explained that he meant eating garlic as a food, not merely using it as a seasoning; and brought Calvin some of his home-grown garlic. The fresh garlic looked like green onions and had a surprisingly mild flavor Calvin found he actually enjoyed. In addition to stirring it into cooked dishes, he placed garlic slices on bread (spread with cholesterol-free margarine) for his noontime sandwich, and minced the tender tops along with more garlic in his dinner salad. Calvin adopted his friend's "garlic farming" method; planting cloves of dried garlic in his backyard flowerbeds and interspersing them with the decorative container-plants on his porch. He was delighted when the first green shoots appeared, assuring the production of a successful crop, and became even more pleased when his next physical check-up produced a blood pressure reading in the normal range. Calvin continues to use a lot of garlic, not only as a precautionary measure, but because he likes its taste.

Herbal Teas—Alfalfa, catnip, cayenne pepper, mint, red clover, sage, sassafras, skullcap, and watermelon-seed teas are considered specifics for lowering blood pressure.

Onions—When eaten daily, either raw or cooked, onions are thought to be antihypertensive—possibly because they help control cholesterol levels.

Potato Broths

- Place the peelings (without sprouts or green portions) from five well-washed potatoes in two cups water and boil for 15 minutes in a covered saucepan. Cool and strain, then drink two cups of the liquid each day.
- Stir two cups chopped potato (scrubbed but not peeled), one-half cup each shredded carrots and celery, and one-half cup of any other green vegetable into three cups of boiling water. Cover and simmer for 20 minutes. Strain and drink while warm, or store in the refrigerator and sip during the day.

Whey—Three times each day dissolve one tablespoon powdered whey (available in health food stores) in one-half glass water and drink. Positive results have been noticeable within three weeks in some cases.[76]

Nerve Massage

Firmly press and knead the area between the eyebrows for three minutes every day.

With firm, circular movements, massage the hollows in the back of the neck at the base of the skull for several minutes each day.

Gently pinch and knead the areas above, below, and on either side of the Adam's Apple for 30 seconds each day.

Bend the left arm so that it forms a 90-degree angle and massage the hollow of the inner elbow for 30 seconds daily. Repeat with the right arm.

Massage all parts of the thumb, the two fingers next to it, and the webs between the fingers on both hands once each day.

Nerve Pressure

Place the index fingers in each ear and press in the direction of the eyes for one minute each day.

Several times daily, wind rubber bands around the thumbs and first and second fingers of both hands. Leave in place for three to 20 minutes, removing at the first sign of numbness.

Three times a day, pull the middle fingers of both hands for 20 seconds.

Once each day, press the following points three times for 10 seconds each:

- Use the thumb and index finger to squeeze the vertical groove on the back of the ear about one-third of the way up from the bottom of the lobe.
- Use the thumb and index finger to press gently 1-1/2 inches on both sides of the Adam's Apple.

- Hook the index fingers along the inside of the ribs two-thirds of the distance down from the lowest end of the breastbone and press inward and upward on the slight notch that can be felt.
- Press just below the fingernail of the middle finger, on the side toward the thumb. Repeat with the other hand.
- Press 1-1/2 inches toward the elbow from the large crease on the inner wrist, directly below the middle finger on each hand.
- Press 1-1/2 inches directly below the navel.
- On each foot, press just below the ball of the foot in line with the third toe.

Sources (See Bibliography)

3, 4, 13, 22, 24, 25, 34, 52, 53, 62, 63, 64, 67, 68, 76, 78, 81, 84, 88, 89, 92, 104, 134, 152, 154, 165, 173, 174, 180, 184, 190, 193, 204, 208, 228, 229, 243, 249, 250, 252, 254, 256, 257, 261, 266, 280, 282, 288, 289, 291, 297, 301, 303, 315, 319, 333, 334, 335, 348, 349, 353.

BLOOD PRESSURE—LOW (HYPOTENSION)

Considered by many to be a blessing rather than a malady, relatively little attention has been given low blood pressure. As a general rule, 100/60 constitutes low blood pressure for an adult, but many insurance companies accept a systolic reading (upper figure) as low as 80 to be compatible with good health. Following injuries producing shock or extreme blood loss, blood pressure may temporarily fall to dangerously low levels. Chronic hypotension may be caused by physical disorders such as anemia, internal bleeding, low blood sugar, tuberculosis, an underactive thyroid, or a heart condition—all of which require medical diagnosis and treatment. Most cases of hypotension, however, originate from nutritional deficiencies.

Postural Hypotension—evidenced by momentary faintness or dizziness when rising abruptly from a reclining or sitting position—may be a symptom of low blood pressure, but may be due merely to an inefficient internal mechanism that is slow to make the changes in blood pressure required to accommodate these sudden movements. Temporary episodes of postural hypotension may occur in connection with viral infections or influenza. Rising gradually and avoiding abrupt changes of position often prevents problems with this form of low blood pressure. Deep breathing and improving circulation by hot and cold morning baths followed by brisk rubbing with a coarse towel are sometimes helpful, as is rapidly stroking the entire body for several minutes twice each day.

Diet and Supplements

When no underlying physical disorder is responsible, low blood pressure can usually be corrected with a few weeks of supplemented diet. A low-protein diet or lack of certain vitamins and minerals can cause the walls of the blood vessels to lose their elasticity, become flabby, and expand. Since the volume of blood remains the same, the pressure against the arterial walls is reduced and fewer nutrients can penetrate into the tissues—thus producing fatigue, weakness, and a feeling of lightheadedness. A high-protein diet that stresses organ meats, potatoes baked in their skins, leafy green vegetables, soybeans or flour, and wheat germ helps restore elasticity to the arteries, stimulates the adrenal glands, and helps normalize blood pressure. (Desiccated liver powder or tablets may be used by those who do not enjoy eating liver or kidney.) Bell peppers, brewer's yeast, cabbage, citrus fruits, cucumber, dandelion greens, dates, leeks, onions, peas, raisins, sweet potatoes, tomatoes, and whole grains also are recommended. Including generous amounts of salt for the first week or two is suggested.[89] Folk practitioners swore by beets and beet juice. One 6-ounce glass of beet juice plus one serving of beets each day was their prescription for lagging blood pressure. Skullcap tea with a bit of cayenne pepper was another folk remedy for raising low blood pressure, but as little liquid as possible should be taken with meals to encourage nutrient absorption. In addition to a daily multi-vitamin-mineral tablet to help compensate for decreased nutrient assimilation, these individual supplements have been found helpful.

> **B Complex**—One comprehensive, high-potency tablet daily. Even a mild deficiency of any of the B vitamins can produce low blood pressure. An additional 10 to 50 milligrams of B-1 helps regulate an erratic heartbeat. A deficiency of pantothenic acid inhibits the production of adrenal hormones, which causes an overabundance of salt and water to be excreted, thus decreasing the volume of blood and creating low blood pressure. 100 to 500 milligrams of pantothenic acid daily is suggested.
>
> **Vitamin C**—1,000 to 3,000 milligrams taken in several divided doses during the day. The adrenal glands require copious amounts of this vitamin to function properly.
>
> **Calcium and Magnesium**—Up to 1,000 milligrams of calcium and 500 milligrams of magnesium, depending on the amount of milk and dairy products included in the daily diet. Both minerals are needed for healthy heart action.
>
> **Vitamin E** (see Caution, page 6)—100 to 800 IU daily. Besides decreasing the need for oxygen and relieving the fatigue caused by oxygen-starved tissues, vitamin E tends to normalize blood pressure.
>
> **Potassium**—A deficiency of this mineral can cause a slow, irregular pulse. Supplements may be required to maintain the proper sodium-potassium balance if liberal amounts of salt are used in the diet. (See Blood Pressure—High for a dietary comparison chart.)

Nerve Pressure

Pressing each of these points for 10 seconds, releasing for 10 seconds, and repeating three times for a total of 30 seconds pressure once each day has been found to normalize some cases of low blood pressure.

- Press inward and upward under the center of the back of the skull.
- Hook the left index finger as far up as possible on the inside margin of the left rib cage and press inward and upward.
- Press 2 inches toward the front of the body from the center of the right underarm, in the center of the breast muscles.
- Press 1 inch below the tip of the breastbone.

Sources (See Bibliography)

25, 34, 76, 81, 82, 88, 89, 110, 173, 184, 190, 254, 261, 288, 289, 301, 302, 315, 353.

BOILS, ABSCESSES, FURUNCLES, CARBUNCLES, STIES, FELONS, AND WHITLOWS

Among the most miserable of mishaps, boils were one of the Ten Plagues chosen to afflict ancient Egyptians for having enslaved the Hebrews. Sometimes called an abscess or furuncle, a boil is a pimple-like infection that originates in a hair follicle; usually it is due to the presence of staphylococcus bacteria. A carbuncle is a large boil, or a cluster of smaller ones, which affects the underlying layers of skin and muscle. Sties are little abscesses that form between the roots of the eyelashes. A felon or whitlow is a painful abscess on the tip of a finger or toe, triggered by an injury to the base or side of the fingernail or toenail.

Improving nutrition and correcting any vitamin deficiencies can shorten the duration of the boils and strengthen the body's defenses against further outbreaks. When sties or other boils first erupt, they may sometimes be checked by holding a small piece of ice against the spot. Once a boil has developed, warm, moist compresses help bring it to a head so it can break, drain, and heal. Squeezing or pinching only aggravates the condition. Lancing should be performed by a physician, but *Dr. Taylor's Self-Help Medical Guide* [315] suggests opening small boils that appear ready to burst by using a needle sterilized with alcohol, then inserting a small rubber band (also cleansed with alcohol) as a drain. One end of the rubber band should be allowed to extend so it can be removed after two days. The boil should be covered with a bulky dressing to absorb the drainage.

Diet and Supplements

A high-protein diet with generous amounts of fresh fruits, vegetables, and whole grains helps combat the infection and improves the body's natural resistance. Apricots, bananas, citrus fruits, liver, onions, and tomatoes are considered especially beneficial. Drinking one or two glasses each day of the juice from beets, carrots, cucumbers, lettuce, and spinach (in any combination) has been found helpful. Including a tablespoon or so of unprocessed bran in the diet and drinking eight to 10 glasses of water every day will help avoid the constipation that frequently accompanies this malady. At least one tablespoon of cold-pressed vegetable oil should be used daily to provide the essential fatty acids, but an outbreak of boils may be brought on by too many rich foods—so anything greasy, spicy, or sweet should be avoided during the attack.

Some individuals have a genetic need for extra vitamins A and C, and the mineral zinc, and will be beset by boils if they do not take large amounts. The formula recommended by Lendon Smith[305] is 50,000 units A, 1,000 milligrams C, and 50 milligrams zinc each day. Other authorities suggest the following optional supplements:

Vitamins A and E (see Caution, page 6)—25,000 units A plus 100 to 600 IU of E daily. A deficiency of vitamin A has been shown to increase susceptibility to boils. Vitamin E protects vitamin A from oxidation within the body. The combination speeds healing. Applying an A + E ointment (or vitamin E oil) to the boil and covering with a bandage may be helpful. Once the drainage appears complete, squeezing on vitamin E from a pierced capsule may prevent scarring.

B Complex—One comprehensive, high-potency tablet daily. All the Bs help combat the stress of infection. Vitamins B-1, B-2, B-6, biotin, folic acid, niacin, and pantothenic acid aid the body's production of antibodies. Taking 10 to 1,000 milligrams B-6, 100 to 4,000 milligrams pantothenic acid, and 500 to 5,000 milligrams vitamin C in divided doses each day for several days has cleared painful boils for some individuals.

Vitamin C—500 to 1,000 milligrams each two hours for several days, then 500 to 1,000 milligrams once each day. Research has shown massive doses of vitamin C to be as effective as antibiotics in destroying harmful bacteria.[350]

Tissue Salts—3X-potency tablets, as directed:

- During an attack of boils, take alternate doses of two tablets of Ferr. Phos. and Kali. Mur. at hourly intervals, plus two tablets of Silicea three times a day.
- When the boil comes to a head and is ready to drain, take three tablets of Silicea every two hours. If the discharge is foul smelling, take the same amount of Kali. Phos. with the Silicea.
- If the boils continue to drain without healing, change the remedies to Calc. Sulph. and Nat. Sulph., two tablets of each at two-hour intervals.
- For carbuncles, add four tablets daily of Calc. Fluor. to the dosages recommended for boils.
- For external compresses: in one-half cup hot water, dissolve three doses of whatever tissue salts are being taken internally.

Zinc—15 to 50 milligrams daily to promote healing.

Folk Remedies

Folk medicine dealt with boils for thousands of years before the advent of doctors and antibiotics. While some of the old remedies (such as applying scraped beefsteak or rubbing a sty with a gold wedding ring) are no longer advised, many of the remedies utilize vitamin therapy (citrus fruits are rich in vitamin C and carrot poultices contain vitamin A), and warm compresses are prescribed by physicians as well as folk practitioners.

Bread—Stale bread soaked in hot milk and applied as a poultice was a standard remedy. The Pennsylvania Dutch preferred poultices made from breadcrumbs and honey.

Egg—The skin of a raw egg was used to "draw" a boil to a head. A poultice of mashed, hard-cooked egg white was also considered helpful.

Flour—A poultice of warm milk and flour (with one tablespoon salt added to each cup of flour, if desired) was a basic remedy. During the early 1800s, flour and ground ginger made into a paste was often used.

Fruit—Placing raw figs over boils was advised by Hezekiah. (*Isaiah 38:21*) Over 2,400 years later, folk healers are still using the same treatment but recommended splitting the figs and soaking them in hot water for a minute or two before applying. Eating at least one dozen oranges or grapefruit daily was an early specific for boils and carbuncles. To relieve the pain of a felon, a hole was cut in a lemon and the finger inserted. For a boil, a thick slice of lemon was applied, then covered with a bandage. Poultices of crushed raw cranberries were another option.

Herbs—Instead of water, drinking teas made from cayenne pepper, comfrey root, red clover, sarsaparilla, sassafras, or slippery elm is recommended. Herbs may be applied externally as fomentations of strong comfrey tea, or as poultices made from sage leaves or a combination of triple-strength sassafras and slippery elm teas thickened with cornmeal.

Hot Compresses—A boil is often brought to a head more quickly when a continuous wet dressing is applied. Plain hot water for sties (or a solution of one tablespoon epsom salts or table salt to one cup water for other boils) may be used to moisten the bandage. Felons can be soaked in the mixture. Frequent changing of the dressing helps insure localization of the infection.

Pekoe Tea—For an incipient sty or boil, moisten a teaspoonful of black pekoe tea wrapped in cloth (or a teabag) with boiling water and apply while very warm. Secure with a loose bandage and leave in place several hours. Repeat with fresh tea, if necessary.

Vegetable Poultices (Mix with castor oil or vegetable oil, if desired; apply warm and renew at least twice each day.)—Cabbage leaves dipped in hot water, ground raw cabbage, grated raw or cooked carrots, cooked minced garlic, the green blades of leeks finely chopped and added to a little milk or lard, chopped raw or cooked onions (blended with either of the oils or with blackstrap molasses), grated raw or cooked white potato, or thin slices of raw pumpkin.

Case History

Steven F. didn't want to tell his grandparents about the sore on his behind. Besides having promised his mother that he wouldn't be any bother for the elderly couple, the 12-year-old was too modest to even describe the location of the sore. However, the sore was getting sorer, might be "catching" (like measles, or something even worse), and was taking all the fun out of this vacation visit. Steven waited until he was alone with his grandfather, then hesitantly explained the terrible problem. "All you have is a carbuncle," declared his grandfather after taking one look at the inflamed lump. "Let's go concoct a magic potion to make it disappear." Together they chopped an onion, added a little water, waited while the mixture cooked, then stirred in a tablespoon of sugar. Steven yelped when his grandfather applied the hot poultice. He wondered if the "magic potion" would give him a burn as well as a sore to worry about, but he obediently allowed the process to be repeated before bedtime and again the next day. By the following night the carbuncle had come to a head and burst, and in a few days all the soreness was gone. The remainder of his visit was so much fun that Steven still remembers it as his "magic vacation."

Sources (See Bibliography)

13, 27, 28, 52, 53, 62, 68, 81, 82, 89, 98, 122, 142, 151, 152, 156, 168, 174, 176, 184, 190, 226, 227, 228, 236, 243, 254, 256, 272, 282, 288, 305, 315, 319, 333, 349, 350.

BRONCHITIS

Bronchitis can be serious enough to warrant immediate medical attention for the elderly or those with chronic lung or heart conditions, but is commonly a relatively mild malady. Acute bronchitis is a temporary inflammation of the bronchial tubes. It may develop as a result of a cold, viral infection of the nose or throat, or inhalation of exhaust fumes, industrial pollutants, or tobacco smoke. It may be accompanied by a fever for three to five days. (A physician should be consulted if the fever persists longer as it might be an indication of pneumonia.) The accompanying cough usually lingers for several weeks. Chronic bronchitis is a long-continued, recurring form of the ailment that is generally limited to people with a background of allergies. Infection seeks out chronically irritated membranes, and, if untreated, chronic bronchitis can progress into emphysema.

During a bout of bronchitis, cigarette smoking and all known allergy-provoking substances should be avoided. Staying indoors with the windows closed, getting plenty of rest, and using a humidifier or inhaling steam is recommended. The cough is nature's way of getting rid of the poisons which started the problem. Cough expectorants rather than cough suppressants should be used, but in moderation. Large quantities may stimulate a reflex action in the stomach and act as an emetic. To help drain mucus from the lungs, lie face down over the side of a bed with the chest leaning down to the floor. Cough while turning the head from side to side, then blow the nose.

Case History

George C. had coughed until he was ready to collapse. When he telephoned his doctor for assistance with this latest bout of bronchitis, the nurse offered two helpful suggestions for relieving the tenseness and improving breathing ability.

1. Lie in a fetal position, cover your body and head with a thermal blanket or sheet (nothing airtight, asphyxiation is not the object), and imagine the peace and security of having returned to the womb.

2. Run the hot water until the bathroom is filled with steam. If time permits, soak in a tub filled with comfortably hot water. If time is limited, take a hot shower.

Both these remedies were effectual in relieving the tenseness engendered by prolonged coughing, but George still could not sleep at night. Sitting in a recliner chair or propping himself up on pillows in the bed merely aggravated his breathing problem. In desperation he sat on the floor to watch television, faced the recliner, and rested his head on a pillow he had placed on the seat of the chair. Awakened several hours later by the bleeping sound of the television station's sign-off, George realized that he had found his own emergency solution for getting some much-needed sleep during bronchitis attacks.

Diet and Supplements

A nutritious diet with plenty of liquids is recommended. Water and juices help loosen and cut the phlegm. All kinds of fruits and vegetables and their juices (especially apricots, citrus, papaya, pineapple, beets, carrots, celery, cucumber, green pepper, onions, and tomatoes) are beneficial. Spicy foods such as horseradish and hot peppers stimulate the production of watery secretions in the lungs—which makes it easier to cough up mucus. A report in *Medical World News* (February 20, 1978) suggested that those with bronchitis eat at least one very spicy meal each day—hot enough to cause a tingling tongue and runny nose. When spicy foods cannot be tolerated by the stomach, gargling with 10 to 20 drops of hot pepper sauce in a cup of warm water may stimulate mucus flow. The proverbial chicken soup with plenty of garlic, pepper, and possibly curry powder, increases expectoration and helps clear the air passages.

Some physicians advise staying away from foods believed to produce mucus: dairy products, eggs, chocolate, sugar, coffee. For bronchitis cases where food allergies may be a factor, eliminating milk and/or wheat has proven helpful. If antibiotics have been prescribed, acidophilus yogurt should be eaten daily (or acidophilus capsules taken with each meal) to help restore the friendly flora in the intestines. Other suggested supplements:

Vitamin A—25,000 units one to three times daily for one month, then limited to 25,000 units per day. Vitamin A has a marked anti-infectious action.

B Complex—One comprehensive, high-potency tablet daily to combat the stress of illness and help build antibodies; plus at least 100 milligrams each B-6 and pantothenic acid for their antihistamine, anti-mucus action. These B vitamins are especially helpful when taken in combination with vitamin C.

Bee Pollen—1,000 milligrams or up to one teaspoon of pollen granules daily. Bee pollen has been particularly helpful for those with allergy-related bronchitis.

Vitamin C and Bioflavonoids—3,000 to 5,000 milligrams C plus 200 to 600 milligrams of bioflavonoids daily. Patients with bronchitis have responded almost miraculously to massive doses of the vitamin-C complex in conjunction with B vitamins. In acute conditions, 1,000 milligrams of vitamin C may be taken every hour or two for its antibiotic action.

Calcium—800 to 1,000 milligrams daily if milk and dairy products are being avoided.

Vitamin E (see Caution, page 6)—100 to 600 IU daily. Vitamin E is necessary for the absorption of vitamin A and, in addition, reduces the amount of oxygen required by the tissues.

Tissue Salts—In all cases of bronchitis, taking one 12X tablet of Ferr. Phos. twice each day is recommended to help carry oxygen to the lungs. For acute bronchitis with fever, the remedy is one 6X tablet of Ferr. Phos. every half hour until the temperature is normal.

- When there is soreness in the chest and larynx: take three tablets of 6X Ferr. Phos. each four hours, and three tablets of 6X Calc. Sulph. between those doses.
- For chronic bronchitis with thick phlegm: twice daily take one tablet each 12X Ferr. Phos. and Nat. Mur.
- For chronic bronchitis with a dry, painful cough: three times daily take one tablet each 12X Ferr. Phos. and Nat. Mur.
- For an expectorant: take three 6X tablets of Kali. Mur. every two hours. If the cough is accompanied by fever, substitute Kali. Sulph. in the same potency.

Zinc—15 to 50 milligrams daily. Zinc helps correct the inflammation and speeds recovery.

Folk Remedies

Asparagus—Liquefy a can of asparagus in an electric blender and store in the refrigerator. Take one-fourth cup each morning and evening. If desired, dilute with water for a hot or cold beverage. Improvement in chronic bronchitis has been noticeable in two to four weeks.[3]

Castor Oil and Turpentine—Warm two tablespoons castor oil, add one tablespoon turpentine. Rub on the chest at bedtime and cover with flannel. In severe cases, discomfort may be relieved by applying the mixture several times a day.

Cough Syrups (expectorants)

- Cook fresh blackberry juice with equal amount of sugar to make a syrup. Take in tablespoonful doses as needed.
- Mix equal parts honey and freshly grated horseradish. Take one tablespoonful every morning. Or, let the mixture stand overnight, squeeze through cheese-cloth, and take one tablespoon of the syrup each hour.
- Combine fresh lemon juice with an equal amount of honey and take by the spoonful whenever needed.
- Mix equal parts lemon juice and olive oil. Take one teaspoonful each morning.
- Chop a large onion into a bowl of honey and let stand for 10 hours. Strain to remove the onions, then add one tablespoon apple cider vinegar. Take a spoonful three times a day, or as needed.

Cranberry-Pear Juice—Boil fresh cranberries in water for 10 minutes. Whir in an electric blender with an equal amount of pear juice and drink several glasses each day.

Fig Drink—Boil four chopped figs in two cups of water for six minutes. Cover until cool, then store in the refrigerator. Sip half a cup of the liquid each morning and night.

Herbal Teas—Fenugreek seed tea is one of the oldest remedies for bronchitis. Make the tea by steeping one tablespoon of the seeds in one cup boiling water until aromatic and golden. Drink one cup each hour during the first day, then four cups each day to flush mucus out of the body. Other teas considered beneficial: camomile, chicory, comfrey, dandelion leaf, ginger, horseradish, licorice root, parsley, peppermint, rose hips, rosemary, saffron, sage, savory, slippery elm.

Milk and Honey—Stir one or two tablespoons raw honey into a cup of scalded milk and sip slowly to relieve bronchial distress.

Onions

- Fry finely cut onions in lard and apply to the chest at night. Cover with folded cloth and keep the rest of the body warm, using heating pads or hot water bottles if necessary.
- At least once each day, eat several slices of onion with tomato and minced garlic.

Nerve Massage

Hold the right foot with the left hand and use the right hand to rub the entire area directly beneath the toe pads. Use a circular, rolling motion, starting under the big toe. If there is any tenderness, massage it out. Repeat with the left foot.

Nerve Pressure

Unless otherwise indicated, press each point three times for 10 seconds each to bring short-term relief from bronchial distress.

- Press over the bridge of the nose with the fingers and thumb.
- Press in and up under the bony shelf on the cheeks adjoining each side of the nose above the nostrils.
- Use the two index fingers to stretch the lips from the corners of the mouth.
- With the thumb and fingers, pinch the area along the spine at the back of the neck. The pinches should be fast "nipping" motions and should be made up and down the neck for one minute.
- Extend the left arm, palm up. Press at the inner hollow of the elbow 1 inch toward the thumb. Repeat with the right arm.
- Press a point 1½ inches toward the elbow from the center of the largest crease on the inner wrist. Repeat on the other arm.

- Squeeze the sides of the thumbnail on each hand with the thumb and index finger of the opposite hand. Or, wear rubber bands around the thumbs and first fingers of both hands until they start to turn blue or become numb.
- Press against each side of the breastbone, between the collarbone and the first rib.
- Press a point on the sternum in the center of the chest.
- Press a point the width of one hand directly above the navel.

Sources (See Bibliography)

3, 6,7, 13, 34, 40, 53, 62, 63, 64, 68, 92, 142, 152, 156, 159, 165, 168, 173, 174, 184, 190, 226, 227, 228, 243, 256, 260, 277, 288, 297, 315, 316, 319, 330, 333, 335.

BRUISES, "BLACK EYES," AND SPRAINS

The typical black-and-blue mark of a bruise usually results from a bump or blow that ruptures small blood vessels to cause internal bleeding without breaking the skin. The escaped blood darkens from lack of oxygen; then gradually is resorbed, allowing the discoloration to fade away. Sprains are injuries to soft tissues surrounding the joints. They are most commonly caused by twisting or wrenching ankles, fingers, wrists, or knees and stretching or tearing ligaments, muscles, tendons, or blood vessels; a sprain may be accompanied by a bruise.

The first treatment for either mishap is the application of ice and pressure. Vigorous massage should be avoided to prevent further injury to the tissues and more internal bleeding. No pressure should be applied to an injured eye, but alternating ice with squeezing or pressing at brief intervals for 15 to 30 minutes minimizes the pain, swelling, and discoloration of other bruises and sprains. In severe cases, an x-ray may be necessary to make sure that no bones have been chipped, fractured, or dislocated.

Minor bruises heal without additional treatment. Sprains should be elevated and immobilized with a sling, strapping, or elastic bandage for at least 24 hours, with frequent applications of ice. Once the swelling has stabilized, soaking the sprained joint in contrasting-temperature baths for 30 to 60 minutes several times daily (or using moist compresses of cracked ice alternating with hot towels) is beneficial. Some gentle motion is essential to prevent the muscles from atrophying, but activity should not be forced as long as it causes pain. A sprained ankle should be wrapped with a nonelastic bandage for all walking until the supporting tissues have healed. A crutch or cane may hasten recuperation.

Light massage plus the application of heat will improve blood circulation and may be used for a bad bruise as well as a sprain. For the swelling due to bruises or sprains, Dr. Airola[13] recommends drinking fresh pineapple juice or taking the pineapple enzyme, bromelain, in tablets. Taking any or all of the antioxidants (see page 3) helps control the free radicals released when bruising occurs. An assortment of liniments, poultices, and compresses of towels wrung out of various liquids were folk remedies for both bruises and sprains. Applying either strong sage tea or diluted vinegar was a popular treatment. The 1879 edition of *Housekeeping in Old Virginia*[324] advised a liniment made from one egg beaten light and shaken well with one cup each apple cider vinegar and spirits of turpentine, but this is not advised for black eyes!

Compresses

- **Sage and Mint**—Steep one teaspoon dried sage with one-half teaspoon dried mint in one cup boiling water for 10 minutes. Add one tablespoon apple cider vinegar. Saturate a small towel and apply as warm as can be tolerated.
- **Salt and Vinegar**—Dissolve two tablespoons salt in three-fourths cup hot water, then mix with three-fourths cup apple cider vinegar. Use a small turkish towel to apply a wet compress to relieve congestion and promote better healing.
- **Tea**—Wring a small towel out of strong, hot pekoe tea. Place over the painful area to reduce swelling and relieve discomfort.

Poultices

- **Bran**—A paste of boiling water and unprocessed bran, applied hot and covered to retain the heat, was used to remove inflammation from bruises and sprains.
- **Oregano**—Moisten two tablespoons dried, ground oregano with hot water. Let stand, covered, for 10 minutes. Add more hot water to make a paste, then apply to the sore area as a pain reliever.

Specifically for Bruises

Diet and supplements

Spontaneous bruising, or purpura, usually indicates a lack of vitamins C and E. Nutritional deficiencies may cause bruises to appear from slight bumps or even from the pressure of clothing. Daily doses of 2,000 milligrams vitamin C, 100 to 500 milligrams of bioflavonoids, plus 100 to 400 IU vitamin E (see Caution, page 6) often strengthen the capillaries and correct the problem. Eating generous amounts of citrus fruits and green, leafy vegetables is helpful, but supplemental vitamin K may be necessary in some cases.

Tissue Salts

- **To reduce both discoloration and swelling**—Take 3X Ferr. Phos. and Kali. Mur. at 10-minute intervals for one hour after the bruising occurs, then reduce to two or three times a day.
- **For flesh bruises**—Dissolve equal amounts of the same two tissue salts in water and apply as a cool lotion.
- **For bruises of the shins or other bones**—Use a lotion made from Calc. Fluor. tablets and water. The lotions should be covered with a bandage to retain the moisture.

Folk remedies for bruises

In the 1800s, kerosene, turpentine, or bread soaked in vinegar was applied to bruises when ice was not available. A modern folk-solution is to use a package of frozen food or a can of chilled beverage. Any cold application will serve its purpose in half an hour or so, but raw beefsteak is no longer recommended for black eyes. After the initial chilling, heat can be used to lessen the pain and help absorb the blood under the skin. The *American Frugal Housewife*[73], first published in 1829, advised a poultice of wet brown paper dipped in molasses for healing a bruise and taking down inflammation. The more intrepid steeped a handful of tobacco in warm water for several hours, applied the tobacco to the bruise and drank several spoonfuls of the water. Other suggestions to use after the cooling period:

- Stir one-fourth cup apple cider vinegar into one quart of hot water. Soak the bruised part for 15 minutes several times a day to reduce swelling.
- Dip cloths in hot water or tea and foment the part for 30 minutes each night and each morning. Sprinkling the cloths with dried thyme or turmeric was believed to enhance the effect.
- Make a poultice of moistened camomile, comfrey root, dandelion, or slippery elm tea leaves and apply to the bruise.
- Chop together equal amounts of raw salt pork and boiled onions. Apply warm to a thickness of ½ inch and cover with a bandage.
- Apply a poultice of alum, bread mixed with water or milk, minced raw ham, or chopped fresh parsley mixed with butter.

Specifically for Sprains

Diet and supplements

Including fresh vegetables and citrus fruits in the diet and taking at least 250 milligrams of vitamin C with each meal is suggested to aid the formation and healing of connective tissue in ligaments. The lingering pain from stretched or torn ligaments may be alleviated by taking 100 to 800 IU of vitamin E (see Caution, page 6), 50 milligrams B-6, and several calcium tablets in addition to a multi-vitamin-mineral tablet each day for a week or so.

Tissue Salts—If available when the sprain first occurs, one 6X tablet each of Calc. Fluor., Calc. Phos. and Mag. Phos., taken every 20 minutes for two hours may lessen the pain and binding of muscles. Following each dose with a drink of hot liquid increases the effectiveness.

Folk remedies for sprains

Hot Applications

- Wring a small towel out of warm vinegar and foment the sprain for five minutes every four hours.
- Apply towels wrung out of hot milk several times daily.
- Bathe the sprained part in hot water, then foment with a solution of one or two tablespoons of salt in one cup each alcohol, vinegar, and water.

Liniments—For the deep-seated congestion of sprains, folk medicine recommends both soothing and stimulating applications.

- Steep fresh rosemary in vegetable oil for a week in a covered jar, then store in a cool place. When needed, warm and massage over the sprained area.
- Simmer one tablespoon cayenne pepper in two cups apple cider vinegar for 10 minutes. While still warm, spread over the sprain.

Poultices and compresses

- Make a compress of apple cider vinegar mixed with unprocessed bran, oatmeal, or breadcrumbs.
- Stir ground caraway seeds into boiling water and cook until the mixture thickens, then cool slightly and bind over the sprain.
- Apply a poultice of grated raw carrots.
- Steep comfrey tea leaves in alcohol and apply as a compress.
- Beat salt into the white of an egg and apply to form a cast over the sprain. Or, blend two tablespoons of ground ginger with the white of an egg and ½ teaspoon salt. Spread on gauze and lay over the affected part. Or, combine one tablespoon each honey and salt with one egg white. Beat until stiff, then let stand for an hour. Anoint the sprained part with the liquid produced from the mixture and bind well with a bandage.
- Mix grated raw onion with granulated sugar to form a paste. Apply to the affected region.
- Stir enough ground black pepper into half a cup of boiling apple cider vinegar to make a thick paste. Spread on a piece of gauze the size of the painful area and place the paste next to the skin. Remove after three hours and wash off any pepper remaining on the skin.
- Soak strips of newspaper in vinegar, apply to the sprained part, then cover with an airtight material such as a plastic bag.

Nerve pressure

To relieve the pain of a sprain anywhere on the body, press just below each outside anklebone for 10 seconds, release for 10 seconds and repeat three times for a total of 30 seconds pressure.

Sources (See Bibliography)

7, 13, 52, 53, 62, 68, 73, 81, 89, 98, 142, 152, 154, 156, 165, 168, 173, 174, 176, 190, 206, 226, 227, 228, 252, 254, 288, 297, 315, 318, 324, 333, 353.

BURNS AND SCALDS (See Also Sunburn)

Burns are classified according to degree. A first-degree burn causes pain and redness but no blisters. Second-degree burns are characterized by blisters and are equally painful. A third-degree burn may be painless when it first occurs because the nerve endings are destroyed when all layers of the skin are burned. Medical attention should be obtained for serious burns but immediately submerging even a severe burn in cold water, or covering it with a cloth kept wet with ice, can keep a first-degree burn from becoming a second-degree burn, or a second-degree burn from becoming third degree. Dousing a scalded area with cold water before removing the clothing prevents the hot cloth from burning deeper.

Case History

Roberta R. was thinking about the appointment she had in an hour, and was hurrying to finish their dinner casserole before it was time to go. Her son's scream of pain startled her out of her reverie. Bobby, who had been perched on a stool to watch her cook, had put his hand on the hot stove burner as he attempted to slide down to the floor. Roberta quickly emptied a tray of ice cubes into a mixing bowl, added a little cold water, and immersed Bobby's burned hand in the mixture until the pain subsided and the tears ceased. Then she looked at the little hand, scarlet with the imprint of the stove burner. She feared that her momentary inattention would result in terrible blisters and possibly scar her son for life. As calmly as possible, however, Roberta plunged Bobby's hand back in the ice water, washed his tear streaked face, and prepared to leave for her appointment. She filled Bobby's plastic sand pail with ice cubes and water, wrapped it in a towel and braced it with pillows beside his car seat. While she buckled him in she explained that the cold water would keep his hand from hurting, but that he must take his hand out of the water once in a while so it would not turn into an ice cube. They made a game of "out and in" as Roberta paused at each stop light, then carried the ice water with them into the office building. Onlookers may have wondered about the three-year-old walking beside his mother with his hand in a yellow plastic bucket, but the treatment was successful. Bobby's hand healed in a remarkably short time, without either blisters or scars.

For a chemical burn of the eye, immediately flood the eye with water or milk for 10 minutes, then get medical assistance. To prevent shock from severe burns, elevate the burned part and sip one-half cup cool water mixed with one teaspoon salt and one-half teaspoon baking soda. Persons with electrical burns may require immediate artificial respiration because of the shock. As reported in *Journal of Preventive Medicine* (Spring 1974), massive amounts of vitamin C (at least 1,000 milligrams immediately, then 1,000 milligrams each hour for several hours) helps prevent shock.

Small, superficial burns usually respond quickly to the application of an ice cube followed by a thin layer of aloe vera gel, Vaseline, or similar substance. Minor burns should have at least 30 minutes of the cold-water treatment. More serious burns require two to 24 hours of cooling. Early folk-medicine practitioners recommended immersing in cold milk or covering the burned area with cold-milk compresses when ice was not available. All authorities are in agreement about the importance of cooling as the first step, and that cotton should never be placed in contact with burned skin. But what is best to put on a burn **next** is still being debated. Some doctors recommend vitamin E, various ointments, compounds or sprays, and a bandage. Others claim that burns heal more rapidly if nothing touches them but air.

Diet and Supplements

Medical nutritionists suggest a high-protein diet plus oral supplements to combat stress, support the adrenal glands, and accelerate healing. Several of the vitamins may be applied topically for reducing discomfort and speeding recovery.

Vitamins A and D—Up to 100,000 units of A and 1,000 IU of D daily for a few days to fight infection and promote healing of severe burns. Applying a vitamin A-D-E ointment is helpful as healing progresses.

B Complex—One comprehensive, high-potency tablet twice a day for one week to compensate for the stress of serious burns. Taking an additional 200 milligrams PABA with each meal during the painful period often eases the discomfort. Local applications of PABA ointment soothes the pain of minor burns.

Vitamin C—1,000 milligrams per day to 1,000 milligrams per hour for the first few days for extensive burns. Including bioflavonoids with the vitamin C has proven helpful. Vitamin C helps prevent infection, aids healing, and improves the tensile strength of connective tissue. Medical studies have demonstrated the effectiveness of taking 250 to 1,000 milligrams of vitamin C four times daily and spraying the burned area with a solution of 2,500 milligrams vitamin C crystals dissolved in one cup water.

Vitamin E (see Caution, page 6)—100 to 1,000 IU daily plus topical applications. Drs. Evan and Wilfred Shute of Canada have had amazing success, even with massive burns, by applying vitamin E oil, covering the injury with a bandage, and having the patient take at least 600 IU of vitamin E orally each day. In addition to minimizing blistering, speeding healing, and helping to prevent scarring, the vitamin E reduces pain. It may be applied every hour or so, as needed. The oral supplements have been found more effective when combined with vitamin C. Both should be continued for several weeks after healing appears complete, then gradually reduced. If a healed burn has produced an itchy scar, local applications of vitamin E oil often brings quick relief.

Tissue Salts—Immediately following the accident, take one 3X tablet each Ferr. Phos. and Kali. Mur. at 10-minute intervals for one hour. For severe burns, Kali. Phos. should be included to help prevent shock.

Zinc—50 to 100 milligrams daily for two to four weeks to stimulate healing.

Folk Remedies (To be used following the immediate cooling)

Aloe Vera—One of the oldest and best known treatments for burns, bottled aloe vera gel may be purchased in health food stores. When a fresh plant is available, the blades can be split (after dethorning) and held in place over the burned area with gauze.

Apple—Grate a pared, cored raw apple and mix with salad oil to form a paste. Spread over the burn and refresh as it dries. Apple butter may be used in the same manner. Both have been found soothing and are believed to help prevent scarring.

Apple Cider Vinegar—Pour apple cider vinegar over the burn to stop the pain. Or, combine equal parts of vinegar, brandy, and water, then apply constantly until the pain is gone. Keep the burn covered with a vinegar-soaked bandage.

Baking Soda—Sprinkle baking soda over the surface and bind lightly with a soft cloth. Or, make a paste of the soda (combined with flour, if desired) blended with egg white or water to cover the burned area.

Cornmeal and Charcoal—Apply a poultice made with two parts cornmeal and one part powdered charcoal (tablets, not briquettes) moistened with milk.

Eggs

- Cover the burned region with a beaten raw egg, then apply alcohol to "cook" the egg and form a protective film. Or, beat the egg with two tablespoons castor oil or olive oil, spread the mixture on soft cloth, and apply over blistered burns.
- Beat the white of an egg (with or without one tablespoon of lard), apply to the burn, and let remain for one hour.
- If the throat is burned from hot liquid, beat an egg white with water and sip slowly.

Flour—Cover a superficial burn with flour and wrap with soft cloth to exclude the air. Or, cover the burn with lard or molasses before sprinkling with flour. Most physicians recommend that blisters be left intact for protection against infection, but if the blisters do break, wheat flour may be sprinkled over the raw flesh.

Honey—Probably the most ancient remedy for burns, raw honey has been found to have antibacterial properties and is now used in some hospitals. It can be applied directly to the skin to stop pain. Adding bee pollen granules to the honey is believed to speed healing. Slavic folk healers stir flour into the honey. Lelord Kordel[191] suggests equal parts of honey and wheat-germ oil blended with enough comfrey tea leaves to make a thick paste. The honey mixtures may be covered with a dry bandage, if desired, as honey does not stick to either the wound or the gauze.

Oatmeal—Apply a poultice made of oatmeal and cold water.

Oil—Before vitamin E oil was available for burns, good results were reported from the use of other oils. Cod liver oil, garlic oil, and sesame oil in particular were used to ease the pain of burns. In the 1880s, "Oil of Brown Paper" was made by saturating a piece of thick brown paper with oil, burning the paper on a clean plate, and applying the oil that dripped down.

Soap—Dissolve 1 ounce of pure white soap, scraped or sliced, in one-half cup boiling water. Mix with bread to make a poultice for burns.

Sugar—When sprinkled on the surface of deep, oozing burns, granulated sugar is believed to encourage healing by pulling out the excess moisture.

Tea—Steep three pekoe tea bags in two cups boiling water for 15 minutes. When cool, apply the liquid to the burned area as a compress. Or, make a poultice from slippery elm tea by combining the dried tea with enough boiling water to make a paste. Spread between two pieces of cloth and apply to the burn, renewing several times with fresh tea.

Vegetables—For minor burns, the application of mashed cabbage leaves, ground carrots, slices of raw onion, or pureed raw pumpkin or turnips was used to bring relief. For more severe burns, grated or ground raw white potato placed over the burn under a bandage and changed once each day was said to encourage healing from the inside without leaving a scar.

Yogurt—Plain yogurt, reapplied as it dries, often provides swift relief from painful burns and is reported to speed healing.

Nerve Pressure

Pressing inward and upward just below each eyebrow an inch out from the nose is believed to activate natural healing. Apply pressure for 10 seconds, release for 10 seconds, and repeat for 30 seconds of pressure once each day.

Sources (See Bibliography)

3, 6,7, 13, 19, 28, 52, 53, 66, 68, 69, 73, 78, 81, 86, 89, 98, 113, 122, 128, 142, 150, 151, 152, 153, 156, 168, 173, 174, 181, 191, 215, 226, 227, 228, 252, 256, 261, 276, 288, 289, 297, 299, 300, 304, 305, 312, 315, 318, 324, 325, 330, 333, 335, 345, 350.

BURSITIS

The joints of the body are surrounded by thin liquid-filled sacs (bursa) that act as shock absorbers. Injury, infection, arthritis, gout, or the habitual use of a joint can lead to painful inflammation of these sacs. Any of the 140 joints can be affected by bursitis, but shoulders, "tennis elbow," or "housemaid's knee" are the most common. If the inflammation continues or there are repeated attacks, calcium deposits (which may require surgical removal) may accumulate in the joints. Strangely enough, these deposits result from calcium deficiency rather than over-ingestion of dairy products.[88,353] A lack of the B vitamins or magnesium may also be a factor in the formation of these calcium deposits.

Cold applications for 30 minutes every four hours usually helps relieve the pain. (Ice therapy goes deep enough to reach the inflamed bursa, heat seldom does.) The joint should be immobilized until the acute pain subsides, then moist heat packs and gentle exercises are in order to prevent adhesions or permanent immobility. For bursitis of the shoulder, a painless exercise is to lean forward and let the arm swing back and forth like a pendulum, eventually raising the arm higher and higher without pain. To avoid recurrence, giving the over-worked joint a rest by using the other arm to open doors, hold a book, etc.—and following some of these natural remedies—may be effective.

Diet and Supplements

Diet is rarely considered in connection with bursitis but some doctors recommend reducing purines (see Gout). Eating six small meals daily (each one containing 25 grams of protein), and accompanying each meal with acidophilus yogurt or capsules is often advised. Foods high in calcium and B vitamins—such as brewer's yeast, liver, and wheat germ—may forestall bursitis or its reappearance. Including generous amounts of citrus fruits and chloride-rich foods (avocado, endive, kelp, oats, tomatoes, watercress) plus one tablespoon unsaturated vegetable oil daily also may be of help.

Vitamin A—At least 10,000 units daily to hasten recovery.

B Complex—One comprehensive, high-potency tablet daily. Taking 25 to 100 milligrams B-2, B-6, and pantothenic acid, plus 400 to 800 micrograms of folic acid each day often helps prevent the formation of calcium deposits. Additional B-6 (four 50-milligram tablets during the day) for three weeks has eliminated pain for some bursitis sufferers.

The injection of 1,000 micrograms (1 cc) of B-12 daily for seven to 10 days has proven the most successful treatment for acute bursitis. With a doctor's prescription and instructions, these shots can be self-administered and provide more rapid relief than an equal amount of oral supplementation. The pain is usually relieved after the first day but continuing the injections at less frequent intervals for six weeks is suggested to reduce or prevent calcium deposits or a recurrence of bursitis. Accompanying the B-12 with 50 milligrams of oral B-1 each day often improves its effectiveness.

Vitamin C and Bioflavonoids—1,000 milligrams vitamin C every hour during the first one to three days, then 2,000 to 6,000 milligrams (in divided doses) each day for several weeks. Taking 600 to 1,200 milligrams of bioflavonoids per day, in three divided doses, enhances the effect of vitamin C in relieving the inflammation and speeding recovery.

Vitamin D—1,000 to 2,000 IU natural vitamin D daily during the acute phase, then 800 IU each day to assist in the absorption of B-12 and calcium, and help prevent a return of the bursitis.

Dolomite—Three tablets twice each day during the acute period to supply both calcium and magnesium. Since a deficiency of either of these minerals can trigger bursitis, or its return, continuing to take two dolomite tablets daily is recommended.

Vitamin E (see Caution, page 6)—100 to 1,200 IU daily during the acute phase, then 300 IU each day to help prevent the formation of calcium deposits or scar tissue in the affected joint.

Tissue Salts—Three tablets 3X-potency Nat. Mur. taken three times each day with one teaspoon of apple cider vinegar stirred into a glass of water.

Folk Remedies

Apple Cider Vinegar and Honey—Stirring two teaspoons each apple cider vinegar and raw honey into a glass of water and sipping at each meal is believed to prevent and correct the calcium precipitation that may instigate bursitis.

Camomile Tea—Drinking strong camomile tea, especially at bedtime, often helps ease the pain of bursitis.

Olive Oil—A daily massage of the sore joint with warmed olive oil has relieved soreness and prevented the return of bursitis for some individuals.

Potato Juice—Slice one scrubbed, raw potato into thin slices and place in a large glass. Fill with cold water, cover, and let stand for eight to 12 hours. Strain out the potatoes and drink the liquid on an empty stomach. If preferred, the potato juice may be made in an electric juicer and diluted half-and-half with water.

Poultices—(Before applying any of these remedies, rub the affected area with olive oil to protect the skin.)

- **Cayenne Pepper**—Boil one tablespoon cayenne pepper in two cups apple cider vinegar for 10 minutes. Cool until comfortably warm, then wring out a handtowel in the liquid and apply to the sore joint.
- **Comfrey**—Place a handful of comfrey leaves, fresh or dried, in a saucepan and cover with water. Bring to boiling, cool slightly, and spread between pieces of gauze to apply to the painful area.
- **Flaxseed**—Sprinkle one-fourth pound crushed flaxseed in two cups boiling water and stir until smooth, then stir in one tablespoon olive oil. Spread between layers of gauze and apply to the sore joint.

Sea Water—Two to three teaspoons per day. When continued for six to nine months, this amount of bottled sea water (available in health food stores) has cured cases of chronic bursitis.[135]

Nerve Pressure

Apply pressure for 10 seconds, release for 10 seconds; repeat three times once each day.

For bursitis in any joint of the body—Press a point in the center bottom of each foot, just in front of the heel prominence.

For bursitis in either shoulder—use the pressure point nearest the painful side.

- Press a point just above the collarbone, 1½ inches to either the left or right of center.
- Press the upper margin of the collarbone, 4 inches to either the left or right of center.
- Using the thumb of the opposite hand, press the front tip of the shoulder.
- Press just below the end of the collarbone as it meets the shoulder prominence.
- Press the center of the spine an inch below the shoulders.

Sources (See Bibliography)

3, 4, 7, 13, 19, 35, 52, 53, 67, 81, 84, 88, 89, 110, 135, 152, 156, 168, 173, 180, 181, 189, 254, 261, 288, 293, 297, 312, 315, 316, 325, 353.

CATARACT

There are over 30 types of cataracts with at least 100 different varieties. The most common, senile cataract, was once considered a normal part of the aging process. Now it is believed by many experts to be the result of a lifetime of marginal malnutrition. Surgical removal of cataracts may restore clear vision but orthomolecular physicians and research scientists are questioning the necessity for all the over 400,000 cataract operations performed every year in the United States. Vitamin supplements (vitamin B-2 in particular) have proven successful in retarding and even clearing some cataracts. Folk medicine, nerve massage, and nerve pressure offer remedies that are credited with miraculous cures. Since prevention or regression of a cataract is much to be preferred over surgery, some of these natural methods may be beneficial when used to augment the diagnosis and care of an ophthalmologist.

Diet and Supplements

The eyes are nourished by the body's blood supply, so proper nutrition is an important factor in the prevention and treatment of cataracts. While no single nutrient has proven effective in either preventing or curing cataracts, the response has been favorable, and rapid, when the entire team of nutrients was supplied at the first sign of a cataract. Optimum eye nourishment requires high-quality protein plus sufficient vitamins and minerals. The diet should include green vegetables, especially leafy ones; fruits, including citrus and cantaloupe; milk and dairy products; organ meats; whole grains; and polyunsaturated oils. Two daily glasses of vegetable juices (at least 8 ounces carrot juice plus any combination of beet, celery, cucumber, parsley, and spinach) help provide adequate nourishment for the optic nerves and muscles. Dr. Rinse's famous daily food supplement has proven beneficial for the prevention and cure of cataracts.[250] For a simplified version: combine two teaspoons each brewer's yeast, lecithin granules, and raw wheat germ with three-fourths teaspoon bone meal and two teaspoons unsaturated oil. Blend with yogurt or cereal and milk, adding brown sugar or honey, if desired.

Incomplete absorption of the milk sugar, galactose, provokes or speeds the development of cataracts for some individuals. Elevated blood sugar combined with impaired vitamin C absorption due to lack of insulin is considered responsible for the high proportion of cataracts among diabetics. Some food additives have been indicted as possible contributory factors in the development of cataracts. The nitrates and nitrites in processed meats are still under investigation. Laboratory tests have shown that sorbitol (used as a sweetener and moisturizer in packaged food products) aggravates cataracts in animals. Atherosclerosis (see Hardening of the Arteries) blocking blood vessels to the eyes may promote cataracts. Deficiencies of vitamins A, B, C, E, and/or calcium may also contribute to the formation of cataracts.

> **Vitamin A**—50,000 to 200,000 units per day for a few months. Vitamin A is essential to eye health, and, when combined with 1,000 milligrams of vitamin C daily, has been reported effective in clearing cataracts.
>
> **B Complex**—One comprehensive,high-potency tablet daily. Cataracts are not always the result of a lack of B-2, but additional supplements of 15 to 100

milligrams daily have brought marked improvement in just a few days and reversed many cataracts after nine months. B-6 is necessary for proper assimilation of the amino acid, tryptophane, from proteins. An extra supplement of 10 to 100 milligrams B-6 plus an equal amount of pantothenic acid has proven beneficial in many cases.

Vitamin C and Bioflavonoids—500 to 15,000 milligrams vitamin C plus 100 to 1,000 milligrams bioflavonoids per day. Vitamin C deficiency has been implicated in the formation of cataracts. When taken along with vitamin A, B-2, and complete proteins, both slowing and clearing of cataracts has resulted. Bioflavonoids not only enhance the action of vitamin C but, according to experiments at the National Eye Institute in Maryland, actually prevent the formation of cataracts.[6]

Calcium and Vitamin D—1,000 milligrams calcium plus 400 to 1,000 IU natural vitamin D daily. Insufficient or poorly assimilated calcium is believed indirectly involved in cataract formation; vitamin D is necessary for calcium absorption.

Vitamin E (see Caution, page 6)—100 to 600 IU daily. Vitamin E therapy has cleared cataracts from the eyes of children in six months[3] and, with the addition of adequate selenium and other nutrients, has been equally successful with adults.

Lecithin—One tablespoon granules or 10 1,200-milligram capsules daily. The onset of cataracts may be triggered by cholesterol narrowing the blood vessels to the eyes. The emulsifying action of lecithin has been credited with correcting this condition.

Selenium—150 to 200 micrograms daily. A lack of selenium, particularly when accompanied by a deficiency of vitamin E, has been linked to all types of cataracts, including those of diabetics.

Tissue Salts—Four daily tablets of 6X Calc. Fluor. plus two of 6X Silicea have been reported helpful for cataracts and the connective tissues involved.

Exercise

The Edgar Cayce readings suggest that this head-and-neck exercise be performed twice daily to slow the development of cataracts. With the neck fully stretched, bend the head forward, backward, to the right, and to the left, three times, then rotate the head three times each to the right and to the left.

Folk Remedies

Apple Cider Vinegar and Honey—With each meal, sip a mixture of two teaspoons each apple cider vinegar and honey stirred in a glass of water. This is believed to improve calcium and protein absorption and either retard or reverse cataract growth.

Camomile Tea—Use cooled, strained camomile tea as eyedrops or an eyewash each night and morning.

Epsom Salts—A mild solution of ordinary epsom salts used as an eye wash is said to be helpful during the early stages of cataract formation.

Honey—A drop of raw honey in the corner of the eye (or rubbed around the edge of the eye) each night has been reported to begin improvement in two months, and, when combined with proper nutrition, to eventually cure cataracts.

Oils—Drop cod liver oil in the eye or rub it around the edge of the eye each night for a month. If no improvement is noticed, linseed oil (from a pharmacy) should be used instead. Complete cures are attributed to this remedy.[76,322]

Potato—Spread peeled, grated raw potato between pieces of gauze and place over the closed eyelid for an hour or more daily.

Sea Water—Place two or three drops of sea water (from a health food store) in the eye each morning and night, then swallow a spoonful of the water.

Nerve Massage

At least once every day, massage the area at the bottom of the second toe and the one next to it, as well as the base of the index and middle fingers, on the side on which the cataract is located. Then massage the center of each foot from the ball of the foot to the beginning of the arch.

Nerve Pressure

Once or twice each day, press each point for 10 seconds, release for 10 seconds, and repeat for a total of 30 seconds pressure for each treatment.

- With the thumbs, press upward under the eyebrows on each side of the bridge of the nose.
- With the index finger, press the small notch in the bone surrounding the eye—about 1/4 inch from the lower outside corner of the eye.
- With the index fingers, press the back of the jawbone (just under each ear) and pull forward.

Sources (See Bibliography)

3, 6, 8, 13, 34, 63,64, 68, 76, 78, 84, 88, 89, 92, 154, 165, 173, 179, 181, 184, 189, 236, 243, 249, 250, 254, 260, 261, 282, 293, 322, 331, 349, 350.

COLD SORES, FEVER BLISTERS, AND CANKER SORES

Cold sores or fever blisters are caused by the virus Herpes Simplex, Type 1 or Type 2. Both types of viruses produce similar symptoms. They can afflict the soft membranes of the lips, mouth, nose, or even genital areas. Canker sores *(apthous stomatitis)* usually appear inside the mouth. They are considered virus infections, are difficult to distinguish from true herpes, but may not be of herpetic origin. Most people pick up the herpes virus in infancy but it remains dormant unless the body's defense mechanisms are weakened by allergy, antibiotic medications, colds, emotional stress, exhaustion, gastrointestinal upsets, menstrual difficulties, or sunburn. Usually a self-limiting malady, the annoying skin disturbances often disappear in a week or two even without treatment. The herpes virus, however, cannot be expelled—it returns to its dormant state within the body.[149] During the active phase, the three things to guard against are:

- Secondary infection from bacteria. (Keep the sores clean and avoid scratching or rubbing.)
- Spread of the virus to a new site on the body. (Wash hands after touching the sores and before rubbing the eyes or inserting contact lenses.)
- Exposure of others to the virus (Avoid such direct-contact activities as kissing and, in case of genital lesions, sex.)

A few years ago the orthodox advice was to leave these sores alone and treat them only with contempt, but the following natural remedies have been shown to shorten the duration and help prevent recurrence.

Diet and Supplements

Acidophilus—Two to five capsules or tablets taken with meals or milk three times a day. Numerous clinical tests have shown both canker and cold sores to quickly respond to this treatment. Since *Lactobacillus acidophilus* inactivates but does not destroy the herpes virus, a maintenance dosage of at least six capsules daily is recommended for those who are frequently troubled by this mishap. Eating acidophilus yogurt is especially helpful if the sores are inside the mouth. Homemade yogurt, made with acidophilus culture and eaten within a few days is suggested in preference to commercial yogurt which may not contain *L. acidophilus*. Prolonged chilling or the addition of sugar can reduce the number of living lactobacilli. Acidophilus milk and kefir are beneficial but the concentrated capsules have been found more effective.

B Complex—One or two comprehensive high-potency tablets daily, plus optional individual B vitamins. 100 milligrams of niacinamide with each meal often corrects canker sores. Taking 500 milligrams of pantothenic acid at the first sign of a sore and every hour or two for a day may abort its formation, or at least shorten its duration. Some cold sores have quickly cleared when the pantothenic acid was taken with 50 milligrams B-6 and 500 milligrams vitamin C. 50 to 350 micrograms B-12 taken twice daily have cleared cold sores in a day or two, and have also been effective for herpes genitalis. A study reported in *Journal of Oral Pathology* [Vol. 7, 1978] showed that the B-12 plus an iron supplement and 5 milligrams of folic acid three times a day gave definite improvement and prevented recurring canker sores in 87 percent of those tested.

Vitamin C—150 to 1,000 milligrams every hour when either a canker or cold sore threatens, then at least 2,000 milligrams daily until healing is complete. Taking calcium along with the vitamin C and avoiding sugar has been successful in some cases. Applying vitamin C powder to sores on the lips or in the mouth often causes them to dry up within a few hours.

Vitamin E—Every four hours, squeeze the oil from a pierced capsule directly on the sores. According to the *British Dental Journal* (Vol. 148, 1980), covering the vitamin E oil with powdered vitamin C is even more effective.

Lysine—300 to 1,500 milligrams daily. Large amounts of this amino acid have stopped the pain of fever blisters overnight, prevented spreading of the sores, and speeded healing. In the smaller, maintenance dose, lysine has successfully prevented recurrences. *Medical World News* (October 1, 1979) explained that another amino acid, arginine, is necessary in order for the herpes simplex virus to reproduce, and lysine nullifies this effect of arginine. Avoiding foods high in arginine (chocolate, coconut, corn, gelatin, nuts, oats) may be helpful. Taking 1,000 milligrams of lysine with two acidophilus capsules each day has brought improvement within two days and complete cures in two weeks.[52]

Zinc—30 to 100 milligrams daily. Zinc speeds healing and has cleared canker sores as well as herpes 1 and herpes 2. To hasten healing even further, zinc tablets may be pulverized and applied to the sores with a moist cotton swab.

Case History

Greta C. had been troubled with fever blisters since childhood. Fearing that these painfully ugly sores could prove hazardous to her new position as an account executive, she tried all the medications prescribed by her dermatologist; but the blisters persisted in cropping up and were slow to heal. When a tender, puffy lip indicated the approach of another sore—just a few days before she was to speak at an important conference—Greta asked her secretary to try to schedule an appointment with a different doctor. None were available on such short notice, so, as a possible alternative, the secretary offered Greta a health magazine containing an article about the amino acid lysine, its interaction with arginine, and its ability to combat fever blisters and canker sores. The magazine also described the healing properties of zinc. Greta was so desperate she decided to experiment with the natural remedies. On her way home she bought lysine and zinc, along with some red clover tea (see Folk Remedies, below) suggested in a booklet she picked up at the health food store. The incipient blister never developed, Greta's presentation was successful, and by avoiding arginine-containing foods and continuing a maintenance dosage of lysine, she has avoided further problems with the embarrassing blisters.

Folk Remedies

Alcohol—A drying lotion of two-thirds cup pure alcohol mixed with one-third cup water and applied with cotton may be helpful for cold sores.

Buttermilk—Drink buttermilk as a beverage and apply it externally to help dry and heal cold sores.

Ice—Holding a piece of ice tightly against a freshly erupted cold sore for 45 minutes is said to bring about healing within a day or so.

Pomegranate—Dry and grind pomegranate rinds, then boil one tablespoon in one and one-half cups water until reduced to one cup. Strain and keep on hand to apply to canker or cold sores.

Potato—Including liberal amounts of unsalted baked potato in the diet is believed to speed the disappearance of fever blisters and canker sores.

Red Clover Tea—For either canker or cold sores, drink one cupful after each meal. For fever blisters, apply triple-strength tea to the sores several times daily.

Sage and Ginger Tea—Stir one teaspoon powdered ginger into one cup sage tea. Drink several cups at intervals during the day. This is said to work overnight for cold sores.

Salt Water and Brandy—To abort an incipient fever blister: dissolve as much salt as possible in one-half cup boiling water. For three hours, keep the sore spot covered with a cloth saturated with the hot solution, renewing as soon as it cools. Then rinse with brandy every hour or so and keep covered with a bit of gauze.

Soda—Rinsing the mouth with a weak solution of baking soda and water may alleviate the pain of canker sores.

Whipping Cream—an application of cold, heavy cream may provide relief from the pain of cold sores.

Sources (See Bibliography)

3, 4, 52, 53, 62, 81, 89, 142, 149, 152, 156, 168, 174, 226, 228, 229, 251, 252, 254, 261, 270, 288, 300, 305, 325, 350.

COLDS AND INFLUENZA, COUGHS AND SORE THROAT

Colds can be instigated by any of 200 viruses; influenza set in motion by any of three other virus groups. Both are "caught" from contact with microscopic droplets of virus-laden mucus either in the air surrounding someone with the malady or by touching a recently contaminated object and delivering the virus to the eyes or nose. The viruses must then incubate for 24 to 48 hours and are usually destroyed by the body's immune system. Anything that lowers natural resistance—chilling, emotional upsets, fatigue, etc.—allows the virus to multiply and a cold or flu can result. (Stomach or intestinal flu is caused by gastrointestinal bacteria or viruses unrelated to true influenza. "Imitation colds" or a cough that lingers after other cold or flu symptoms have abated may be caused by allergic reactions, especially to dairy products.)

Influenza symptoms are intensifications of cold symptoms, plus muscle aches and fever, and the same remedies are applicable to both. Rest, with lots of liquid and little food, allows the body to concentrate its defensive efforts against the invading viruses. Deliberate relaxation (see pages 9-10), both physical and mental, hastens recovery. With or without treatment, colds and flu generally run their course in a week or two. If complications appear or fever persists, medical help should be obtained to prevent or correct any secondary infection such as strep throat or pneumonia. There is no "cure" for the common cold. Antibiotics are of no avail against viruses, and flu shots are now recommended only for the elderly or those with respiratory ailments. But recent scientific studies show that nutritional supplements can either abort or shorten the duration of colds and influenza—and folk remedies offer symptomatic relief from this most common of mankind's maladies.

Diet and Supplements

The human constitution has changed very little since 400 B.C. when Hippocrates stated, "If you feed a cold you will have to starve a fever." A light diet—including the proverbial chicken or vegetable soup—is still recommended for the first few days of a bout with either a cold or influenza. If fever is present, at least 10 glasses of liquids per day are suggested to replace the fluid lost through perspiration. Refuting the traditional hot-toddy remedies, studies have shown that alcohol increases nasal irritation and congestion. Water, diluted citrus or grape juice, or herbal teas, are thought to be more beneficial.

When vitamins and minerals are inadequately supplied, immune defenses go down, allowing germs to multiply and prolong illness. The well-known nutritionist, Adelle Davis[89], recommended this "antistress formula" for upper respiratory ailments. Take with "fortified milk" (see Index) at every meal and before going to bed: at least 500 milligrams vitamin C, 100 milligrams pantothenic acid, and at least 2 milligrams each vitamins B-2 and B-6. *Earl Mindell's Vitamin Bible*[229] suggests 25,000 units vitamin A one to three times each day for five days, 1,000 milligrams vitamin C three times a day, 400 IU vitamin E one to three times daily, and three acidophilus capsules three times daily. Combinations or individual supplements recommended by other authorities are:

Vitamin A—25,000 to 160,000 units daily until well, then 10,000 to 25,000 units each day for at least one month to prevent recurrence. Carlton Fredericks[128] recommends 200,000 units daily for five days for those who do not respond to treatment with vitamin C. Robert Atkins[24], however, has found 100,000 units vitamin A per day plus 1,500 milligrams vitamin C every two hours to be the most effective remedy. After five days of this combined dosage, the amounts should be reduced by one half for another five days.

B Complex—One comprehensive, high-potency tablet daily to combat the stress of illness. An additional 100 to 500 milligrams B-6 plus 400 to 3,000 milligrams pantothenic acid, taken in divided doses daily, aids the immune system and has an anti-mucus effect, especially when used in conjunction with vitamin C.

Bioflavonoids—200 to 600 milligrams daily to increase the effectiveness of vitamin C and to prevent the swollen tissues and inflammation accompanying a cold.

Vitamin C—500 to 10,000 (or more) milligrams daily in divided doses. Although there is controversy over its merits, vitamin C is widely accepted as both a preventive and cure for colds and influenza. There is scientific evidence that 4,000 to 10,000 milligrams vitamin C, taken during the course of each day, will prevent colds in 95 percent of the population.[171] Once a cold is suspected, the generally accepted dosage is 1,000 milligrams each hour for one or two days. Doctors Cathcart and Pauling[24, 251] recommend as much vitamin C as can be tolerated without causing diarrhea, with individual tolerances varying from 250 to 60,000 milligrams per day. Even if the cold or flu is not aborted, continuing to take large amounts of vitamin C inhibits virus multiplication and speeds recovery. Some experts have found that adding 500 milligrams of the amino acid, lysine, or one-half cup wheat germ, to the daily quota of vitamin C is more effective than the A + C combination recommened by Dr. Atkins. Regardless of the amount taken, vitamin C should be continued in gradually smaller doses for several weeks following recovery to prevent a recurrence.

Case History

Rhonda N. did not have time for the cold that threatened on Friday afternoon—she was in charge of the branch office that was to open on Monday. Rhonda went home early, sipped a hot toddy, and took to her bed in hopes of forestalling the incipient malady. Sniffly-nosed and raspy-throated, Rhonda was still in bed when a friend telephoned the next morning. When the sympathetic friend asked if she was taking vitamin C, Rhonda assured her that she had taken a 100-milligram tablet the night before, and another one when she awakened. Startled by her friend's suggestion that she increase the vitamin-C dosage to 1,000 milligrams per hour, Rhonda argued that so much vitamin C would be dangerous—the RDA was only 40 to 60 milligrams per day. An explanation of vitamin C's virus-inhibiting properties convinced Rhonda that it was worth a try. She took 1,000 milligrams of vitamin C each hour for the rest of that day, and every time she roused during the night. On Sunday, Rhonda felt so much better that, still fearful of an adverse reaction, she reduced the dosage to 1,000 milligrams of vitamin C at two-hour intervals. This amount proved to be sufficient. By Monday morning Rhonda's cold had disappeared, and she could enjoy coping with the responsibilities of her new office.

Calcium and Vitamin D—1,000 to 2,000 milligrams calcium plus 400 to 1,000 IU natural vitamin D, taken in divided doses with vitamin C each day for several days. Vitamin D is necessary for calcium absorption, which, in turn, is required for assimilation of vitamin C.

Vitamin E (see Caution, page 6)—100 to 800 IU per day to insure efficient utilization of vitamin A, complement vitamin C, and increase the flow of nourishing blood.

Lecithin—One tablespoon granules (or 10 1,200-milligram capsules) taken every eight hours for two days has been known to abort viral colds and flu when taken at the onset.[315]

Tissue Salts

- At the first sign of a cold, take one tablet 6X Ferr. Phos. every 15 minutes for one hour, then three tablets every two hours. If accompanied by aching and chilling, take 3X Nat. Sulph. at 30-minute intervals. For watery running of nose or eyes, take one 3X tablet Ferr. Phos. every two hours, plus one 3X Nat. Mur. tablet each hour.

- When there is stuffiness and/or clear mucus, take three doses daily of Kali. Mur. in the 6X potency. If mucus is thick or yellow, take one 12X Kali. Sulph. three times a day. If the mucus is hard, substitute Silicea for the Kali. Sulph.
- For convalescent aches and weariness: take 12X Kali. Mur. and Kali. Sulph. alternately, twice each day, plus one 12X tablet Kali. Phos. at bedtime.

Zinc—30 to 50 milligrams daily. There is considerable evidence of zinc's infection-fighting capabilities. Since the body loses zinc when a cold is present, supplements are recommended. Zinc tablets dissolved in hot water for use as a throat spray not only inhibit the local viruses but strengthen the entire immune system.

Folk Remedies

Once the patient was snuggled into a warm bed, neither European nor American folk practitioners worried about possible nasal irritation from alcohol, and laced their libations liberally. The "Silk Hat Cure," popular during the 1800s, consisted of placing a tall silk hat on the right-hand bedpost, then lying quietly and sipping brandy until there appeared to be silk hats on both bedposts. Many of the other old remedies made use of the nutritional and medicinal properties of available foods and herbs. Even the "Conserve of Roses"[311] prescribed for colds in 1669 would have contained vitamin C. One-half pound of rose petals was to be simmered with two pounds dark sugar before being eaten plain, stirred into milk, or spread on toast.

Apple Cider Vinegar and Honey—Stir two tablespoons each vinegar and raw honey in a glass of hot or cold water. Drink three glasses during the day and another at bedtime. This mixture may also be used as a gargle.

Cinnamon—Place several sticks of cinnamon in a clean tin can over a medium flame. Let the cinnamon burn and inhale the fumes. (Said to cure both colds and flu.)

Citrus Fruit

- Add one teaspoon dried, grated grapefruit rind to each cup of herb tea. When the fresh fruit is available, cut two large, unpeeled grapefruit in small pieces and simmer in one quart water for 30 minutes. Strain and add honey to taste, then drink the entire quart of liquid each day.
- Dilute the juice of a lemon with an equal amount of water and drink three or four times a day.
- Stir the juice of one lemon, one tablespoon honey, one-fourth cup rum, and/or one teaspoon bee pollen into a cup of boiling water and sip slowly.
- To the juice of one lemon, add one minced garlic clove (or one-fourth teaspoon garlic powder), one-fourth teaspoon vitamin C powder (1,000 milligrams vitamin C), and one-eighth to one-half teaspoon cayenne pepper. Stir in boiling water or herb tea to make one cup. Sweeten with honey, if desired.
- Pour two cups boiling water over two tablespoons whole flaxseed and steep for three hours. Strain, add the juice of one lemon, and sweeten with brown sugar. Add a little water if the mixture is too thick to drink.

- Orange rinds, thinly pared and rolled inside out, then thrust into the nostrils, were a cold remedy during the reign of Queen Victoria.

Garlic—So well known for its anti-infection capabilities that it is called Russian Penicillin, garlic in many guises is recommended for the treatment of colds and influenza. The *Mother's Book of Daily Duties,* published in 1850, advised bottling three-cents-worth of garlic with one cup of rye whiskey and taking a tablespoonful of the mixture several times a day for chills and fever accompanying a cold.

- At the onset of a cold, place a piece of garlic in each side of the mouth between teeth and cheek. The garlic should be scored with the teeth once in a while, but not chewed.
- To stop colds as soon as they appear: mince and swallow three or four garlic cloves daily, or take three garlic perles three times a day for two days.
- Combine garlic oil with an equal amount of water—add a little onion juice, if desired—then take one-half teaspoonful every four hours.
- Steep 1 pound chopped garlic in one pint brandy or vodka for two weeks. Take 10 to 15 drops an hour before each meal.
- For colds with nausea and headache: simmer one teaspoon each coriander seeds, minced garlic, and sliced gingerroot (or one-half teaspoon ground ginger) with one tablespoon honey in two cups water until reduced to one cup. Strain and sip throughout the day.

Herbal Teas—Camomile, catnip, cayenne, dandelion leaf, elder, fenugreek, ginger, horehound, lemon grass, licorice root, peppermint, rose hips, rosemary, saffron, sage, sarsaparilla, savory, scullcap, and slippery elm are recommended. A combination said to cure a cold in 24 hours when taken freely: one teaspoon each bay leaf, cinnamon, and sage steeped in one cup boiling water. For a cold with fever: mix catnip tea with fresh cherry juice. For a cold with headache: boil 10 cornhusks in water for 30 minutes. Strain and drink.

Horseradish—For a cold with tightness in the chest, take one tablespoonful horseradish mixed with enough honey to be palatable.

Ice—An Eskimo remedy for a drippy nose is to immerse it in snow or ice water. Oriental folk healers secure a piece of ice on the bottom of the big toe three times a day to cure a cold by activating an acupuncture point.

Milk

- At the onset of a cold, stir one tablespoon butter into one cup scalded milk. Make the surface black with ground pepper and drink while hot.
- Stir one-fourth to three-fourths teaspoon ground cinnamon or ginger into one cup scalded milk. Add honey to taste and drink immediately.
- Stir one tablespoon honey, one teaspoon butter, and one-half teaspoon garlic powder into one cup scalded milk. Sip just before bedtime.
- Simmer six chopped figs in one quart milk for one hour. Drink a cup of the liquid three times a day.

- Whisk one egg yolk with one tablespoon sugar and one-half cup sherry. Stir in one cup boiling milk, then season to taste with cinnamon and nutmeg. Drink hot, just before retiring. The egg may be omitted and the mixture strained, if desired.
- Stir one cup molasses into one cup hot milk. Let stand for 10 minutes, then strain and drink before retiring.

Nasal Spray or Drops—For a sophisticated variation of the old-fashioned "sniff hot salt water" remedy: dissolve one-fourth teaspoon each vitamin C powder, garlic oil, and salt in one-half cup warm water. Pour into a spray bottle, or dropper bottle, and squirt a little in each nostril.

Nutmeg—As recorded in his diary of 1660, Samuel Pepys' cold remedy was to go to bed and take a spoonful of honey mixed with a grated nutmeg. Stirring grated nutmeg into a cup of hot pekoe tea sweetened with honey and laced with a shot of brandy was another option.

Onion—For tightness in the chest: sweeten onion juice with sugar and take one teaspoonful each hour. For a cold with hoarseness: simmer three chopped onions with two tablespoons oatmeal in one cup water. Stir in one tablespoon butter, season with salt and pepper, and eat just before bedtime.

Poultices and Plasters for Chest Colds

- Mix equal parts dry mustard and flour with enough warm water to make a paste. Spread between layers of cloth. Grease the chest, then apply the plaster and let it remain until the chest turns red.
- Blend dry mustard with the white of an egg to make a paste. Wring a small towel out of hot water and spread the mixture on one half. Fold over and apply to the chest. The plaster can be refreshed by dipping the towel in hot water and reapplying.
- Mix one-third cup dry mustard with one-half teaspoon each ground black pepper and ground ginger. Add warm water to produce a soft paste. Grease the chest, then spread the mixture between layers of gauze and apply.
- Blend two tablespoons lard with one tablespoon turpentine. Rub on the chest and throat, then cover with a woolen cloth.
- Spread cooked, mashed onions between pieces of cloth to make a poultice. While still warm, place on the chest and leave overnight.
- Dip a piece of flannel in boiling water, sprinkle with turpentine and lay over the chest as hot as can be tolerated.

Soda and Lemon—Stir one teaspoon baking soda in one-half cup boiling water. Stir the juice of one-half lemon into one-half cup cool water. Combine the mixtures by pouring one into the other, then into a glass. Drink as soon as the foaming subsides. Repeat every two or three hours during the first day of a cold.

Whiskey and Honey—Mix half-and-half, then take one tablespoonful every hour.

Witch Hazel—For a head cold, spray both the throat and nasal passages with witch hazel.

Nerve Massage

- Using the thumbs, massage across the entire length of both eyebrows for one minute.
- For a cold with runny nose: start at the top of the nose and massage down to the base of the nostrils with small circular motions. Repeat seven times.
- With the thumb and fingers, gently massage the area on each side of the Adam's Apple, from the collarbone to the base of the jaw, for three minutes twice each day.
- Place the fingers in the hollow at the base of the skull and massage for three minutes several times during the day.
- Massage the hollows on the underside of the knees for two minutes, then massage the kneecaps for the same length of time.
- Massage the big toe and the pads on the sole of the foot below the toes on both feet.

Nerve Pressure (Press each point three times for 10 seconds each)

- For a head cold: press the point where the jawbone ends just below the earlobe, and the center of the lower jawbone directly beneath the outer corners of the lips.
- Press a point in the center of the breastbone.
- Press a point 3 inches above the navel, then a point 2½ inches below the navel.
- With the arm extended, palm up, press a point in the hollow of the elbow 1 inch toward the thumb. Repeat with the other arm.
- Press the point on top of the hand where the bones of the thumb and index finger join. Repeat on the other hand.
- Press just below the ball of each foot, in line with the third toe.
- For sneezing: press a point directly under the center of the nose. Or, press the point between the eyes where the eyebrows would meet. For running nose: squeeze the same point eight times, or press at the outer base of both nostrils.

Cough Remedies

Doctors generally agree on the benefits of stopping a dry cough but believe a productive one should not be suppressed as it helps rid the respiratory system of harmful substances. (See Bronchitis for additional expectorants.) For instant relief from a dry, irritating cough, folk healers recommended smoking equal quantities of ground coffee and pine sawdust in a clean pipe and swallowing all of the smoke possible.

Anise Seeds

- For coughing with hoarseness or loss of voice: boil one-half cup anise seeds in one cup water for 20 minutes. Strain and sweeten with honey. Add one-quarter cup brandy or cherry vodka. Take two tablespoons each half hour.
- Simmer one teaspoon each anise seeds and dried thyme in two cups of water for 10 minutes. (If desired, one teaspoon each horehound and licorice root may

be included.) Strain, then dissolve one cup brown sugar or honey in the hot liquid. Bottle and sip one tablespoonful every hour, or as needed.

Honey

- Mix honey and apple cider vinegar half-and-half. Sip as needed to relieve coughing.
- Stir two tablespoons honey and one-half teaspoon cayenne pepper into a mixture of one-fourth cup each apple cider vinegar and water. Take by the teaspoonful as needed.
- Combine equal parts of honey, olive oil, and rum. Shake well before using. Take one tablespoonful three times a day. Or, mix one cup honey, one-half cup olive oil, and the juice of one lemon. Take one teaspoonful every two hours.
- Stir honey into the water left from cooking turnips. Sip to relieve coughs and hoarseness.

Horseradish—Mix one-half teaspoon horseradish with two teaspoons honey and take to stop a coughing spasm. Or, steep two tablespoons each horseradish and crushed mustard seeds in two cups boiling water for 20 minutes. Strain, then stir in enough honey to make a syrup.

Juices—Sip hot grapefruit juice sweetened with honey. Or, mix one-half cup either carrot or cherry juice with an equal amount of honey and take by the teaspoon as needed.

Juniper Berries—To clear a persistent cough, eat eight or 10 dried juniper berries each morning before breakfast.

Lemon

- Chop one lemon and stir into one cup honey. Heat and take one tablespoonful as often as needed. Or, mix one tablespoon lemon juice with two tablespoons raw honey and take a little at a time.
- Boil three whole lemons for 15 minutes. Without peeling, slice them over 1 pound of brown sugar in a saucepan. Simmer until thick, then stir in one tablespoon almond oil. Take a spoonful whenever a cough is troublesome.

Milk

- Stir one teaspoon each honey and sesame seed oil into a cup of warm milk. Sip to stop an irritating cough.
- Boil three chopped dried figs in one cup milk and let stand for one hour. Reheat and drink while warm to soothe a cough.
- Combine equal amounts of barley, oats, and rye. Simmer in milk until well done. Strain and sip the liquid to ease coughing spasms.

Nerve Massage—Massage the thumb and first two fingers on both hands.

Nerve Pressure (Press each point for 10 seconds, release, and repeat three times.)

- With the index fingers, press inward and upward against the underside of the cheekbones adjoining the nose just above the nostrils.

- To stop a coughing spasm, press hard on the roof of the mouth.
- To stop nervous coughing, press the upper lip beneath the nose.
- With the index finger, press in and pull down on the top of the breastbone at the hollow of the throat.
- To stop a fit of coughing, press both sides of the right thumbnail. Or, use the left thumb to press firmly on the lower joint of the right index finger.

Oil—To calm nighttime coughs, swallow one teaspoon vegetable oil just before retiring.

Okra—Cut very fine and cook with any recipe for cough syrup to act as a sugar substitute for thickening. The mucilaginous property of okra also softens and helps eliminate mucus. Okra, liquefied in an electric blender with the water in which it was cooked, may be sipped or used as a soothing gargle to stop coughs.

Onion

- Mince or slice raw onions and layer in a dish with sugar or honey. Cover and let stand eight to 12 hours, then take one teaspoon of the liquid each two hours.
- Cook minced onions or leeks in enough milk or wine vinegar to cover. Strain, add an equal amount of raw honey to the liquid, and take a teaspoonful each hour.

Case History

Randy B. was about to have his life ruined by a lousy cough. His relatives were spending only a few days with them at their summer cabin, and the overnight fishing trip he and his older cousins were planning was the most exciting thing that had ever happened to him. Except...it might not happen. Despite all the cough drops he had devoured, Randy's hacking cough persisted. His mother was afraid the cough might mean he was "coming down with something," and was insisting the outing would be too risky for him. Then Randy's aunt came to his rescue. She remembered her grandmother's remedy for coughs, and offered to concoct a facsimile from the ingredients on hand. She chopped an onion, covered it with milk, and simmered it to a mush. They had neither honey nor a sieve, so she stirred in an equal amount of granulated sugar; and accepted the suggestion of adding one drop of turpentine to the teaspoonful Randy was to take each hour. The mixture did not taste as good as a cough drop, but the results were miraculous. Randy's cough blared forth less and less frequently, and he was allowed to accompany his cousins for his first "grown-up," overnight excursion.

- Boil 1 pound chopped onions in one quart water with one and one-half cups brown sugar and one-half cup honey for 45 minutes. Strain and bottle. Take one tablespoonful as needed.

Tissue Salts

- For a hacking cough, take 12X Kali. Mur. four or five times a day.
- For an irritating cough with difficulty in expelling phlegm, take 12X Silicea three or four times each day.

- For a tickling cough, take 6X Mag.Phos. and Silicea alternately during spasms.

Whiskey

- Dissolve one teaspoon sugar in one teaspoon whiskey. Take to stop a coughing spasm.
- To one cup boiling water, add three tablespoons whiskey and one tablespoon butter. Drink as hot as possible.
- Dissolve four sticks horehound candy in a pint of whiskey. Take by the teaspoon as needed.
- Mix equal parts of whiskey and hot pepper sauce. Add honey to make a syrup and take by the spoonful.

Sore Throat Remedies

Bran—Boil one-half pound unprocessed bran in one quart water for 30 minutes. Strain, add honey to taste, then sip throughout the day.

Brandy and Sugar—Dissolve one-quarter cup brown sugar in an equal amount of brandy and sip to relieve a sore throat.

Coconut Milk—Sipping coconut milk has been found to help some cases of sore throat.

Compresses and Poultices

- Secure a strip of woolen cloth around the throat and leave on overnight.
- Apply a cold compress to the throat. Cover with plastic to keep airtight and leave in place for four hours or overnight.
- Mash one-half cup tofu with two tablespoons whole wheat flour and blend in one teaspoon grated fresh ginger. Spread on a strip of cloth and place the tofu mixture next to the throat. Cover with another cloth to hold in place. Replace every two hours.

Gargles

- **Aloe Vera**—Blend one-quarter cup aloe vera gel(available in health food stores) with one-quarter cup water and gargle to stop pain.
- **Apple Cider Vinegar, Lemon Juice, or Pekoe Tea**—Use any of these liquids as a gargle each hour. Dilute half-and-half with water, if desired.
- **Beets**—Juice raw beets (or liquefy in a blender with a little water) and gargle to soothe irritated membranes.
- **Brewer's Yeast**—Combine one-quarter cup brewer's yeast with one tablespoon honey and stir in one cup water. Gargle every 20 or 30 minutes.
- **Currants**—Simmer one tablespoon dried currants in one cup water for 10 minutes. Add one-half teaspoon ground cinnamon and cover for 30 minutes. Strain and use warm as a gargle.
- **Honey**—Boil one teaspoon honey with one cup water for a gargle. If the throat is extremely tender, swallow two teaspoons of the mixture each hour. For an uncooked variation: combine one-fourth cup each raw honey, apple cider

vinegar, and water for a gargle. If desired, the water may be omitted and a spoonful of the mixture swallowed six times a day.

- **Pomegranate**—Boil two tablespoons dried, grated pomegranate rinds in three cups of water until reduced to two cups. Strain, cool, and use as a gargle as often as needed.
- **Prune Juice**—Sipping a small amount of prune juice is often helpful for a sore throat.
- **Sage and Cayenne**—Popular during the 1800s, this gargle has character! Steep two teaspoons each dried sage and ground cayenne pepper in one cup boiling water. Stir in two teaspoons each honey, salt, and vinegar. Strain and bottle, then gargle four to 12 times daily. A variation considered an infallible cure was to substitute sugar for the honey and increase the vinegar to one-half cup. One or two teaspoons of the mixture was to be swallowed while gargling. (Modern studies have shown both salt and sugar do have an osmotic effect which pulls liquid out of the swollen tissue in the throat.)
- **Salt**—Stir one or two teaspoons of salt in a glass of hot water and gargle every three or four hours. Using one teaspoon each salt and baking soda was preferred by some folk practitioners.

Honey and Bee Pollen—Mix equal parts honey and bee pollen granules, then sip from a teaspoon to soothe a sore throat. Or, stir one tablespoon honey with one teaspoon bee pollen in a glass of freshly boiled water and sip slowly.

Lemon

- Apply fresh lemon juice externally to the throat area of the neck.
- Mix the juice of one lemon with boiling water to make one cup. Add honey to taste and sip slowly.
- Blend equal parts of lemon juice, honey, and egg white. Sip by the teaspoonful to ease sore-throat distress.
- Bake an unpeeled lemon in a 350-degree oven until it begins to crack open, about 30 minutes. Take one teaspoon of the juice, sweetened with honey, if desired, every hour. As an alternative, the juice from the roasted lemon may be stirred into a glass of hot water, sweetened with honey, and sipped.

Lysine—1,000 milligrams of this amino acid has aborted sore throats when taken at the onset.

Nerve Massage—Rub the underside of the big toe on each foot.

Nerve Pressure

- Using a piece of clean cloth for a firm grip, pull the tongue out as far as possible and move from side to side for one or two minutes.
- With the right thumbnail, press the bottom outside corner of the left thumbnail for seven seconds. Release and repeat three times, then apply the same sequence of pressure to the right thumbnail.

Onion—For laryngitis, eat a raw onion. For an inflamed throat, mix onion juice with honey and take by the teaspoonful. For a sore throat accompanied by hoarseness, eat onions boiled in molasses.

Pineapple—Eat fresh pineapple or drink fresh pineapple juice. (The bromelain it contains is believed to destroy the dead tissue in the throat without affecting the healthy tissue.)

Sources (See Bibliography)

3, 6, 7, 9, 10, 13, 24, 27, 28, 29, 34, 52, 53, 62, 63, 64, 67, 73, 78, 86, 89, 98, 111, 113, 116, 121, 122, 128, 142, 151, 152, 156, 159, 165, 168, 173, 174, 176, 180, 181, 184,. 190, 215, 226, 227, 228, 229, 234, 247, 251, 252, 261, 269, 272, 277, 280, 288, 289, 293, 297, 299, 305, 311, 314, 315, 318, 319, 324, 325, 330, 333, 335, 344, 345.

COLITIS AND DIVERTICULAR DISEASE (See Also Constipation and Diarrhea)

Inflammation of the intestinal walls has become so common in the United States that diverticular disease is believed to affect one-third of the population over 40 and three-fourths of those over 70. Colitis (irritable bowel, mucous colitis, spastic colon) occurs in the large bowel. "Enteritis" can refer to an inflammation of the entire intestinal tract or of only the small intestine. "Ileitis" is inflammation of the last section of the small intestine. Persistent irritation can create "ulcerative colitis" —bleeding sores in the lining of the colon.

Colitis may precede diverticulitis; the two conditions often seem to blend into one another. Small pouches or sacs (diverticula) form when the lining of the colon bulges into the intestinal tract. These pouches may be hereditary and are harmless unless stagnant food particles become trapped in them, causing inflammation or infection to develop and produce diverticulitis or diverticulosis. The symptoms (abdominal cramps and pain, occasional nausea, and constipation alternating with diarrhea) are similar. So is the treatment. Any persistent abdominal pain or abnormal occurrences in the bowel should receive immediate medical attention as complications could necessitate surgery.

Medical texts list the cause of these maladies as unknown, but the theories are many. There is usually a correlation between colitis and emotional stress, depression, or anxiety. Relaxation therapy (see pages 9-10) often helps reduce intestinal spasms and the resulting damage. Hurried and irregular meals, overwork, allergy, and abuse of laxatives are other possible causes. The big news on this subject is that medical scientists have indicted our civilized diet with its high proportion of refined carbohydrates as the principal cause of diverticular disease. Most physicians now recommend plenty of roughage from whole grains, fruits, and vegetables rather than the bland, low-residue regimen previously prescribed. Nutritional supplements are considered especially important as the body uses its reserves to combat the stress of the inflammation and rebuild tissue. The irritation and bouts of diarrhea prevent the body's manufacture of B vitamins and the full absorption of new nutrients from food.

Diet and Supplements

Fiber is the key word in dietary prevention and control of diverticular disease. It has been reliably established that the low-fiber diets formerly recommended were actually a cause rather than a cure. A diet high in fiber not only helps prevent diverticular disease but alleviates pain and corrects existing intestinal problems—even diarrhea—and forestalls recurrent attacks. (Recent clinical studies have shown a success rate of 88 percent for chronic colitis and diverticulitis sufferers.[156])

Unprocessed bran is the naturally magical substance which augments the fiber from fruits and vegetables. Wheat bran is most frequently recommended but corn or oat bran, or glucomannan, is preferred by some authorities. Bran absorbs approximately eight times its own weight in water to transform it from roughage to "softage." The optimum amount required varies with each individual—two to four tablespoons per day is the average. Beginning with two teaspoons and gradually increasing to no more than one-half cup per day is suggested. Adding bran to meals containing other forms of natural fiber produces soft, bulky stools that move rapidly through the colon without causing irritation or requiring the contraction of intestinal muscles. These contractions can force fecal material into the diverticula or form high-pressure segments of the bowel that can explode to cause peritonitis—which may happen when harsh laxatives are used.

Pectin (contained in apples, bananas, and some other fruits) has absorptive qualities similar to those of grain fiber, gently draws bacteria and other debris away from the intestinal walls, soothes irritated membranes, and helps restore muscle tone. Pectin is available as a supplement to accompany "fruitless" meals.

An ample fluid intake is vital for intestinal well-being. Fruit and vegetable juices are frequently advised—with apple, beet, cabbage, carrot, celery, cucumber, papaya, and pineapple leading the list. Herbal teas made from camomile, caraway, comfrey, peppermint, sage, or slippery elm have proven beneficial—as have the folk remedies of two teaspoons each apple cider vinegar and raw honey, or one tablespoon aloe vera gel, stirred in a glass of water to be sipped with each meal.

Bowel irritation from poorly digested foods can usually be cleared by eating small, frequent meals; eating slowly; and chewing food thoroughly. When this is not successful, taking papaya enzymes or betaine hydrocholoride tablets with each meal may solve the problem for those without ulcers. Reducing the intake of sugar and white flour may be helpful. Any disturbance in carbohydrate metabolism, such as hypoglycemia (see Low Blood Sugar), can result in colitis.[13, 171] Sugar is a gastrointestinal irritant which many nutritionally oriented physicians believe to be at least partially responsible for stimulating the growth of the bacteria that cause diverticulitis.

Greasy or heavily spiced foods, seeds or nuts, popcorn, extremely hot or cold drinks, coffee, alcohol, and tobacco are irritants in some cases. Eggplant, peppers, tomatoes, and white potatoes can instigate the development of diverticulosis for those who are sensitive to the Nightshade Family. Allergenic sensitivity to other foods may cause diverticular disease. Trial periods of individual elimination may reveal the culprits, but allergy tests may be necessary. Medical studies have shown that one out of five coliltis patients is unable to properly digest the milk sugar, lactose, and that eliminating dairy products other than yogurt is an effective treatment for them.[18,52]

During acute attacks, a soft, bland diet may reduce discomfort. Even then, sprouted seeds and grains as well as cooked millet and tapioca are usually well-tolerated. Bananas, cooked pureed carrots, okra, and parsnips are soothing and healing to a disturbed intestinal tract.

Taking one multi-vitamin-mineral tablet (including magnesium, potassium, and phosphorus) each day helps compensate for lack of nutrient absorption. Additional, optional supplements:

Vitamin A—10,000 to 25,000 units daily, if not incorporated in the multi-vitamin. Vitamin A is required for healthy maintenance of the entire colon and also helps prevent or combat infection.

Acidophilus—Two to six capsules with each meal. *Lactobacillus acidophilus* helps improve digestion, provides beneficial bacteria in the intestines, and encourages the body's production of the B vitamins.

B Complex—One comprehensive, high-potency tablet daily plus at least 50 milligrams each B-6, niacinamide, and pantothenic acid, and 1 to 5 milligrams of folic acid. The B vitamins improve digestion, combat stress, and help prevent further damage to the intestinal walls.

Vitamin C—500 to 3,000 milligrams in divided doses daily. Vitamin C strengthens tissues and combats toxic substances that encourage or aggravate diverticular disease.

Dolomite—Six to nine tablets daily. This calcium-magnesium combination soothes intestinal muscles to prevent spasms and is especially valuable in more serious cases of colitis.

Vitamin E and Vegetable Oils—Two to six tablespoons cold-pressed vegetable oil each day for lubrication and tissue resiliency, plus 10 IU of vitamin E per tablespoon of oil to prevent oxidation of the essential fatty acids. Additional amounts of vitamin E, from 100 to 1,000 IU daily (see Caution, page 6), may prevent scar tissue from forming after recovery.

Garlic—Three garlic perles (or one teaspoon minced fresh garlic) daily are recommended for the antibiotic effect.

Zinc—15 to 50 milligrams daily to speed healing.

Nerve Massage

- Massage the palm of the hand at the inner edge of the thumb pad, directly in line with the index finger. Repeat with the other hand.
- Massage the shinbones of both legs, from just below the knees to mid-calf.
- Massage the sole of each foot just in front of the heel prominence, rubbing toward the outside of the foot.

Nerve Pressure

Once each day, press just in front of each ear at the end of the cheekbones. Maintain pressure for 10 scconds, release, and repeat three times.

Poultices for Acute Attacks

- Saturate a towel with hot water, salt water, or a strong epsom-salts solution. Apply to the painful area and keep warm with a heating pad, or repeat the hot applications, for two or three hours.
- Heat chopped red beets. Wrap in cloth and place over the abdomen with a protective covering.
- Saturate a towel in apple cider vinegar, sprinkle with coarse salt, and fold over so the salt is encased. Place over the abdomen, cover with plastic, and let remain for four or five hours. Repeat as needed.

Sources (See Bibliography)

13, 18, 24, 46, 52, 53, 54, 63, 64, 76, 81, 84, 89, 106, 128, 156, 171, 173, 174, 175, 181, 184, 189, 226, 227, 229, 243, 254, 261, 269, 272, 274, 288, 293, 297, 301, 303, 315, 316, 321, 325, 332, 334, 335, 353, 354.

CONJUNCTIVITIS, PINKEYE, AND BLOODSHOT EYES (See Also Infection and Vision Problems)

Conjunctivitis is the general term for a number of inflammations or infections of the mucous membrane (conjunctiva) which lines the eyelids and white part of the eye. Pinkeye is often caused by viruses and is a highly contagious malady, as is bacterial conjunctivitis resulting from an eye injury or a cold. Allergic conjunctivitis may be caused by irritation from smog, tobacco smoke, chlorine in swimming pools, or chemical fumes in the air. Infection from the roots of the teeth is sometimes responsible for eye inflammation. In addition to the discomfort of itching, burning, and the feeling of sand under the eyelids, there may be temporary blurring of vision due to excess mucus in the eye.

The presence of infection is indicated if the eyelids are stuck shut after sleep or the eyes "matter" during the day. No eye medications should be used unless specifically prescribed by a physician because drops or ointment containing cortisone-like agents can damage the eyes during viral infections. If the condition does not show improvement after a few days of treatment with natural remedies, medical attention should be obtained. Deep pain or visual distortion could indicate glaucoma or iritis; hemorrhages in the eyes might be caused by high blood pressure.

Bloodshot eyes—tiny, deep-red vessels on the whites of the eyes making them appear pink or red—can be triggered by the same external irritations that cause conjunctivitis, or by sun, wind, alcohol, or lack of sleep. Most orthomolecular physicians believe the underlying cause of this condition to be nutritional deficiencies. Even hemorrhaging of blood vessels in the eyes can often be corrected by supplementing the diet with vitamins C, E, and the B complex. Avoiding obvious irritants and unnecessary use of the eyes, plus wearing dark glasses when outdoors, usually relieves the immediate irritation while vitamin supplementation gradually clears the eyes.

Diet and Supplements

A natural high-protein diet including fresh fruits and vegetables, whole grains, liver (or the desiccated tablets), and yogurt is recommended. Alcohol, coffee, and sugar destroy B vitamins needed for eye health, so should be limited or avoided.

Vitamin A—10,000 units three times a day for one week, then reduced to 10,000 to 20,000 units per day for maintenance. A deficiency of vitamin A can cause conjunctivitis. Besides being an infection-fighter, vitamin A prevents drying and hardening of the mucous membranes and the itchy burning which follows.

B Complex—One comprehensive, high-potency tablet daily, plus 10 to 400 milligrams B-2 per day in divided doses. Vitamin B-2 is primarily responsible for supplying oxygen to the tissues covering the eyes. When there is a deficiency of B-2, the body forms tiny new blood vessels to supply the needed oxygen, making the eyes appear bloodshot. A lack of this vitamin may also cause inflamed, itchy eyelids; discomfort in bright light; and sticky accumulations at the base of the lashes as well as cracks at the corners of the eyes. Both bloodshot eyes and conjunctivitis have shown rapid improvement when large amounts of B-2 were accompanied by vitamin C and calcium supplementation. Additional B-6 (10 to 200 milligrams daily) assists B-2 and the amino acids from protein in transporting oxygen to the eyes.

Vitamin C and Bioflavonoids—500 to 1,000 milligrams vitamin C with half that amount of bioflavonoids twice daily—each two hours if infection is suspected. Vitamin C is vital to the oxygen uptake of the eye lens. When combined with bioflavonoids, it corrects capillary fragility and strengthens artery walls to prevent or help clear eye hemorrhages.

Calcium and Vitamin D—1,000 milligrams calcium plus at least 800 IU natural vitamin D. Some authorities believe there is an underlying calcium deficiency in certain forms of conjunctivitis. In clinical studies, 90 percent of patients with pinkeye showed dramatic improvement with this combination[261], which also relieves the sticky eye-discharge frequently accompanying conjunctivitis.

Tissue Salts—For "sandy" eyelids: take four tablets of 6X Kali. Mur. every hour or two until relieved.

Folk Remedies

Aloe Vera—Blend equal parts of aloe vera gel (available in health food stores) and boiled water. Strain and store in the refrigerator. Warm a small amount to body temperature and put two or three drops in the affected eye three or four times daily.

Castor Oil—For immediate relief of burning caused by irritation, put one drop of castor oil in each eye.

Egg White—To relieve eye inflammation: spread beaten egg white on a piece of cloth and bandage over the closed eye overnight.

Fruit and Vegetable Poultices (To be applied over closed eyelids)

- Applying a poultice of warm boiled, roasted, or rotten apples to the eyes was the advice given in *Consult Me*, a medical reference published in 1872.
- For irritated eyes: cover the closed lids with raw cucumber slices.
- For inflamed eyes: pound a leek to a pulp (or use a food processor) and place between pieces of gauze to apply to the eyes. Or, boil and mash a white potato. Stir in finely ground slippery elm tea leaves and apply as a poultice.
- For bloodshot eyes or the feeling of sand in the eyelids: grate a scrubbed, unpeeled white potato and place a large spoonful directly on the eyelid. Cover with a gauze pad and let remain for one or two hours.

Herbal Teas—Wring compresses out of cold camomile, fennel, or slippery elm tea and place over the eyes to relieve inflammation. Or, place a poultice of moistened slippery elm powder over the eyes. Bathing the eyes with half-strength, strained camomile or fennel tea is believed helpful for inflamed eyelids and watering eyes.

Hot and Cold Water—For irritated eyes: saturate cloths in hot water and in ice water, then apply alternately for five minutes as eye compresses.

Lemon—To relieve eye inflammation: each morning before breakfast, drink the juice of one lemon stirred into a cup of hot water.

Onion—For conjunctivitis or eye inflammation: mince one raw onion, stir into a glass of beer, then drink.

Pekoe Tea—Place cold, moist tea bags over the closed eyes. Or, cover with a poultice of wet tea leaves from the bottom of the pot or cup.

Salt Water—For eye irritation: twice each day immerse the face in a basin filled with two quarts of water to which one tablespoon of salt has been added. Open the eyes under the water. Use fresh salt water each day. Or, dissolve one teaspoon salt in two cups warm water and bathe the eyes with an eye-cup several times a day.

Soda—For a soothing eyewash: stir one teaspoon baking soda in one-half cup warm water.

Witch Hazel—To relieve eye irritation: moisten gauze pads with Witch Hazel and place over the closed eyes for 15 minutes.

Nerve Massage

To stop watering eyes: massage the webs between the second and third fingers. Left hand for left eye, right hand for right eye.

Nerve Pressure

- For eye infection: press the underside of the cheekbone, 1½ inches in from the ear, for 10 seconds, then release for 10 seconds. Repeat three times once each day.
- For eye inflammation and granulated lids: squeeze the joints of the first and second fingers of the hand corresponding to the irritated eye. Apply pressure on the upper and lower surfaces as well as on the sides for five minutes at a time once each day.

Sources (See Bibliography)

3, 4, 6, 13, 22, 34, 53, 68, 84, 88, 89, 98, 142, 151, 153, 154, 156, 168, 173, 174, 176, 184, 189, 190, 211, 226, 229, 236, 241, 252, 261, 272, 288, 297, 315, 316, 335.

CONSTIPATION

One of the most common of human complaints, constipation (once referred to as costiveness) is often a self-inflicted mishap rather than an organic malady. "Normal" bowel emptying can vary from four times daily to once or twice a week. Misconceptions regarding the necessity of "daily regularity" can create chronic constipation through the use of laxatives. Most constipation results from either lack of fiber and liquid in the diet or delayed response to nature's call for evacuating the bowel. Emotional stress, with its muscular tension and added requirements for B vitamins, can cause constipation. So can irregular eating habits or lack of exercise. The use of certain antacids or drugs such as ACTH, cortisone, codeine, or other opiates which slow nerve reactions, or diuretics which deplete the body of liquids, may also be responsible for constipation. Spasms in the large bowel (spastic constipation) may occur when there are deficiencies of calcium, magnesium, potassium, or vitamin B-6. Most chronic constipation can be corrected by increasing the proportion of bulky, fibrous foods in the diet and deliberately relaxing away some of the daily tension (see pages 9-10). Any sudden change in bowel habits—bleeding, abdominal pain, or constipation which continues for longer than one week despite natural remedies—should have the immediate attention of a physician or proctologist since several potentially serious ailments of the gastrointestinal tract have similar symptoms.

Diet and Supplements

A modern diet of highly processed foods leaves little residue for the intestines (The chemically refined diets of astronauts in space travel reduce their bowel action to once a week.[84]) Dairy products, (including cheeses and eggs), fish, meats, poultry, sugar, coffee, tea, soft drinks, and alcoholic beverages do not contain any fiber at all, and there is very little in pastas or bakery products made from white flour. (At least nine slices of white bread would have to be eaten to equal the fiber from one slice of whole-grain bread.[189]) Many cases of chronic constipation can be corrected by increasing the daily intake of fruits and vegetables. Whenever possible, the skins should be left on. If unsprayed produce is not available, a five-minute soaking in a solution of one-quarter cup vinegar to a bowl of water, followed by a quick rinse in clear water, will remove 85 percent of the surface spray.[261] Including kefir or acidophilus yogurt or capsules is effective for some individuals. Others require the addition of bran for a permanent return to regularity.

Adequate liquid is necessary for fiber to do its job in the intestinal tract. At least six glasses of water daily is suggested, with one or two of them before bed and before breakfast. Either cool or hot water is considered more beneficial than ice water. The juices from fresh apple, cabbage, carrot, cucumber, lemon, papaya, spinach, or tomatoes are believed especially helpful. *The Complete Handbook of Nutrition*[243] recommends 8 ounces daily of carrot juice plus 8 ounces of any combination of apple, celery, and spinach juice. Milk itself is not constipating, but excessive milk consumption that replaces solids in the diet can lead to constipation.[261] In addition to fluids and fibrous foods, supplementary nutrients have proven of benefit for many people.

> **Vitamin A**—25,000 units daily. Vitamin A helps maintain the health of the mucous membrane lining the intestinal tract and prevents infection from retained stagnant foods.
>
> **B Complex**—One comprehensive, high-potency tablet once or twice each day. Clinical studies have shown that B-vitamin deficiencies can cause constipation, and all are a factor in its correction. Two to three tablespoons of brewer's yeast, or double that amount of wheat germ, offers a daily source of the entire complex. Lecithin capsules or granules provide choline and inositol. The addition of 100 milligrams each B-1, B-6, and niacinamide have proven helpful. From 100 to 500 milligrams pantothenic acid each day has brought back proper elimination in a number of cases—pantothenic acid is a peristaltic stimulant.
>
> **Bran**—Two teaspoons daily to three tablespoons three times a day. Unprocessed bran is a normalizer of bowel function rather than a laxative. Recent studies have shown excellent results with both corn and oat bran, but wheat bran (miller's bran) has been thoroughly tested by many doctors and has proven to be the safest and most effective substance available for alleviating and correcting constipation. Instead of stimulating bowel function through irritation or merely providing the bulk of most other fibrous foods, bran swells up like a sponge as it absorbs eight or nine times its own weight in liquid to form soft, bulky stools. When first adding bran to the diet, it is wise to start with the two daily teaspoons and gradually increase the dosage until the desired results are obtained. (Beginning with larger amounts can cause flatulence for a few days.) Bran should always be taken with plenty of liquid and an upper limit of one-half cup per day should not be exceeded. (An excess could accumulate in the colon to create further constipation or an obstruction.)
>
> **Vitamin C**—Stir one teaspoon vitamin C crystals into a glass of juice and drink immediately upon arising. (Adding one-fourth teaspoon baking soda is

suggested for those with stomach ulcers.) Taken in this form, vitamin C will stimulate a "normal" bowel movement in approximately one hour.

Case History

Marlene K. was seldom troubled by constipation and her limited experience with laxatives had not been satisfactory; but after the second day at a week-long convention, she had a real problem. The flurry of preparations for the trip plus the irregular hours and mealtimes caused more than "irregularity." Recalling the abdominal cramping and numerous dashes to the bathroom brought on by previous "aids to regularity," Marlene asked her roommate if she knew of a laxative that would be "safe" to take without interfering with their planned activities. The roommate opened her cosmetic case, handed Marlene a bottle of vitamin C crystals and a small can of fruit juice, told her to mix a spoonful of the crystals with the juice for results within an hour, and explained that she never traveled without this safe, emergency laxative. As soon as she awoke the next morning Marlene drank the juice-vitamin C combination as directed. It worked as comfortably and quickly as promised, allowing her to relax and enjoy the scheduled breakfast meeting.

Vitamin E and Vegetable Oil—Two tablespoons daily of any cold-pressed unsaturated vegetable oil plus 20 IU of vitamin E to assure absorption. The oil acts both as a natural lubricant for the mucous membrane of the intestine and as an aid to increase the flow of digestive juices from the pancreas to relieve constipation.

Potassium is essential for muscular contraction. Medications such as cortisone or certain diuretics can deplete the body's potassium. A diet high in salt can so upset the sodium-potassium balance that weakened muscles allow constipation. Increasing the intake of fruits and vegetables while limiting sodium consumption often corrects this situation. If potassium supplements are necessary, large amounts should be taken only with medical approval.

Tissue Salts (6X potency unless otherwise directed)

- If there is difficulty expelling the stools: take Calc. Fluor. and Silicea, one dose of each at bedtime and early in the morning. If the bowel movement is difficult and dry, substitute Nat. Mur. and Nat. Sulph. for a few days.
- If there is no desire to defecate: take one dose each 12X Calc. Fluor. and Kali. Phos. at bedtime and again in the morning for several days.
- If there is discomfort in the bowel: take Ferr. Phos. every half hour until relieved.
- If there is no movement and the tongue is white: take Kali. Mur. at bedtime and early in the morning for several days. If the tongue is yellow, substitute Kali. Sulph.
- If all efforts at stool come to nothing: use Nat. Phos. at half-hourly intervals until a bowel movement results.

Enemas

A time-honored remedy for constipation, 220 enemas were taken by Louis XIII of France during his last six months. The ladies of the court and even his dogs were equally well-flushed. Enemas ease the evacuation of waste for immediate relief but now are recommended only as an occasional remedy. Adding a little olive oil and/or a beaten egg yolk to the warm water is often helpful. The folk practitioners' solution was a frothy mixture of soap suds with warm water.

Exercise

Exercises that condition the abdominal muscles are particularly valuable, but any type of exercise stimulates peristaltic activity. A brisk walk each morning may help correct constipation.

Folk Remedies

Apple Cider Vinegar and Honey—Stir two teaspoons of each into a glass of water and take three times daily.

Apples—Eat one raw apple each night before retiring. Or, eat one or two raw unpeeled apples before (or for) breakfast; wait 10 minutes, then drink one or two glasses of cool water. Or, bake apples without sugar and eat one or two for breakfast.

Cabbage—Drink two glasses of fresh cabbage juice before breakfast. Or, shred a small head of cabbage, sprinkle with salt, and place in the container of an electric blender overnight. Add enough water to liquefy, then drink for breakfast.

Cloves—Steep six whole cloves in one-half cup boiling water overnight. Drink the cool liquid before breakfast.

Cornmeal—Stir one teaspoon to one tablespoon cornmeal in a glass of cold water and drink immediately upon arising each morning.

Escarole—Eat raw escarole the first thing each morning. Or, boil it and drink the warm liquid.

Figs and Raisins

- Cook figs in milk. Drink the liquid and eat the figs. Or, stew the figs in olive oil until tender, then add a little honey and lemon juice, and simmer until thickened.
- Boil two tablespoons pearled barley in one quart water until reduced to one pint. Strain and discard the barley. Add one sliced fig, one tablespoon raisins, and one-fourth teaspoon dry licorice root tea to the liquid. Boil for five minutes, then eat the solids and sip the liquid.
- Chop or grind one-half pound each figs, prunes, and raisins. Mix with one-half cup unprocessed bran and press into a shallow pan. Cut into one-tablespoon-size squares, wrap, and store in the refrigerator. Eat one square daily.

Flaxseed—Stir two teaspoons flaxseed into one cup cold water, let stand 30 minutes, and drink. Or, pulverize the flaxseed and swallow it with a full glass of water.

Garlic—A remedy for constipation even before the days of Hippocrates, one teaspoon of minced raw garlic daily is the usual dosage. Combining the garlic with minced onions and/or yogurt may increase the effectiveness.

Herbal Teas—Drinking aloe vera, basil, buckthorn, chicory, dandelion, fennel, ginger, licorice root, or senna leaf tea was thought to relieve costiveness.

Honey—Eating several tablespoons of raw honey every day is an old remedy believed to be even more effective when one teaspoon of bee pollen granules is added and the mixture spread on whole-grain bread. For those who are not diabetic, hypoglycemic, or counting calories, one-half cup honey each day for adults (one-fourth cup for children) is said to relieve chronic constipation.

Olive Oil—Mix one teaspoon each olive oil and lemon juice. Take each morning upon awakening.

Onions—Eat roasted onions at bedtime. Or, fill a jar with fresh vegetable juice, add one minced onion, and let stand overnight. Strain, then take two teaspoons of the liquid stirred into a glass of cold water twice daily, before meals.

Prunes—The most well-known folk remedy, dried prunes, should be soaked for at least eight hours before being used for their laxative effect. Prunes are valuable for their intrinsic fiber, but prune juice has a stimulating action on the bowels and should not be used every day as a substitute for natural bulk.

Pumpkin Seeds and Sunflower Seeds—Eating a handful of either, or both, each day provides mild laxative action plus added nutrients.

Rhubarb—Raw rhubarb stems (not the poisonous leaves or roots) are considered one of nature's best laxatives. Cooked rhubarb has little or no laxative value.

Laxatives

Castor oil was prescribed for constipation on an Egyptian papyrus inscribed in 1550 B.C. Strong laxatives are no longer advised and definitely should not be used if there is pain in the abdomen. Perforation of an acute appendix or rupture of a blocked bowel could result. Stimulant-type cathartics are laxatives that reduce nutrient absorption, destroy friendly bacteria, and irritate the delicate linings of the intestinal tract. They usually remove not only the waste matter that should be eliminated but also the still-liquid material in the tract above it. This prevents a normal bowel movement for the following day or so and creates the impression of further constipation. Laxatives can become addictive as their regular use weakens or nullifies the normal defecation reflex. The use of mineral oil as a stool softener is no longer recommended because it has been found to block absorption of the fat-soluble vitamins, and may even be absorbed into the lungs to cause a form of pneumonia.

Nerve Massage (Massage Each Area for Two Minutes Each Day)

- Massage a spot on both cheekbones parallel with the nostrils, 1½ inches toward the ears.

- Massage the area at the base of both nostrils.
- Massage the cleft of the chin.
- Gently massage both sides of the lower part of the Adam's Apple.
- Massage the center of the palm of each hand.
- Rub the inside of each upper leg bone between the knee and the groin.
- Place the palm of the hand on the abdomen just below the navel and rotate in a clockwise motion as firmly as is comfortable.
- Massage the sole of the right foot just under the pad of the little toe, and the bottom of each foot under the arch toward the heel pad.

Nerve Pressure (Press each point for 10 seconds, release, and repeat three times.)

- Press the spine in the center of the back of the neck. At the same time, press on the navel.
- At least three times during the day, press a point the width of one hand directly above the navel.
- Press 3 inches above and below the navel, approximately 2 inches toward the left side. Press another point 1½ inches directly below the navel.
- Press directly below the inside of the nail on each of the big toes.
- Press a point on the sole of each foot in line with the third toe, just below the ball of the foot.

Sources (See Bibliography)

3, 5, 13, 18, 19, 28, 44, 52, 53, 54, 62, 63, 64, 67, 68, 69, 76, 81, 84, 88, 89, 92, 103, 106, 122, 142, 152, 154, 158, 160, 168, 173, 174, 180, 184, 189, 208, 214, 226, 227, 229, 243, 252, 253, 254, 260, 261, 269, 274, 288, 289, 303, 314, 315, 316, 325, 330, 332, 333, 334, 335, 344.

CORNS AND CALLUSES

Thickenings of the outer layers of the skin caused by persistent friction and pressure, corns are usually cone-shaped with the point directed inward. Soft corns occur between the toes. The horny tissue of a callus spreads over a surface area but can become painful. A "Plantar's Wart" on the bottom of the foot may have a hard surface similar to a corn or callus but contains blood vessels and nerve endings, so professional removal may be required if home remedies do not suffice (see Warts).

Protruding corns can be protected by a corn pad cut into the shape of a horseshoe, or a spot-type bandage with the gauze center next to the corn. Correctly fitted shoes may take care of calluses, especially if vitamin A supplements are added to the diet. Soft corns between the toes may be helped by wrapping a strip of turpentine-saturated cloth or a few strands of lamb's wool around the base of adjoining toes.

Most foot specialists caution against using over-the-counter "corn cures" as the acid they contain can destroy healthy tissue surrounding the corn to cause potentially dangerous ulcerations. Corns may be rubbed down to surface level with a pumice stone, but bathroom surgery is generally unsuccessful as well as hazardous. Any painful foot condition which does not respond to natural remedies should receive the attention of a podiatrist.

Diet and Supplements

An insufficiency of vitamin A, vitamin E, or potassium may encourage corns and calluses. Increasing the proportion of fruits, vegetables, and whole grains in the diet may prevent their formation or recurrence. Bananas and carrots are especially beneficial. Sprinkling paprika on all suitable foodstuffs provides extra vitamin A—1,273 units per teaspoon.[189] Using a salt substitute containing potassium may also be helpful. Drinking a mixture of two teaspoons each apple cider vinegar and raw honey in a glass of water with each meal provides some added potassium, as does drinking apple or cranberry juice daily.

> **Vitamins A and E**—25,000 to 50,000 units vitamin A plus 100 to 800 IU vitamin E daily (see Caution, page 6) for several months often corrects the problem of calluses and helps prevent corns. Rough, cracked calluses (particularly those on the heels) may be softened and cleared by rubbing with vitamin E oil or the contents of a vitamin E capsule each night.
>
> **Tissue Salts**—Take two 3X tablets of both Kali. Mur. and Silicea three times each day.

Folk Remedies

> **Aloe Vera Gel**—To soften callused heels: rub with aloe vera gel each night and morning.
>
> **Bread and Vinegar**—To remove stubborn corns: crumb bread into a teaspoon of vinegar. Let stand 30 minutes to make a paste, then apply to the corn before retiring at night. Repeat each night until the soreness is gone and the corn can be lifted out.
>
> **Castor Oil**—Massage castor oil into corns and calluses twice each day. Cover with a soft bandage, if desired.
>
> **Cranberry**—Bind the cut side of half a raw cranberry over the corn each night. (According to the *American Frugal Housewife,* written in 1829, this will draw out a corn in less than a week.)
>
> **Foot Baths**—to soften corns and calluses, and relieve pain:
>
> • Soak the feet in comfortably hot water. Dry thoroughly, then rub with fresh lemon juice.
>
> • Soak the feet in hot water in which oatmeal has been boiled.
>
> • To a basin of hot water add as much salt as will dissolve. Soak the feet in this solution, then in plain hot water.
>
> **Garlic**—Secure a slice of raw garlic to the corn each night.

Lemon—To soften and eventually loosen a corn, place the pulp side of a small piece of lemon over the corn each night and bandage to keep in place. Or, thrust the toe into a lemon and tie in place overnight.

Mustard—To remove a corn: Place two tablespoons dry mustard in a basin. Stir in enough hot water to cover the corn. Soak the foot, then rub the corn. If not loose enough to be lifted out, applying vinegar may speed the procedure.

Onion

- To remove stubborn corns in three weeks: tape a piece of raw onion over the corn each night.[335]
- For either corns or calluses: apply a salve made from equal parts of roasted onions and soft soap.
- Soak a slice of onion in vinegar for several hours, then bind a section over the corn at night. Or, cook onion with vinegar, mash, and apply to the corn at least twice each day.

Soda and Vaseline—Cover the corn with an ointment made by mixing equal parts of baking soda and pure petroleum jelly.

Turpentine—The 1886 edition of *Dr. Chase's Recipes or Information for Everybody* recommends binding cotton over the corn and saturating it three times daily with turpentine.

Sources (See Bibliography)

3, 52, 68, 69, 73, 98, 142, 152, 160, 168, 174, 181, 189, 190, 226, 227, 229, 261, 288, 318, 333, 335, 353.

DANDRUFF

Flakes that form on the scalp and float off as the hair is brushed or combed indicate the mildest form of seborrheic dermatitis. In more serious cases, the sebaceous glands become so overactive that the scales and itching may extend to the eyebrows, ears, nose, chest, and even the pubic area. All forms are most prevalent between the ages of 20 and 40 (glandular secretions peak, then dwindle with age) and often strike dark complexions more severely than light. "Snowflakes on the shoulders" or "that little itch" are not a disease—no one has ever perished from terminal dandruff—but they may be mishaps with a message. Severe dandruff can lead to baldness (which see) and may be an outward symptom of internal difficulties which should be corrected. Allergies (particularly to milk), emotional upsets, hormonal imbalance, or illness may trigger sudden onsets of dandruff. The basic remedies fall into two categories: correction of the cause through nutrition and supplements, and immediate control by the use of natural shampoos and tonics.

Diet and Supplements

Dandruff may be instigated by a lack of vitamins A, E, and minerals, or too high a ratio of animal fat to polyunsaturated oils. However, clinical studies have shown that most cases of dandruff are related to poor metabolization of refined carbohydrates and the resulting deficiency of B vitamins. According to most authorities, alcohol, sugar, and white flour should be eliminated or at least limited. Natural, complex carbohydrates in fruits, vegetables, and whole grains supply their own B vitamins. Refined carbohydrates contain no B vitamins, yet require them for metabolization, so the necessary B vitamins must be drawn from body tissues. This can cause a deficiency resulting in dandruff. Including fruits and vegetables such as apples, beets, broccoli, cabbage, carrots, grapefruit, Romaine lettuce, and prunes has proven helpful. Taking two to three tablespoons of brewer's yeast daily, plus vitamin and mineral supplements, often clears the problem. The antioxidants (see page 3) are especially beneficial—unless controlled, free radicals can cause an internal chain reaction culminating in dandruff.

> **Vitamin A**—25,000 to 100,000 units daily for one month. A deficiency of vitamin A can cause the cells in the lower layers of the skin to die and accumulate as dandruff.
>
> **B Complex**—One comprehensive tablet with each meal. An additional 100 to 300 milligrams of PABA daily has cleared intractable dandruff that had spread to the eyebrows and sides of the nose.[53,325] Adding 100 milligrams each B-2, B-6, niacinamide, and pantothenic acid each day has solved the problem for others. Supplementing the diet with vitamin B-12, orally or by injection, may be necessary for some individuals.
>
> **Vitamin E and Vegetable Oils**—Two tablespoons unsaturated, cold-pressed vegetable oil plus 20 to 1,200 IU vitamin E daily (see Caution, page 6). When protected from internal oxidation by vitamin E, the essential fatty acids in the oil may correct dry, flaky dandruff. Vitamin E also assists the assimilation of vitamin A to help control the showers of dandruff flakes. To stop the itching and scabs of dandruff, apply vitamin E oil to the scalp twice each week before going to bed, then shampoo out the following morning.
>
> **Selenium**—50 to 200 micrograms daily. Selenium enhances the action of vitamin E and helps prevent the hardening of tissues through oxidation that can result in scaly dandruff.
>
> **Tissue Salts**—For two or three weeks, take two doses per day of both Kali. Sulph. and Nat. Mur. in the 12X potency.
>
> **Zinc**—30 to 50 milligrams daily. In some instances, zinc supplementation has halted the itching and scaling of dandruff within one week.[53]

Shampoos and Rinses

Shampooing daily with a mild, unmedicated shampoo diluted half-and-half with water has proven more satisfactory for many than using harsh, medicated shampoos.

(They can instigate an overproduction of oil and more dandruff.) Dandruff may result from disturbed pH of the skin and an over-alkaline condition that can be corrected by adding diluted lemon juice or vinegar to the final rinse after shampooing. If commercial conditioners or cream rinses are used, they should be applied just to the hair, not the scalp. For oily hair with profuse dandruff, rubbing cornmeal or unprocessed bran into the scalp and brushing it out will provide a dry shampoo.

Egg shampoos

- Once each week, beat one raw egg lightly with a fork and rub it into the scalp as a substitute for shampoo. Rinse well with lukewarm water.

Case History

Whitney B. felt her efforts toward establishing a glamorous image were being defeated by her persistent dandruff. The dark sweaters she wore to accentuate her fair skin and blonde hair also accentuated the dandruff dust, and destroyed the chic effect she was striving to achieve. Whitney tried over-the-counter dandruff remedies without success. The white flakes kept falling on her shoulders. Then she read a magazine article touting the wonders of natural hair-care treatments, and decided to do some experimenting. She bought a bottle of natural jojoba shampoo, and, by combining two of the suggestions in the article, finally bested her problem dandruff. Twice each week, Whitney beat a tablespoon of sea salt into a raw egg, rubbed the gooey conglomeration on her scalp and hair, and let it remain for five minutes. After thoroughly rinsing out the gritty mixture, she washed her hair with the natural shampoo. The results were fantastic. Even after her dandruff disappeared, Whitney continued to use the egg-salt treatment once every week. Besides guarding against a reappearance of the ugly little flakes, she wanted to maintain the radiant sheen it imparted to her hair.

- Use the white of an egg as a shampoo—afterwards, rub the scalp with Vaseline.
- Simmer 1 ounce of white oak bark tea in one cup water for 15 minutes. Strain, then stir in 1 ounce pure liquid castile soap. When ready to shampoo, combine two tablespoons of the mixture with one egg and one teaspoon honey. A little cream, mashed avocado, peach, or apricot may be added, if desired.

Rinses

- Rinse freshly shampooed hair with strong catnip, celery seed, or wintergreen tea.
- Pour one-fourth cup apple cider vinegar over the hair as a final rinse. Let dry, then rub castor oil into the scalp before combing the hair.
- Mix the juice of one lemon, or one tablespoon vinegar, with one glass of water for use as a final rinse.

Tonics

Apple cider vinegar

- Mix one teaspoon apple cider vinegar in one cup water and apply to the scalp with a cotton ball, or comb through the hair, three times daily.
- Combine equal amounts of apple cider vinegar and water. Apply to the scalp with cotton before shampooing.
- Twice each week, warm one cup vinegar, pour over the head and wrap in a towel for one hour before shampooing.
- Shake one cup vinegar, one cup water, and two tablespoons bee pollen granules in a glass jar. Apply to the scalp with cotton pads before shampooing.

Castor Oil—Rub castor oil into the scalp before going to bed, then shampoo out in the morning.

Glycerine and Rosewater (available in pharmacies)—Rub into the scalp twice each week.

Lemon Juice—Massage the scalp with fresh lemon juice and allow to dry before shampooing.

Mint—Simmer two tablespoons dried mint (or one-half cup fresh mint leaves) with one cup water and one-half cup vinegar for five minutes in a covered saucepan. Let stand to cool. Strain and store in a glass jar. Rub into the scalp before shampooing.

Rosemary and Sage—Pour two cups boiling water over 1 ounce each dried rosemary and sage. Let stand for 24 hours, strain and store in a glass container. Massage into the scalp as an anti-dandruff treatment.

Vaseline—Apply to the scalp twice each week, rubbing in well. Wait at least one hour before shampooing.

Witch Hazel—Combine one tablespoon each witch hazel and water with one teaspoon strained lemon juice. Dab on the scalp with a cotton ball after shampooing.

Sources (See Bibliography)

13, 52, 53, 68, 84, 88, 89, 92, 142, 152, 153, 168, 184, 215, 227, 228, 229, 246, 252, 253, 254, 261, 276, 293, 305, 315, 325, 334, 353.

DIABETES

Diabetes was described in 1500 B.C. in Egyptian writings but was not given the name "diabetes mellitus" until the mid-1600s. Currently affecting approximately 10 million Americans, diabetes is becoming even more prevalent. The incidence increased by over 50 percent between 1965 and 1973, and is continuing to rise by about

6 percent each year.[41] Only one-tenth of these diabetics are considered "insulin-dependent"—usually those with juvenile-onset diabetes—while most of the remainder are maturity-onset diabetics who can maintain control through nutritional methods and/or oral agents.

Heredity is a major factor in its onset. It is estimated that one of every three Americans carries the gene of diabetes. But some combination of allergic response, dietary imbalance, lack of exercise, obesity, stress, or a virus such as mumps or German measles must be added to the genetic tendency before pancreatic failure to produce insulin adequate for processing carbohydrates results in diabetes. The possible combinations of these factors helps explain the difficulties involved in attempting to discover a cure for the malady.

Routine medical examinations usually detect diabetes before there are any of the obvious symptoms of frequent urination, increased thirst, recurring infections, or weight change. Insulin injections may be prescribed on a temporary basis during periods of illness, pregnancy, or stress; or on a regular schedule for those who cannot produce their own insulin. Diabetics whose pancreas secretes insulin which is not efficiently utilized may require one of the oral anti-diabetic drugs. Insulin shock, which can result from an overdose of insulin or from lowered blood sugar caused by stress or lack of food, can be forestalled by eating a small amount of sugar or candy, or drinking sweetened orange juice.

Home monitoring of sugar levels is advisable, but it is most important for all diabetics to see their physicians frequently. Uncontrolled diabetes can lead to serious disorders. With proper medical attention, dietary control, and adequate exercise, however, most diabetics can enjoy a normal life without undue restrictions.

Diet and Supplements

With or without the aid of oral drugs or insulin injections, diet is still a vital part of the treatment for diabetes. Dietary recommendations have undergone many alterations during the millennia. In 1797 a diet of nothing but meat and rancid fat was believed to be the solution and, in 1900, an all-carbohydrate "oat cure" was used in Germany.[338] One basic rule holds fast—diabetics should avoid, or severely limit, all sugars and foods containing sugar. Eating too large a proportion of refined carbohydrates puts an unnatural strain on the pancreas, although it may require as long as 20 years to culminate in diabetes.

While it is true that the carbohydrates in all foods are transformed into glucose by the body, the speed with which the conversion is accomplished makes a difference in the amount of insulin required. Official diabetic diets are gradually being revised to include more fruits, vegetables, dried legumes, and whole grains. The validity of "food exchange" lists is being questioned since it has been discovered that foods with identical calories and carbohydrates may call for varying amounts of insulin.

Recent research at the University of Colorado and the University of Toronto (reported in the public media in July, 1983) indicates surprising variations in blood-sugar reactions to individual foods. In these university tests, carrots, corn, honey, parsnips, white potatoes, white rice, and wheat bread were shown to have much faster blood-sugar response than apples, dried legumes, fructose, ice cream, milk (whole or skim), oatmeal, oranges, peanuts, spaghetti, sponge cake, tomato soup, or yogurt. Earlier tests at Stanford University demonstrated that the amount of insulin secreted varied from 45 units one hour after a dose of sugar, through 27 units after a dose of potato starch, to only 12 units following a dose of rice starch.[24] Other research programs have shown that celery with its green leaves, cucumber, garlic, green beans, Jerusalem artichokes, and onions contain natural hormones that increase insulin production for diabetics.[13,227]

Studies reported in the *British Medical Journal* [May 29, 1982] found that fiber and pectin improved glucose tolerance by delaying absorption of carbohydrates and reducing insulin requirements. Most fruits, especially those with edible skins and seeds, are excellent sources of fiber and pectin. Dried peas and beans are high in fiber. Soybeans are particularly valuable as they contain more protein and fewer assimilable carbohydrates than other legumes. Among the grains, buckwheat, millet, and oats are thought to be especially beneficial. Although high in fiber, sweet potatoes and dried fruits should be used with caution because of their sugar content. Avocados are also well supplied with fiber but are not recommended for diabetics as they depress the release of insulin.[129] Taking two pectin capsules and/or a few teaspoons of unprocessed bran with meals provide both pectin and fiber.

Fructose has an advantage over honey or other sugars because it does not require insulin in order to reach the liver, but it should be used in small amounts as it is eventually converted to glucose by the body. Many food processors have disguised the easily recognizable forms of sugar by listing them as corn syrup, dextrose, glucose, lactose, maltose, sucrose, etc., so labels must be read with care. Moderate use of artificial sweeteners is generally approved of for all diabetics except those who are pregnant. The natural juices of apples, grapes, pineapples, or prunes are not recommended as they may raise blood sugar too rapidly.

Alcohol is forbidden by some authorities and is not for all diabetics. (It may cause a reaction with anti-diabetic agents.) Most physicians, however, approve of a drink or two before or with dinner and/or a bedtime snack. Sweet wines and liqueurs should be avoided. Indulgence in ale or beer may require a reduction in the amount of bread eaten at the following meal. (Some brands of light beer contain only 2 grams of carbohydrate; regular beer or ale has 10 grams per 8-ounce glass. One slice of wheat bread equals 11 grams of carbohydrate, but it is not recommended that more than one slice per day be sacrificed in such an exchange.) The caffeine in coffee, chocolate, tea, and many soft drinks stimulates the liver into releasing stored sugar that requires extra insulin. Accompanying any form of caffeine with food can help reduce its effect but decaffeinated coffee and the limitation of other forms of caffeine is suggested.

The low-carbohydrate, high-fat diets advised for the past 50 years may have contributed to diabetic complications resulting from clogged arteries and poor circulation. According to Dr. Julian Whitaker, director of the National Heart and Diabetes Treatment Institute in Huntington Beach, California, excess fats (especially saturated ones) prevent insulin from lowering blood sugar. Most complex carbohydrates, on the other hand, help insulin function normally. Drastically increasing the proportion of raw foods in the diet has succeeded in reducing insulin requirements for some diabetics. An Oriental diet consisting only of lean meat, fish, raw vegetables, and unsaturated oils has shown remarkable results when adhered to for from one to four weeks.[333]

With the exception of substituting complex carbohydrates for the simple ones of sugar and refined flour, a diabetic diet allows approximately the same nutrient proportions as any other normally healthful diet. The American Diabetic Association recommends that 43 percent of the calories be carbohydrates, with 34 percent fat and 23 percent protein. Many nutritionally oriented physicians suggest much less fat and a higher proportion of complex carbohydrates, with an upper limit of 100 to 150 grams of carbohydrates per day. Dr. Robert Atkins,[23] however, believes the upper limit for carbohydrates should be 40 grams each day. Individual doctor's instructions and personal experimentation may be the best solution.

To correlate calories with grams: 1 gram of either carbohydrate or protein equals 4 calories. Each gram of fat equals 9 calories. For weight maintenance, adults require 10 calories per pound of body weight every day plus 3 calories per pound for light activity, 5 calories per pound for mild activity, and 10 calories per pound for strenuous exertion.[154,230]

If no diabetic diet has been prescribed, the dietary regimen for Low Blood Sugar (which see) may be used as a guide. Although hypoglycemia is the result of over- rather than under-production of insulin, the nutritional method for controlling fluctuations in blood sugar is the same for both.[128,171] Clinical tests have shown that eating small, frequent meals, and eating them slowly, helps control blood sugar. Each meal or snack should include both carbohydrates and protein in order to avoid abnormal demands for insulin and maintain proper blood sugar levels. Insulin-users should never attempt even a one-day fast as skipping meals may induce insulin shock.

Even the wisest of diabetic diets is seldom sufficient without supplements, most of which have therapeutic as well as nutritional benefits, but no pronounced dietary change should be undertaken without medical approval.

> **Vitamins A and D**—5,000 to 10,000 units of A plus at least 400 IU natural vitamin D daily. Diabetics are poorly able to utilize the vitamin A in fruits and vegetables as it occurs in the form of carotene, which their bodies have difficulty in remaking into assimilable vitamin A.
>
> **B Complex**—One comprehensive tablet daily. B vitamins are necessary for carbohydrate metabolism. An additional 50 to 100 milligrams B-6 each day is often helpful in maintaining the health of the pancreas. B-6 also reduces foot pain, burning, and numbness for diabetics with neuropathy. Studies show that families in which several members suffer from diabetes have an unusually high hereditary requirement for B-6.[88]
>
> Injections of B-12 may be necessary for those who have neuropathy and/or cannot absorb this vitamin when taken orally. Up to 1,000 milligrams choline plus 600 to 1,500 milligrams inositol have proven beneficial to diabetics who

have nerve damage. Choline plus desiccated liver may help control blood glucose levels for those who have become insulin resistant. Vitamin B-15, rarely included in combination supplements, has been shown to have a favorable effect on blood sugar levels when 50 milligrams were taken daily.[24]

Vitamin C and Bioflavonoids—1,000 to 5,000 milligrams vitamin C plus 100 to 1,000 milligrams bioflavonoids daily. Diabetics, especially when on insulin therapy, lose vitamin C more readily than do nondiabetics. Vitamin C helps make better use of insulin, helps prevent allergic reactions and offset possible side effects from artificial sweeteners, aids in preventing retinopathy or other vascular complications, and, like insulin, helps metabolize carbohydrates. Taking bioflavonoids along with vitamin C enhances its effectiveness and is believed helpful in preventing the onset of diabetic cataracts. Massive amounts of vitamin C should not be taken for a few days preceding a medical examination as they might interfere with test readings.

Chromium—1,000 to 2,000 micrograms daily for six months, then 200 micrograms each day. Considered one of the most valuable supplements for diabetics, chromium is essential for the metabolism of carbohydrates. It is the active component of the glucose tolerance factor (GTF) which helps insulin maintain the blood-sugar balance. Taking two or three tablespoons brewer's yeast daily potentiates the effect of chromium supplements and, according to the *American Journal of Clinical Nutrition* (April 1980), has improved glucose tolerance and reduced insulin requirements.

Vitamin E (alpha tocopherol)—100 to 1,200 IU daily. Diabetics are advised to start with 100 IU daily and add 100 IU each month until at least 400 IU are taken each day (see Caution, page 6). Decreases in vitamin E intake should be gradual, also. Vitamin E improves the action of insulin and has enabled some diabetics to reduce their insulin dosage, but its primary function is to combat the degeneration of blood vessels and assist the tissues affected. Hospital tests have shown amazing results with large amounts of vitamin E, particularly when accompanied by at least 3,000 milligrams of vitamin C each day. Slow-to-heal sores, even small patches of gangrene, have been completely healed with two months of oral vitamin E supplementation plus topical applications of vitamin E oil.[261,302]

Vitamin F—Two tablespoons cold-pressed unsaturated oil (or the equivalent in capsules) each day. Unsaturated fatty acids are believed extremely important for diabetics.

Magnesium—200 to 500 milligrams daily. Magnesium is necessary for maintaining the health of the pancreas, activates six of the nine enzymes known to be involved in the metabolism of carbohydrates, and helps protect against heart disease as well as retinal problems for diabetics.[24]

Manganese works in conjunction with chromium as part of the glucose tolerance factor. If it is not included in a daily vitamin-mineral tablet, some supplementation may be helpful. Blueberries, brewer's yeast, garlic, and onions are good natural sources of manganese.

Potassium—Essential for preventing a sodium imbalance which can lead to high blood pressure and arterial problems, potassium deficiency can also cause blood sugar elevations. However, medical approval should be obtained before taking the frequently recommended dosage of one 99-milligram tablet three times a day. Potassium is included in some diuretics and salt substitutes, and a low-sodium diet may make supplementation unwise. Fresh fruits and vegetables, and their juices, offer excellent dietary sources of potassium.

Seaweed and Spirulina—Three kelp tablets (or up to one teaspoon kelp granules) daily has long been recommended as a source of trace minerals for diabetics. The recently publicized Spirulina contains vitamins and protein as well as minerals, to help make any necessary weight loss easier to achieve.

Tissue Salts—Nat. Phos. and Nat. Sulph. are suggested for diabetics. Two to four tablets of each in the 6X potency may be taken twice daily to stimulate pancreatic action.

Zinc—15 to 50 milligrams one to three times daily. Zinc increases the potency of insulin and plays a role in insuring its effectiveness. A deficiency of zinc has been related to the onset of diabetes.

Drugs and Medications

No medication or drug should be taken unless medically prescribed. Barbiturates, hypnotics, and sedatives can affect insulin release and the effect of oral anti-diabetic agents. Amphetamines, Dilantin, ginseng, Inderal, marijuana, or other drugs or narcotics can alter the absorption of sugar.[230]

Exercise

Physical activity improves glucose tolerance and lowers blood sugar. Sedentary persons require much more insulin than those who are active, but any program of physical activity should be geared to individual tolerance and have medical approval. Prolonged, strenuous exercise may temporarily increase glucose levels, raise blood pressure, and trigger more hemorrhaging for those who already have retinopathy. Diabetics who engage in vigorous physical activity during the working day may require no further exercise, but often the fatigue felt at the end of an inactive day can be overcome by a brisk walk or other mild exercise. Walking for 30 minutes after every meal has lowered blood sugar counts in many cases.[194] Snacking before, and every 20 minutes during, exercise helps maintain blood sugar levels.

Folk Remedies

For centuries, folk healers have advised drinking one to three cups of blueberry leaf tea daily as a treatment for "sugar diabetes." Other recommended teas are: alfalfa, comfrey, dandelion root, juniper berry, uva ursi, and wintergreen. Most of the old remedies have been negated by modern research, but following the instructions given in the 1852 edition of *Ladies' Indispensable Assistant* for steeping 2 ounces of fresh ginger in a quart of good wine and drinking two or three glasses every day might be pleasant. Two remedies that have been scientifically substantiated are:

- **Garlic**—Tests have shown garlic to be as effective as oral drugs in clearing the bloodstream of excess glucose. Minced fresh garlic, garlic juice or oil, or a 5-grain capsule with each meal has produced remarkable results for some diabetics.[13]
- **Green Beans,** particularly the skins of the pods, contain hormonal substances closely related to insulin. When the pods are made into tea, one cup equals one unit of insulin. The suggested dosage is one cup with each of three daily meals.[12]

Hot Baths

A daily 30-minute soak in a hot bath with some seaweed or sea salt, followed by a tepid shower, is believed to help remove sugar and acid accumulations from the body. Brief foot baths, alternating between warm salt water and clear cold water, may aid circulation. Longer soaking should be avoided as it may soften the skin so much that breaks or skinned spots could easily develop.

Nerve Massage

When performed daily, nerve massage has been reported to stimulate the release of insulin, so blood-sugar levels should be carefully monitored.

- Massage the center of the palm, then the thumb and the two fingers next to it on each hand.
- With the thumb, massage the pad under the little toe on the right foot.
- Massage a strip across the sole of each foot midway between the center of the arch and the pad beneath the big toe.

Nerve Pressure

To stimulate and encourage the distribution of insulin, press each point for 10 seconds, release for 10 seconds, and repeat three times once each day.

- Press the underside of the protuberance at the center back of the skull just above the neck.
- With the arms bent, press the tip of each elbow.
- Press halfway between the top of the right hipbone and the navel.
- On each leg, press just below the center-front of the knee at the point where the separate leg bones can be felt.

Obesity

The chances of developing diabetes double with every 20 percent of excess weight. Weight control is of particular importance in cases of maturity onset diabetes.

Tests have shown that the number of insulin receptors (which allow glucose to enter the cells and reduce the need for insulin) decreases with obesity and increases as weight is lost.[175,230] When weight is maintained at slightly below the "ideal" on the official height-and-weight charts, many diabetics have found their own insulin production adequate without the outside help of oral agents or insulin injections.

Smoking

Studies have shown that smoking can increase insulin requirements by as much as 15 to 20 percent for diabetics. Inhaling cigarette smoke constricts the smaller blood vessels and is especially dangerous for those who have a tendency toward vascular disease. Before the advent of low-tar, low-nicotine cigarettes, a maximum of 10 cigarettes per day was considered safe for diabetics. Tests on the effects of "light" cigarettes are still inconclusive, so moderation in their use is recommended.

Sources (See Bibliography)

3, 4, 6, 9, 12, 13, 23, 24, 25, 34, 37, 38, 41, 42, 48, 52, 53, 54, 63, 64, 65, 68, 84, 88, 89, 103, 105, 110, 126, 128, 129, 136, 137, 144, 146, 156, 159, 165, 171, 173, 174, 175, 176, 189, 190, 197, 199, 200, 208, 227, 229, 230, 238, 250, 252, 254, 256, 257, 261, 269, 273, 280, 286, 297, 299, 300, 301, 302, 304, 305, 315, 316, 333, 338, 354.

DIARRHEA, DYSENTERY, AND GASTROENTERITIS

When irritated or inflamed, the mucous membrane within the bowel fails to absorb liquid from food material. This results in runny, frequent bowel movements—diarrhea. Possible causes are legion: allergy, antibiotics, bacterial infection (amebic dysentery), emotional stress, fatigue, food poisoning, overuse of enemas or laxatives, nutritional deficiencies, overindulgence in food or alcohol. Viral gastroenteritis (intestinal flu) adds cramps, vomiting, and possibly fever to the discomfort of diarrhea, but is a self-limiting malady. Ample fluids and symptomatic relief of the diarrhea are the generally accepted treatments.

Travelers to areas where hygienic conditions and bacterial flora are unfamiliar are often attacked by bacillary dysentery (Aztec two-step, Casablanca crud, Delhi belly, Montezuma's revenge, tourist trots, etc.). It may be possible to avoid this temporary misery by drinking a little lemon or lime juice before meals or by taking three acidophilus capsules during each meal—with liquid other than unpasteurized milk or the local water. Eating sparingly of cooked or well-washed foods, limiting alcohol consumption, and getting sufficient rest are other helpful suggestions.

The onset of diarrhea is usually abrupt and the duration mercifully brief. Vomiting may accompany the malady, and, in aggravated attacks, blood appears in the eliminations from the rupture of small blood vessels in the lining of the intestines. If diarrhea continues for more than a few days, medical attention should be sought. Dehydration through fluid loss can be extremely serious, particularly for children. When medical help is not available, *Dr. Heimlich's Home Guide to Emergency Medical Situations*[156] suggests sipping a solution of one cup water, one teaspoon sugar, and one-fourth teaspoon each baking soda and salt to help restore minerals and fluid. Chronic cases should be medically evaluated as even a mild form of perpetual diarrhea could indicate the presence of an ulcer or other disease of the digestive tract.

Diet and Supplements

During bouts of diarrhea, extra liquids should be sipped throughout the day to help compensate for the losses in frequent, watery stools. Sixteen ounces daily of a mixture of apple, carrot, celery, parsley, and spinach juices are recommended by Gary and Steve Null in their *Complete Handbook of Nutrition*.[243] Some acute cases have been cleared with a two-day diet of nothing but rice and mashed bananas or applesauce made in a blender from raw apples. An alternative two-day regimen is to eat only stir-fried fresh vegetables such as broccoli, brussels sprouts, cabbage, cauliflower, mustard greens, and turnips.[334] Other authorities advise a low-carbohydrate, high-protein diet of meat broths, soft-cooked eggs, custard, junket, and other concentrated foods to slow down intestinal activity. Buttermilk, cheese, kefir, and yogurt are usually well-tolerated (even by those who suffer from diarrhea after drinking sweet milk) and help restore the beneficial flora to the intestinal tract.

Fruits, vegetables, and whole grains contain fiber and pectin which help "bind up" the foods eaten so they form soft, bulky stools. Cooked grains such as barley, buckwheat, millet, oats, and rice are considered beneficial. Pectin and bran are similar in many ways. Both absorb many times their own weight in liquid to help correct diarrhea. Pectin absorbs and eliminates harmful organisms while promoting the growth of beneficial bacteria. Taking a spoonful of bran or two pectin capsules with each meal is often helpful. Bananas have proven more effective than apples in recent tests, but both are rich in pectin and have long been favorite diarrhea remedies. Berries, especially blackberries, are believed helpful, as are ripe papayas and fresh pineapple juice.

Diarrhea causes foods to pass through the body so rapidly that very few nutrients are assimilated. Within the first few hours of an attack, colossal amounts of vitamins and minerals are washed out of the body. These should be replaced as quickly as possible to speed recovery. A daily multi-vitamin-mineral tablet is usually recommended in addition to any or all of the following supplements.

B Complex—One comprehensive, high-potency tablet daily, plus an additional 50 to 100 milligrams B-1, B-6, niacin, and pantothenic acid. The lack of any of these vitamins, or folic acid, can cause diarrhea or its recurrence. Taking 100 milligrams of niacinamide (not niacin, which may cause flushing) with each meal for two weeks has brought rapid improvement in many acute attacks and cleared some long-standing cases of chronic diarrhea.[89] Extra amounts of pantothenic acid (up to 500 milligrams daily) have been known to bring back proper elimination for some individuals.

Vitamin C—1,000 to 3,000 milligrams daily, more if well-tolerated. Vitamin C washes out of the body along with other water-soluble vitamins and minerals and is needed to combat infection or allergic reactions. When massive doses are taken, the digestive tract in some individuals may rebel to cause a form of diarrhea which can easily be controlled by reducing the dosage.

Magnesium—500 milligrams daily for adults, 100 to 200 milligrams for infants. A deficiency can trigger the onset of diarrhea or cause it to continue. In bottle-fed babies or persons on ulcer diets, diarrhea may be induced by excess calcium, which creates a magnesium deficiency.

Potassium—If many potassium-rich bananas are being consumed, supplementation may not be necessary, but 100 to 1,000 milligrams for several days is often recommended.

Tissue Salts—The tissue salt advised depends on the condition of the stool.

- If greenish: take three tablets 6X Nat. Sulph. each hour.
- If yellow: take three tablets of 6X Kali. Sulph. each hour.
- If brown: take three tablets 6X Nat. Phos. each hour.
- If fetid smelling: take three tablets each 12X Kali. Phos. and Silicea three times a day.
- If contains blood and slime: take three tablets 6X Kali. Mur. each hour and check with a physician if the condition continues.
- If contains frothy water and slime: take three tablets 6X Nat. Mur. each hour.
- If contains undigested food: take three tablets 12X Ferr. Phos. each hour.

Enemas

Incongruous as it may seem, one or two enemas can be both soothing and beneficial during an attack of diarrhea. A little baking soda, garlic juice, or salt may be added to warm water, or white oak bark tea may be used as the liquid. The enema should be retained as long as possible to allow the intestinal tract to absorb some of the fluid.

Folk Remedies

Before the days of refrigeration, diarrhea and dysentery were so common they were known as "summer complaint." Modern physicians usually discourage the use of alcohol, milk, spices, and tea during attacks, but they were favorite ingredients in old-fashioned folk cures.

Alcohol

- Sipping 2 to 4 ounces of blackberry wine, blackberry brandy, or a hot brandy sling is credited with stopping diarrhea within the hour.
- Beat the yolks of three eggs with one-fourth cup sugar. Add one-half cup

brandy and one teaspoon grated nutmeg. Refrigerate and take one teaspoon every two or three hours.

- Dissolve one tablespoon salt in one cup brandy. Take one teaspoon two or three times a day.
- Steep 3 ounces whole allspice in one pint brandy. Sweeten with sugar. Adults were advised to take one-half cup each hour; children, one tablespoonful diluted with water.
- Combine one cup each cherry brandy and rum with ¼ pound brown sugar and 1 ounce peppermint. Take by the spoonful two or three times a day.
- Simmer equal parts of rum, molasses, and olive oil until the consistency of honey. Take by the tablespoonful each hour until improvement is noticed, then once every two or three hours.
- Sip wine in which cinnamon sticks have been steeped.
- Combine one quart blackberry juice with 1 pound granulated sugar or one cup honey. Add one tablespoon each allspice, cinnamon, cloves (optional), and nutmeg. Simmer for 15 minutes, then add one cup brandy, rum, or whiskey. Take one cup three or four times a day—half that amount for children.

Apple Cider Vinegar

- To avoid gastrointestinal upsets, folk practitioners advise adding two teaspoons of apple cider vinegar to a glass of water and drinking it before eating any questionable food. If diarrhea does occur and is accompanied by nausea, two teaspoons of this mixture can be taken every five minutes until relief is felt, then one-half cup with each meal for several days.
- For simple diarrhea, take one teaspoon apple cider vinegar in a glass of water with meals, between meals, and again at bedtime. Or, dissolve as much salt as possible in one-half cup vinegar. Take one tablespoonful with hot water every hour until relieved. Or, add one tablespoon apple cider vinegar and one teaspoon salt to one-half cup warm water. Sip slowly. Repeat in 30 minutes, if necessary.
- Mix one tablespoon each black pepper and salt. Stir in one-half cup each apple cider vinegar and water. Take one tablespoon every 30 minutes.

Apples—Grate raw, cored apples and let stand until darkened, then eat as much as possible. If the condition has not improved, repeat in a few hours.

Bananas—Mashed raw bananas are a standard folk-cure for diarrhea.

Blackberry Juice—Simmer one cup blackberry juice with one-half teaspoon allspice, one-half teaspoon cayenne pepper (optional) and one-fourth teaspoon grated nutmeg. Sweeten with brown sugar, if desired. Take one-fourth cup every few hours—one teaspoon to one tablespoon for infants and children.

Blueberries—For chronic diarrhea, eat a small dish of fresh or frozen blueberries with two or three meals each day.

Bread—Combine two tablespoons raw honey with one teaspoon bee pollen granules. Spread on a slice of whole-grain bread and eat slowly. Or, soak one slice of dry rye bread in one cup boiled water for 15 minutes. Strain, then sip the liquid. Taking several cups throughout the day is said to ease diarrhea within 24 hours.

Carob—One tablespoon carob powder mixed with food at each meal was an old folk-treatment for diarrhea. Recent clinical studies substantiate the remedy. One teaspoon to one tablespoon of the fiber-and-pectin-rich carob powder stirred into one cup milk or water and taken at frequent intervals controlled 60 percent of infectious diarrhea and 95 percent of noninfectious cases.[75]

Carrots—Carrot soup may have moved out of the folk-remedy category. Hospital tests showed that strained "baby food" carrots corrected diarrhea in 24 hours or less for adults as well as infants. Besides vitamins, minerals, fiber, and pectin, carrots contain at least six antifungal substances that can destroy the harmful agents in some types of diarrhea.[261] For homemade carrot soup: cook 1 pound carrots in one cup water. Whir in a blender, then add three-fourths teaspoon salt and enough boiled water to make one quart. Take small amounts every half hour.

Castor Oil—For chronic diarrhea instigated by allergy, doctors in India have found five drops of castor oil in a little fruit juice before breakfast to be effective.[76]

Charcoal—Munching charcoal from wood-burning stoves or campfires is another old remedy that has been updated. Activated charcoal tablets are now available in pharmacies and health food stores. (Charcoal briquettes are not safe for human consumption.) Taken according to label instructions, the tablets have been amazingly effective in mopping up harmful, diarrhea-causing bacteria and toxins in the intestines.[53]

Cold or Hot Packs—Some natural healers recommend placing an ice pack on the middle and lower back for 10 minutes, removing it for 10 minutes, then replacing it for another 10 minutes. Others prefer 30-minute hot packs on both the lower back and abdomen. An alternative advised in the early 1800s was "flannel wet with brandy, powdered with cayenne pepper, and laid upon the bowels to afford great relief."[73] Another option was a "whiskey poultice." One teaspoon each of all available spices were to be mixed, moistened with whiskey, and applied to the abdomen as a poultice.

Egg White—Combine one egg white with the juice of half a lemon. Beat until frothy. Pour over chipped ice and eat with a spoon. Or, just beat the white of an egg and down it.

Flour—Boil flour in milk to make a thick porridge and eat with a spoon. Or, brown one cup flour in a skillet. Stir one tablespoonful into enough water to make a paste and take every three hours while the diarrhea persists.

Garlic is another remedy that has progressed from folklore to medical practice. Whether fresh, powdered, or in capsules, garlic is an effective but harmless antibiotic that can soothe, cleanse, reduce inflammation, and often make diarrhea disappear within a very short time. The suggested dosage is one minced clove of garlic (or equivalent) taken with honey, milk or fruit juice at each meal. An additional minced garlic clove taken with hot tea before bed and before breakfast may be helpful.

Herbal Teas—Basil, cayenne pepper, cinnamon, comfrey leaf, ginger, peppermint, sage, slippery elm, roasted sunflower seed, thyme, and turmeric teas all are considered beneficial.

Lemonade—Sip strong, hot lemonade every 30 minutes.

Milk

- Stir one teaspoon butter in one cup boiling milk. Sprinkle with salt and black pepper, then drink while hot. Or, add one tablespoon brandy to one-half cup scalded milk and take by the spoonful. Or, mix one-fourth teaspoon cinnamon and/or nutmeg in a cup of scalded milk. Add one teaspoon brandy, if desired, and sip slowly.
- Squeeze half a lemon or lime into a glass of milk and drink each morning and evening.

Case History

With five children and six grandchildren of her own, Aunt Ruby was the person to call for any health emergency on her street. When the school secretary telephoned to say that Tiffany's mother was unavailable, but that Tiffany had diarrhea, Aunt Ruby picked up the child, cleaned her up, and tucked her into bed. Then Aunt Ruby scalded a cup of milk, sprinkled it liberally with black pepper, and said, "Drink this." Feeling like "Alice in Wonderland," Tiffany did as she was told. By the time Tiffany's mother came home from work, the diarrhea seemed to be under control and they decided to postpone a visit to the doctor until it seemed imperative. No professional assistance was necessary; the hot milk and pepper had been so effective that Tiffany was able to return to school the next day.

Nutmeg—Prompt relief from some cases of chronic diarrhea has been obtained by taking one teaspoon ground nutmeg four times a day.

Pekoe Tea—Steep green or black tea in boiling milk. Season with nutmeg, add brown sugar if desired, and drink while hot. Or, combine one tablespoon pekoe tea with an equal amount of boiled milk and sprinkle with ground cinnamon. Take every 30 minutes for four hours.

Rice or Barley—Boil two-thirds cup either rice or barley in four cups water. Strain out the solids and sip the liquid. Or, brown dry rice in a skillet, add water, cover, and cook until tender. Eaten plain, or sprinkled with cinnamon, this was believed to quell diarrhea in a few hours.

Yogurt—Eating yogurt (plain, with mashed bananas or cooked carrots, and/or sprinkled with allspice and nutmeg) three times a day is said to cure diarrhea within 24 hours. Taking two or three acidophilus capsules with each meal may increase the effectiveness.

Nerve Massage

With deep thumb pressure, massage a spot on the abdomen 1½ inches directly below the navel. Then, massage just below the front of the kneecap to the outside of the shinbone.

Nerve Pressure (Press each point for 10 seconds, release, and repeat three times.)

- Press directly below and to the corner nearest the thumb of the fingernail on the index and middle finger of each hand. Then, press the hollow of each inner elbow, 1 inch to the outside of center.
- On both feet, press the web of skin where the big toe and the second toe meet. Then press the bottom of each foot, just in front of the heel.

Sources (See Bibliography)

4, 5, 6, 7, 8, 13, 18, 24, 27, 52, 53, 55, 62, 68, 73, 75, 76, 78, 88, 89, 92, 98, 99, 106, 142, 152, 156, 165, 168, 173, 174, 176, 181, 189, 190, 208, 226, 229, 243, 251, 253, 254, 261, 269, 288, 293, 297, 309, 314, 315, 318, 319, 325, 328, 330, 333, 334, 345.

EARACHE

Simple earache, otitis media, is a middle-ear inflammation. It may be a reflection of pain from an aching tooth but usually results from fluid buildup in the Eustachian tubes. Supine bottle-feeding may be responsible for this condition in infants. In adults, the usual instigator is allergy or an attack of the flu or a cold. One form of prevention is to blow the nose gently through both nostrils. (Closing one nostril can force germ-laden mucus into the Eustachian tube and invite ear infection.[174])

Taking all the vitamin C possible (6,000 to 15,000 milligrams in divided doses during the day) and accompanying any prescribed antbiotic with acidophilus yogurt or capsules frequently forestalls this type of earache. If an earache persists or if infection is suspected, medical attention is advised to prevent complications and possible hearing loss. (See also Infections.)

Sudden changes in ear pressure from high-altitude driving or flying, or undersea diving, can create a vacuumlike effect which forces the flexible walls of the Eustachian tubes together to cause a sense of blockage or earache, and possibly an infection of the middle ear. Chewing gum, or yawning and swallowing, often counteracts the pressure. If this is not successful, pinching the nose shut, closing the mouth and blowing out the cheeks may force air into the passages to relieve the pressure. Extreme changes in altitude are not recommended when tissues are swollen from a cold or allergy. When unavoidable, taking the B-6 + pantothentic acid + vitamin C combination suggested for Hay Fever (which see) may shrink the mucous membranes enough to help prevent "airplane earache."

Outer-ear infection, otitis externa or "swimmer's ear," can result from inadequate drying of the ear after bathing or swimming, or from overzealous attempts to clean the ear. Wearing a tight bathing cap and/or ear plugs while swimming may prevent an earache, but deep diving should be avoided by those who are prone to such attacks. When water does get into the ear, inserting a "wick" of twisted facial tissue may absorb the moisture. Reclining with the affected ear pointed down may let the droplet run out. Hopping up and down with the head tilted to the side while alternately pressing and releasing a cupped palm over the ear, or using the heel of the hand to tap above the blocked ear, often forces out the liquid. Another option is to insert a few drops of diluted alcohol to encourage all of the liquid in the ear to quickly evaporate.

The old adage about never inserting anything smaller than an elbow into the ear passage has merit. When left to its own devices, earwax usually takes care of itself (see Hearing Loss). Attempting to remove it or foreign objects from the ear with cotton swabs, hairpins, or tweezers can be injurious and may predispose to infection. If an inanimate object gets into a child's ear, pull downward on the earlobe with the ear pointed down while the head is shaken. (For adults, pull up and back on the earlobe.) If an insect should go exploring, shining a flashlight across the ear in a dark room should entice it into crawling out. If not, a few drops of warm baby oil or diluted alcohol may drown the intruder so it can be dislodged with a downward tilt and shake of the head.

Whatever the cause of the earache, unless it is an infection or a perforated eardrum, applying heat and experimenting with the following remedies may bring relief.

Compresses and Poultices

Herbal Teas—Wring a cloth out of hot camomile or slippery elm tea and apply to the painful ear. Cover with a dry cloth.

Mustard—When the pain is severe, make a paste of dry mustard and flour moistened with egg white or water. Spread between pieces of gauze and place behind the ear. Dissolving a tablespoon of dry mustard in a basin of hot water and soaking the feet at the same time may be helpful.

Onion—Tie slices or sections of hot, roasted onion over the ear.

Salt—Heat table salt in a skillet, then wrap in cloth and place under the ear while the head is resting on a pillow. If possible, sleep with the hot compress.

Drops and Insertions

Black Pepper—Dip a small piece of cotton into warm corn or olive oil, gather into it a pinch of black pepper, then insert in the ear.

Cabbage—Roast cabbage stalks, then squeeze a few drops of the liquid into the ear.

Castor Oil or Olive Oil—Heat and place a few drops in the ear. Or, mix equal parts of the oil and hot milk. Place several drops in the affected ear each hour.

Case History

Ricky and Robby were twins who did everything together, but, thought their mother, developing simultaneous earaches seemed a bit much. However, even if the fact that Ricky clutched his right ear while Robby held his left one could be explained by "mirror image," she recalled her own childhood earaches and her mother's comforting ministrations, and decided both little boys should have the full treatment. She warmed olive oil, put a drop in each offending ear, and gently inserted tufts of cotton. The boys' heads were stuffy, so she got out the old "steamer" and set it to hissing in their bedroom. She hoped this would soften the mucus, encourage drainage of sinus and nasal passages, and help relieve any pressure that might be contributing to the earaches. Then she added a modern touch: she stirred one-fourth teaspoon of vitamin C crystals into each of two small glasses of orange juice for the twins before she tucked them in bed. The earaches departed as coincidentally as they had appeared. By the next morning Ricky and Robby were free of pain and eager to rush out to see what excitement the new day would offer.

Garlic

- Puncture a garlic capsule and squeeze the oil into the ear, then cover with cotton. Or, dip a peeled garlic clove in olive oil, wrap in gauze, or leave "as is" and insert in the ear, making sure that the garlic is too large to be drawn into the middle ear. Bandage to hold in place.
- Add a little garlic juice (or onion juice) to warm olive oil to use as drops for an earache accompanying a cold. Or, stir one minced garlic clove into one cup olive oil. Let stand for at least four hours, then strain and place a few drops in the ear every hour.

Glycerin and Witch Hazel (available in drug stores)—Dip a piece of cotton into a warmed, equal mixture of the two and insert in the outer ear.

Honey and Bee Pollen—Combine warmed honey with bee pollen granules and insert a few drops to ease the pain of an aching ear.

Nerve Massage

- Massage the bottom of the foot just below the little toe and the one next to it. Right foot for right ear, left foot for left ear. If tenderness is felt, massaging it out should relieve congestion and pain.
- To stimulate blood circulation and ease earache pain: pull at the earlobe for 10 seconds, then gently rub the hollow behind the lobe. Next, massage around the outside of the ear, including the bony mastoid area behind the ear.

Nerve Pressure (Unless otherwise indicated, press each point for 10 seconds, release for 10 seconds, and repeat three times once each day.)

- Press against the hinge of each jawbone, just touching the front of the ear.
- Press the lower edge of the mastoid (the small bone just behind the ear).
- Exert firm pressure on the tip of the fourth finger on each hand for five minutes. Clothespins or rubber bands may be used to assure steady pressure.

Tissue Salts

- To relieve congested Eustachian tubes: take three tablets 12X Kali. Mur. each hour for several hours.

- If the earache is accompanied by inflammation: take three tablets of 12X Ferr. Phos. alternately with the Kali. Mur.
- If the earache is accompanied by noises in the ear: take three tablets 6X Nat. Sulph. each hour for several hours.

Sources (See Bibliography)

3, 13, 19, 34, 52, 62, 63, 64, 68, 84, 98, 142, 156, 160, 165, 173, 176, 190, 214, 227, 236, 239, 288, 297, 315, 316, 318, 328, 330, 353.

ECZEMA, HIVES, VITILIGO, AND SKIN IRRITATIONS (See Also: Acne, Athlete's Foot, Dandruff, Insect Bites, Poison Ivy, and Psoriasis)

The word "eczema" was coined in 543 A.D. from the Greek term meaning "to boil out" but even skilled dermatologists still have difficulty identifying all the clinical variations which fall under this heading. Atopic eczema, atopic dermatitis, and chronic dermatitis, are skin rashes accompanied by itching and, possibly, by burning, scaling blisters that may crust or weep. Caused by surface irritations, allergic reactions, or nutritional deficiencies which predispose to attack, rather than a virus or infection, eczema is hereditary in the sense that most sufferers come from families with a history of some form of allergy.

Characteristically, atopic eczema first appears in the skin folds at elbows and knees, but the scaly red patches of cracked skin may cover any part of the body. Overindulgence in highly allergenic foods such as berries, chocolate, eggs, nuts, or tomato products may set it off. It may also be the result of anxiety or emotional stress, reaction to medication (primarily aspirin or antibiotics), or an insect bite. Hives (urticaria), with their familiar red wheals or welts, are customarily a reaction to foods or drugs, but can occur from any of the same causes as eczema, and, in susceptible people, even from chemical additives in foodstuffs or overexposure to the sun or extremely cold temperatures.

Contact dermatitis results from an external irritant such as aeorosol spray products, cosmetics, perma-press or woolen fabrics, etc. Substances used in hair dyes, inexpensive jewelry, or tanned leather frequently trigger this reaction. The chemicals in household detergents can cause the swollen tissues and inflammation of "housewife's eczema." Seborrheic dermatitis is often accompanied by acne, may be almost indistinguishable from psoriasis, and, in its mildest form, is common dandruff.

The rash of prickly heat results from obstruction of the sweat ducts and usually disappears quickly with oral vitamin C supplements, soothing baths, talc, and exposure to air. Irritating cracks at the angles of the eyes, mouth, or nose clear up rapidly, as a rule, when additional unsaturated oils are included in the diet and vitamins B-2, B-6, folic acid, and pantothenic acid are taken as supplements. Infant eczema may be precipitated by cow's milk—a switch to goat's milk may relieve the condition. Diaper rash generally responds to frequent changing, gentle cleansing, and covering the area with a coating of Vaseline. Limiting the amount of meat in the infant's diet may also be of help.

Scabies, the most famous of all itching maladies, is a highly contagious skin infection that can be identified by tiny, greyish-white lines where parasites (itch mites) have burrowed into the skin. Warm baths, scrubbing with soap and water, and applying a sulphur ointment may effect control; but prompt treatment by a physician can limit the seven-year-itch to a seven-hour-discomfort.

Erysipelas (St. Anthony's Fire) and impetigo are two other contagious, rapidly spreading skin diseases. They are caused by germs entering the deeper layers of the skin through tiny abrasions or cuts and usually affect the facial areas. Clearly defined patches of swollen, glazed, fiery-red, burning and itching skin with possible blisters and an accompanying fever identify erysipelas. Alternating applications of ice and hot packs help alleviate the burning and take down the swelling. The folk remedy was a poultice of crushed raw cranberries, cooked navy beans, or grated raw potatoes. The poultice was to be left on the skin until dry, removed with a solution of half-and-half lemon juice and water, then replaced with a fresh application. Bathing the affected area with buttermilk, sour milk, or witch hazel was also advised.

Erysipelas is a streptococcus infection but impetigo may involve either staphylococcus or streptococcus bacteria. Impetigo begins with one or more small spots that become pustules and dry into loosely attached, honey-colored crusts, each with a narrow zone of inflamed skin around it. Washing off the crusts with soap and water, then sponging the surrounding area with a solution of one part iodine to 10 parts rubbing alcohol may control the spreading. The suggestions for Infections (which see) may be helpful, but medical care and antibiotic treatment may be needed. Erysipelas in particular can be serious, even life-threatening, for infants or the aged. Neglected impetigo can cause scarring or loss of skin pigmentation.

Vitiligo is the term for a spotty lack of skin color that can occur from unknown causes. It is often associated with a lack of hydrochloric acid in the body and can sometimes be remedied by taking betaine hydrochloride tablets with each meal. Taking 100 milligrams PABA orally each day, plus five tablets dissolved in a little hot water or pure mayonnaise and sponged over the area, has restored normal skin color for some individuals in a matter of months.[3] Other cases have responded only when 1,000 or more milligrams of PABA, plus a B-complex tablet and at least 100 milligrams of pantothenic acid were taken daily.

Whatever the type of itch, dermatologists and allergists agree scratching creates a vicious cycle that results in more itching and rash as well as possible infection. Avoiding known irritants and experimenting with natural remedies often brings relief. Deliberate positive thinking may allay the causative factors of mental stress (see pages 9-10). Self-help detective work may make it possible to deduce and eliminate the triggers for skin maladies. (Anything new and different, even the elastic in underwear, should be considered.) But if these methods do not clear the condition, skin-testing by a physician may be required to pinpoint the cause of allergy-induced eczema. Medical attention should be obtained for skin eruptions which cannot be contained or are accompanied by a fever.

Diet and Supplements

Almost any food can instigate either eczema or hives. A new food or a familiar one suddenly eaten in abundance (as fresh fruit in season or seafood during a coastal trip) should be suspected and avoided for a week or two, then tried again for verification. Protein deficiency can cause chronic eczema.[88] Sugar decreases the body's ability to fight infection.[353] Constipation (which see) contributes to skin disorders through lack of toxic-waste elimination. A well-balanced diet with ample protein and fibrous foods, but few sweets, is indicated.

A combination of daily supplements which has cleared some cases of eczema in two months is: 50,000 units vitamin A, one high-potency B-complex tablet with each meal and before bed, one or two tablespoons brewer's yeast, 1,200 IU vitamin E (see Caution, page 6), and 30 milligrams zinc; plus local applications of vitamin E oil.[325] Individual supplements or other combinations may prove equally effective.

> **Vitamin A**—20,000 to 75,000 units daily for two months, then 10,000 to 25,000 units for maintenance. Vitamin A is responsible for the health of the skin and helps combat infection. Carotene (a provitamin contained in vegetables for conversion to vitamin A within the body) is now available as a supplement and has effected eczema cures when taken orally and used as an ointment.
>
> **B Complex**—One comprehensive, high-potency tablet daily. Several weeks of this supplementation plus additional amounts of specific B vitamins may be required to correct eczema instigated by B-vitamin deficiencies.
>
> - **B-2**—15 to 100 milligrams daily to correct itching, scaling, and/or a waxlike oozing around the nose or cheeks.
> - **B-6**—200 to 600 milligrams daily to remedy scaly, oily eczema in the eyebrows behind the ears, and around the nose or mouth.
> - **Niacinamide**—Up to 3,000 milligrams daily to alleviate red scaliness around the neck and ankles, as well as other types of eczema.
> - **PABA, Biotin, Choline and Inositol**—Extra supplements of these members of the B-complex family have cleared some otherwise intractable skin conditions. 100 milligrams PABA, 300 milligrams biotin, and 500 milligrams each choline and inositol are the suggested daily amounts.
> - **Pantothenic Acid**—Up to 2,000 milligrams daily. Lack of this vitamin, particularly when accompanied by a deficiency of B-6, can produce a painful, burning type of eczema. When combined with vitamin C, these two vitamins have an antihistamine effect which may prevent or allay hives or allergy-induced eczemas.
>
> **Brewer's Yeast**—One to six tablespoons, or the equivalent in tablets, daily. Possibly due to the as yet unidentified factors in the yeast, some forms of

eczema respond only with this addition. Mixing brewer's yeast with water or milk and patting it over the affected area often relieves itching and speeds recovery. The paste should be applied to freshly cleansed skin, allowed to dry for at least 10 minutes, then rinsed off with clear water.

Vitamin C—1,000 to 5,000 milligrams in divided doses, daily. Vitamin C often gives relief from prickly heat in minutes, preserves the integrity of tiny capillaries beneath the skin, speeds healing, and helps combat allergic reactions and infections. An itchy skin rash may respond to applications of liquid lecithin followed by a dusting of vitamin C powder each morning after bathing.

Vitamin E (see Caution, page 6)—100 to 800 IU daily. Vitamin E has cleared some eczemas on the hands when 300 units were taken daily, and has corrected chronic itching rashes when 600 IU were taken each day along with 50,000 units vitamin A for a few weeks. Vitamin E is especially beneficial when combined with a diet in which calcium, vitamin D, and magnesium are liberally supplied. Applying vitamin E ointment (or the oil squeezed from capsules) has reduced the inflammation of hives, housewife's eczema, and other skin rashes.

Evening Primrose Oil—Eight capsules per day for three months. As reported in *Prevention* (June, 1983), this dosage had a 43 percent success rate for improving both appearance and itchiness for the 99 eczema sufferers involved in a recent British study.

Vitamin F—One to three tablespoons unsaturated oil daily. Used since 1933 to treat many forms of eczema (including cracks in the corners of the eyes, mouth or nose), unsaturated oils plus supplements of B-6 and 10 to 30 IU vitamin E have been found to cure some cases of infant eczema.

Tissue Salts

- **For eczema:** Take three tablets each 3X Ferr. Phos. and Nat. Phos. three times a day. If there are pustules containing hard matter, take an equal amount of both Calc. Phos. and Silicea.
- **For hives:** Take three tablets, three times daily, of 6X Kali. Phos., Mag. Phos., and Silicea while avoiding acid foods.

Yogurt—One daily serving of acidophilus yogurt (or two acidophilus capsules with each meal) has been found to counteract eczema by contributing to the body's manufacture of B vitamins and help restore the friendly bacteria in the intestinal tract following antibiotic therapy.

Zinc—10 to 50 milligrams three times daily for four to six months, then reduced to 15 milligrams twice daily. Mild eczemas have responded to the lower dosage. Severe or chronic cases have shown improvement in three weeks with 150 milligrams zinc plus 1,000 milligrams vitamin C daily.[256,353] Complete cure may require as long as six months. Recovery is often speeded by the inclusion of unsaturated oil in the diet. Since milk sometimes prevents the absorption of zinc, avoiding dairy products and taking calcium supplements for a few weeks may be helpful.

Folk Remedies

Aloe Vera—Cover the affected area with aloe vera gel (available in health food stores) and drink 1 ounce of the gel mixed in a glass of water each day.

Baths—Soap and excess washing tends to further irritate the skin, but soaking for 30 minutes in comfortably warm water with any of the following additions often soothes and relieves itching.

- **Baking Soda**—Add one and one-half cups soda to a tub of warm water.
- **Bran**—Place two cups unprocessed bran in a cotton bag and soak in a bowl of hot water for 15 minutes. Add the liquid to the bathwater and use the bran-filled bag as a washcloth.
- **Cornstarch**—Sprinkle two cups cornstarch in the tub before filling with water, or make into a paste of cornstarch and cold water, then stir into the bathwater. If desired, the cornstarch mixture can be boiled until thick before adding to the tub.
- **Oatmeal**—Tie two cups raw or cooked oatmeal in a cheesecloth bag and let soak in the tub a few minutes. Then gently rub against the skin while squeezing the bag.
- **Oil**—Add a few tablespoons vegetable oil to the bathwater. After drying, cover the affected skin with either plain or mentholated petroleum jelly.
- **Vinegar**—Add one cup vinegar to the bathing water.

Blackstrap Molasses—Twice each day, stir two teaspoons blackstrap molasses in a glass of milk and drink. This is reported to have cleared stubborn eczema on the hands within two weeks.[53]

Herbal Teas

- For eczema or hives: recommended teas were catnip, comfrey, juniper berry, marjoram, slippery elm, or strawberry leaf. One teaspoon of catnip tea three or four times a day was suggested for babies.
- For Erysipelas, several daily cups of ginger or sage tea were advised.

Poultices and Applications

- Sponge the area with a solution of one teaspoon apple cider vinegar in one cup water. (Drinking a glass of the mixture three times daily has cleared some cases of eczema.[293]) If the skin is not too tender, bathe with vinegar which has been boiled to increase its strength.
- Mash (or puree in a food processor) the inner leaves of cabbage and apply as a poultice.
- Mix three tablespoons cornstarch or flour with one tablespoon castor oil or vinegar and apply to the affected area.
- Mash raw garlic (or squeeze the oil from capsules) and rub on the skin afflicted with eczema or impetigo. Taking two garlic capsules with each meal has been reported to speed relief.
- Pulverize dried kidney beans, mix to a paste with water, then apply.

- A compress made with skimmed or powdered milk may bring soothing relief.
- Boil one chopped onion in one cup water. Thicken with unprocessed bran and add one-fourth teaspoon baking soda. Apply as a poultice, changing frequently, until inflammation is reduced.
- Grate raw potato and spread over the itching area. (Eating a raw potato each day is said to cure stubborn eczema.[152])
- Sponge the inflamed area with lemon juice, diluted if desired, or a solution of two teaspoons baking soda in one cup water.

Powders—Arrowroot, baby powder, cornstarch, talcum, or whey powder soothes itching irritations and may be dusted on as often as desired. Arrowroot is believed to be the most gentle. It may be given an appealing odor by allowing a vanilla bean to stand in the covered container, or by mixing in a pinch of cinnamon.

Sources (See Bibliography)

3, 13, 19, 40, 52, 53, 68, 74, 78, 84, 88, 89, 92, 111, 117, 121, 128, 142, 152, 153, 156, 165, 168, 174, 189, 190, 193, 199, 215, 226, 227, 228, 229, 238, 254, 257, 261, 276, 288, 293, 297, 301, 305, 312, 315, 325, 327, 328, 345, 350, 353.

EDEMA (FLUID RETENTION)

Formerly called dropsy, edema refers to swelling caused by abnormal fluid retention in the tissues. It affects both sexes and can appear at any age but is most common among women during their child-bearing years. Occupations requiring standing for long periods, nutritional deficiencies, or excess weight may cause swollen legs or feet; but edema is not a disease, merely a symptom. Chronic episodes of swelling should be checked by a physician as they can be indications of heart, kidney, or other serious problems.

Although diuretic drugs may be necessary in some cases, many authorities believe their sudden flushing of body fluids drains out so many needed vitamins and minerals that unpleasant side effects are often produced. Besides the washed-out-weariness, these drugs block the kidneys' ability to reabsorb sodium and other minerals. When the diuretic is discontinued, the kidneys try to conserve these minerals—which can bring about exaggerated fluid retention and even more pronounced edema. Natural, nutritional methods are more gradual but provide added nutrients and, therefore, a sense of well-being while correcting the edema.

Diet and Supplements

When not the result of heart or other serious conditions, ideopathic (which means "from no obvious physical cause") edema is considered by many medical nutritionists to be a controllable malady caused by a civilized diet. The regulatory mechanisms that control the water balance in the body can be upset by an overabundance of refined carbohydrates (a Low Blood Sugar diet, which see, often clears edema), by a lack of complete proteins, by too much salt, or by either increased requirements for or a deficiency of B vitamins and the essential fatty acids in salad oils. Because sodium is usually retained in the body during edema, salt is customarily restricted. But, since a sodium deficiency can also be dangerous, many physicians prefer supplementing the diet with added potassium rather than completely eliminating salt. (An overbalance of sodium allows fluid to penetrate the cells, causing some of them to burst and create edema—sufficient potassium prevents sodium from entering the cells.) A diet rich in potassium-containing foods such as bananas, lima beans, and apricots, plus a dolomite supplement for added magnesium may be helpful.

Asparagus, beets, carrots, celery, cucumber, green beans, horseradish, leeks, melons of all kinds, onions, parsley, pineapple, pumpkin, and watermelon are foods with diuretic properties. Coffee is often thought of as a diuretic but as much as eight cups per day can be responsible for a form of edema that disappears within one week when decaffeinated coffee is substituted.[9]

Vitamins A and D (natural)—5,000 to 25,000 units A plus 400 to 800 IU of D each day, if not supplied by a daily multi-vitamin tablet. A and D have been found effective in increasing the excretion of salt and urine when taken with calcium, vitamin E, and pantothenic acid.

B Complex—One comprehensive tablet daily, plus additional amounts of B-1, B-6, and pantothenic acid. A deficiency of either B-1 or pantothenic acid can instigate edema, so 100 to 150 milligrams of both are recommended. Vitamin B-6 is the most effective nutritional diuretic because it sets up a sodium-potassium balance to regulate body fluids. The dosage required varies from 50 to 2,000 milligrams daily, in divided doses. 100 milligrams taken four times a day has served to correct many cases of premenstrual fluid retention, but severe edema may require larger amounts.

Vitamin E (see Caution, page 6)—100 to 400 IU daily. Particularly when combined with vitamin A, vitamin E has a diuretic action. A deficiency of vitamin E can cause dead cells to prevent the passage of urine into the kidneys.

Minerals—The amount of potassium required to maintain a balance with sodium depends on the quantities of both obtained from the diet, plus sufficient magnesium to retain potassium in the cells. A research project showed that calcium and potassium produced better results than the use of diuretics.[22] Dolomite provides both calcium and magnesium—two tablets with each meal is the usual dosage. Most salt substitutes and some diuretic drugs contain potassium so supplementation should be undertaken only under the direction of a physician.

Tissue Salts—To eliminate excess water from the tissues, take four tablets of 6X Nat. Sulph. each four hours until relieved. Taking two or three tablets of 6X Silicea each day has been helpful in some cases.

Exercise

Any form of regular exercise—bicycling, jogging, swimming, or walking—improves vascular tone to offer nonnutritional help for edema. Elevating the feet whenever sitting is also beneficial.

Folk Remedies

Garlic—Take one teaspoon minced raw garlic (or the equivalent in capsules) to stimulate fluid elimination.

Gin—fill a jar with crushed, fresh spearmint leaves and cover with gin. Let stand for a day. Strain and bottle, then take by the tablespoon several times a day. Or, take three tablespoons gin (mixed with orange juice, if desired) and repeat the dosage in an hour or so. If this does not remedy the condition, discontinue the treatment.

Herbs

- Drink two to four cups daily of dandelion, juniper berry, parsley, saffron, spearmint, or uva ursi tea. Another favorite remedy was watermelon-seed tea made by steeping two teaspoons dried, ground watermelon seeds in one cup boiling water for one hour.
- Combine 2 ounces bruised juniper berries with one-fourth cup each crushed caraway and fennel seeds. Add two cups gin or whiskey and one-half cup water. Cover and steep for several days, then strain and bottle. Take one tablespoon every few hours.

Honey and Bee Pollen—Combine equal amounts of raw honey and bee pollen granules. Take by the tablespoon or mix with water or juice.

Juices—Cabbage, cucumber, and grapefruit juice mixed in equal proportions is considered one of the best natural diuretics. Raw beet juice (made from the leaves as well as the beets) or pear juice is also believed helpful, as is the juice of one lemon in a cup of hot water. (Sixteen ounces daily of any combination of these juices is the amount recommended.)

Parsnips—Shred raw parsnips and eat three tablespoons three times a day. Or, cook the parsnips with their leaves and eat generously.

Vegetable Cooking Water—Drink the water in which asparagus, celery, or turnips were cooked. Combine with other recommended juices, if desired.

Nerve Pressure (Press each point for 10 seconds, release, and repeat three times once each day)

- Press the center of the breastbone between the collarbone and the second rib.
- Press an inch to the right of the breastbone at the point where it joins the breast muscle.
- Hook the fingers under the bottom of the ribs on both sides and press the slight

notch approximately one-third of the distance up toward the lowest end of the breastbone.

Sources (See Bibliography)

4, 9, 12, 13, 22, 24, 25, 44, 68, 69,76, 78, 81, 88, 89, 98, 126, 142, 151, 152, 156, 165, 173, 184, 187, 189, 226, 227, 228, 229, 243, 253, 254, 257, 261, 288, 297, 330, 333, 349, 350, 353, 354.

FEVER

A symptom rather than a disease, fever indicates the presence of some bodily disorder—most often an infection—but can be caused by almost any illness. Normal temperature fluctuates between 96 and 100 degrees. There is nothing sacred about the figure 96.8. Anything between 100 and 102 degrees is considered a mild fever. There is considerable controversy about the advisability of lowering a fever or letting it run its course. Some physicians regard fever as a second-line defensive and healing force that should not be suppressed unless it goes above 105 degrees. They feel that fever speeds up the body's metabolism to rush white blood cells to the site of the attack, helps antibiotics work, and, that at a temperature over 100 degrees, some bacteria are simply cooked to death. Other doctors believe the discomfort, debilitating effect, and possible dehydration outweigh whatever good is accomplished by fever and suggest temperature-lowering drugs. A temperature higher than 102 degrees, particularly in infants or the elderly, or one that persists, should have medical attention.

Chilling at the onset of a fever may be caused by the constriction of blood vessels temporarily decreasing skin temperature in an effort to raise the internal temperature. Once the fever is achieved, the headache which often accompanies it is also a side effect of the intricate bodily adjustments required for internal temperature elevation. Relief from this dull ache may be obtained by resting with the head slightly elevated, placing a cold compress on the forehead, and applying brief pressure on the carotid arteries (on either side of the windpipe) to restrain the throbbing flow of blood.

The old-fashioned rule was to cover feverish patients with blankets and heat up the sickroom so they could "sweat it out." Since fever indicates that the body is struggling to get rid of heat, today's advice calls for a comfortably cool room with light bed coverings. Temperatures over 104 degrees should be lowered immediately by cooling the body in a tub of cool water, sponging with a two-to-one mixture of rubbing alcohol and water, or by wrapping in a wet sheet. Compresses of towels soaked in a mixture of one quart water, one cup rubbing alcohol, and one tray of ice cubes is another effective cooling method. Applying slices of raw onion or potato to the soles of the feet was a folk remedy for drawing out fever. In an emergency, a cool enema of catnip tea, strawberry leaf tea, or plain water may help bring down the temperature.

Fevers are more apt to be friends than foes and are no longer as frightening as they once were. The cure is treatment and correction of the cause (see Infections and specific maladies) but much can be done to alleviate the discomfort, shorten the duration, and avoid such side effects as dehydration or malnutrition.

Diet and Supplements

To eat or not to eat during a fever is a debatable question, with adamant authorities on both sides. A generation ago it was standard practice to "starve a fever" —which may have annihilated some badly debilitated patients. Fasting on cracked ice and diluted juices is believed by some to lower the temperature by allowing the body to concentrate on taking care of the infection rather than having to digest food. This must have been the logic behind the popular fever-cure of the early 1700s. The instructions were to cut an apple in thirds, write "Father" on the first piece, "Son" on the second, and "Holy Ghost" on the third. Then, without eating anything else for three days, one of the sections was to be eaten precisely at each midnight. Today's treatment calls for a high-protein, high-vitamin diet with all the liquid possible. Most medical nutritionists believe that increased metabolism during fever burns up protein and body tissue more quickly than normal, so ample amounts of nourishing food should be eaten in order for the body to correct the cause of the fever.

Fluid loss during a fever can be substantial even if there is no obvious perspiration. With the fluids go water-soluble vitamins and minerals, so more than plain water is needed to prevent dehydration. Fruit and vegetable juices are recommended, chicken soup is excellent, and the "fortified milk" (see Index) advised for infections provides proteins, carbohydrates, and minerals plus liquid. The caffeine in regular coffee can elevate the temperature or block the fever-reducing properties of aspirin, so should not be used until the fever has abated.

The stress of fever increases the need for B vitamins. Taking one comprehensive B complex tablet daily, plus 50 to 100 milligrams each B-1 and B-6, is suggested. Taking 500 to 1,000 milligrams of vitamin C plus a calcium tablet each hour often accomplishes a rapid lowering of temperature by destroying bacteria or viruses and making the continuation of a fever unnecessary.

Apple Cider Vinegar and Honey—Mix one-fourth cup apple cider vinegar with one-half cup raw honey and three-fourths cup water. Take by the tablespoonful at frequent intervals.

Barley or Oatmeal Water—A favorite folk remedy for fevers: boil one-third cup barley or oatmeal in 10 cups water until reduced to four cups. Strain and sip the liquid during the day.

Herbal Teas—Sipping camomile, catnip, cayenne, elder flower, ginger, sage, or slippery elm tea, flavored with lemon juice and honey, was believed beneficial for those who were feverish. Tea made from the dried petals of marigold flowers was another old remedy for mild fevers. Willow bark tea was used in Greece 2,000 years ago and by the Indians in America. Since it contains the same salicylates as aspirin, it should not be used by those with an aspirin allergy, ulcer, or liver problem. (Salicylic acid reduces fever by acting on the heat-regulating center in the brain rather than on the underlying cause of the fever.[52, 288])

Juices—Two daily glasses of any combination of apple, carrot, grape, grapefruit, or orange juice is suggested.

Raspberries or Strawberries—Eating either of these fruits was believed to quench thirst and quell fevers. Before the advent of electric juicers or blenders, a beverage of strawberries squeezed in water was advised.

Tissue Salts

- For low fever with chilling: take three tablets each 3X Kali. Phos. and Nat. Sulph. every 15 minutes until the temperature drops, then take these remedies in the 6X potency three times a day until recovery is complete.
- For a high fever: take three tablets of 6X Ferr. Phos. every 15 minutes until the temperature begins to drop, then lessen the frequency to once an hour and once every two hours. If Ferr. Phos. does not suffice, take three tablets of 3X Kali. Phos. and, as soon as there is improvement, alternate the Ferr. Phos. with the Kali. Phos.
- If the fever is under control but the temperature rises in the evening: take two doses of three tablets 6X Kali. Sulph. at intervals of two hours.
- If constipation accompanies chills and fever: take four tablets of 6X Nat. Mur. each three hours until relieved.

Nerve Pressure

To relieve fever: press 1/16 inch below the lower corner of the nail on the index finger, on the side facing the thumb. Use the thumbnail of the opposite hand to apply pressure for six seconds and repeat three times on both hands.

Sources (See Bibliography)

4, 7, 12, 19, 37, 43, 52, 53, 54, 68, 75, 76, 88, 89, 142, 156, 165, 176, 190, 196, 226, 235, 243, 253, 270, 288, 297, 311, 314, 315, 318, 344, 345.

FINGERNAIL AND TOENAIL ABNORMALITIES

Nails are affected by general body conditions and are often used for medical diagnosis. Abnormalities of the nails usually indicate nutritional deficiencies but can be caused by exposure to chemicals, extreme cold, medicines, injuries, or illness.

Nails are formed almost entirely of protein, benefit particularly from the sulphur-containing amino acids in egg yolks, and require vitamins and minerals for growth and strength. They derive little help from the incomplete protein of gelatin unless it is combined with meat broth or other protein. Taking one teaspoon of apple cider vinegar three times a day is a folk remedy credited with correcting fragile, peeling nails and clearing white spots on the nails.

> **Breaking Nails**—Constantly breaking nails may be a symptom of an underactive thyroid. A high-protein diet plus vitamins A, B-6, and C encourages the activity of a sluggish thyroid. Taking 500 IU of vitamin E (see Caution, page 6) plus a kelp tablet daily, and using iodized salt helps restore the health of the thyroid gland. If the nails do not improve, medical tests and thyroid medication may be needed.

> **Brittle, Soft, or Peeling Nails**—A lack of complete proteins, excess estrogen, or oral contraceptives can be the cause. Several glasses of milk plus at least three dolomite and/or bone meal tablets daily toughens fingernails. Even better results may be obtained when two tablespoons of cod liver oil or a natural vitamin A and D supplement is added.

> Brittle nails that separate in layers may indicate either iron-deficiency anemia or a deficiency of the B vitamins, and may benefit from the tissue salt, silicea. As reported in *Journal of Clinical Pathology* (November, 1978), supplementation with iron corrected brittle nails in a majority of the cases tested in a British study. Eating sunflower seeds and taking 15 to 50 milligrams zinc each day has strengthened nails, stopped them from peeling off in layers, and made them more flexible within two or three months.[3]

> Drinking raw parsnip juice is said to bring prompt relief from brittle nails. Taking one tablespoon desiccated liver powder mixed with tomato juice has restored nail health in many cases. Another nail-building combination is two tablespoons brewer's yeast plus 500 to 1,500 milligrams choline each day. Eating one egg and a few almonds every day, plus oral vitamin E and external soaks in olive oil, has resulted in strong nails for other individuals.

> **Fungus Problems** under the nails usually clear when two high-potency B-complex tablets are taken daily, large amounts of acidophilus yogurt (or two capsules per meal) are included with the diet, and vitamin E oil squeezed under the nail once or twice each day. Soaking the affected hand or foot in a solution of one tablespoon vitamin C powder and water for 20 minutes before applying the vitamin E has brought even more rapid improvement. Taking 500 milligrams of pantothenic acid each day has reportedly cleared some cases almost overnight.

> **Hangnails**—Frequent hangnails usually indicate that vitamin C, folic acid, and protein are undersupplied. Rubbing the cuticles with fresh lemon juice daily is said to strengthen them. When a hangnail does occur, it should be snipped off with manicure scissors, then rubbed with vitamin E from a punctured capsule to speed healing.

Injuries—Applications of ice will help relieve the pain from a mashed nail and, after the first day, soaking in warm water for 30 to 60 minutes four times daily increases blood flow to aid healing. When a blood clot forms under the nail and medical help is not available, *Dr. Taylor's Self-Help Medical Guide*[315] suggests alleviating the pain and avoiding loss of the nail by using a paper clip. Straighten one end of the paper clip and heat red hot with a cigarette lighter, then gently press the hot paper clip end through the nail into the center of the clot. The nail is insensitive and the blood clot dissipates the heat so there should be little discomfort. After the nail has drained, soak it in warm salt water for 30 minutes several times a day. In *How to Be Your Own Doctor (Sometimes)*[297], Dr. Sehnert recommends simply drilling a hole in the nail with a sterilized pocket knife and covering it with a gauze-type adhesive bandage.

Ingrown Toenails—While generally caused by improper toenail clipping or poorly fitting shoes, there is often a family history of ingrown toenails. Obesity may play a role since flabby skin can engulf the toenail. Trimming the toenails straight across and avoiding tight-fitting shoes are preventive measures. Those who are prone to ingrown toenails may benefit from taking the tissue salt, silicea, each day and/or applying vitamin E oil to the nails at least once each month.

A mild ingrown toenail can be treated by saturating a piece of cotton with castor oil or vitamin E oil and tucking a bit under the corners of the nail, preferably after first soaking the foot in a solution of epsom salts and hot water. Squeezing the contents of a vitamin A capsule on the oil-soaked cotton is often beneficial, as is taking vitamins A, E, and C orally. The pressure at the corners of the nail can sometimes be relieved by cutting a small, V-shaped notch in the center of the nail. A badly ingrown toenail may require treatment by a podiatrist to relieve pain and prevent the development of infection.

Case History

Both Warren F. and his physician were disturbed about the inflammation around the "corners" of the nail on Warren's big toe. Warren was a diabetic; they did not want to risk possible healing problems resulting from podiatric surgery, yet the painful toe was interfering with his job as a plumbing inspector. Warren wore comfortable, well-fitting shoes, and was not overweight; so the ortho-molecular doctor suggested a combination of old and new home remedies. After his daily shower Warren was to gently insert a wisp of vitamin-E-saturated cotton under each irritated nail corner and, at least twice each week, soak his foot in a warm epsom-salts solution. Warren considered the alternatives. He then purchased a bottle of vitamin E capsules with snip-off ends, a box of epsom salts, and a plastic dishpan for foot soaking—and followed his doctor's instructions. The treatment was not as bothersome as he had anticipated: Warren watched the news on TV while his foot soaked in the epsom-salts solution, used a wooden toothpick to poke the vitamin-E-saturated cotton under his toenail, and, in a few weeks, was rewarded with a pain-free toe.

Nail Growth—Nails grow at the rate of about 1/16 inch per week, requiring four to six months to grow to full length if the nail has been shed due to an injury. Stresses such as cold weather, drugs, illness, and inadequate diet retard nail growth. The rate of growth is sometimes used as a measure of protein adequacy in the diet. Nails that refuse to grow despite a high-protein diet plus supplements of A, B, C, D, calcium, and zinc may respond to applications of vitamin E oil from pierced capsules.

Ridged or Furrowed Nails

- **Horizontal**—Crosswise ridges may be formed by the stresses of menstruation, an illness with high fever, or other major physical or emotional trauma, and move upward as the nail grows. Recurrent ridging during menstrual cycles may be prevented by adequate protein, vitamin A, and brewer's yeast.
- **Longitudinal**—Deep, linear ridging may indicate anemia, protein deficiency, or a lack of vitamins A or B-6. If they are not corrected by a high protein diet plus vitamin and mineral supplementation (including the tissue salt, silicea), a medical analysis should be obtained.

Splitting Nails—Eating generous amounts of raw cucumber, or drinking cucumber juice, is believed to help correct the problem. Taking 5,000 milligrams of dolomite daily for three weeks has restored normal nail strength for some individuals.[325] In many cases, splitting nails are associated with a lack of stomach acid and improve remarkably when betaine hydrochloride tablets are taken with each meal.

Spoon Nails—Depressed in the center and high at the edges, these spoonshaped nails often occur in middle-aged women and may be an indication of anemia (which see). They usually regain their normal shape when the diet is adequate and the anemia is treated.

White Spots, Bands, or Opaque Nails—Stress and trauma are factors but are no longer believed the primary cause of the white spots or bands that appear in the nails of many children and a few adults. Usually the result of zinc deficiency, the small spots fade away and the larger ones grow out with the nail when 15 to 150 milligrams of zinc is taken daily. Dolomite tablets have helped in some instances, and, when, the entire nail is opaque, adding supplements of vitamin B-6 have caused the opaque part of the nail to be replaced by healthy pink nail as it grew out.[256]

Sources (See Bibliography)

3, 4, 6, 22, 53, 68, 84, 88, 89, 156, 171, 184, 230, 238, 254, 256, 257, 270, 288, 293, 297, 305, 315, 325, 333, 353.

FLATULENCE (See Also Heartburn and Indigestion)

By far the most common digestive disturbance, intestinal gas may result from swallowed air, air-filled foods such as soufflés or carbonated beverages, or may develop from decomposing food in the intestines. Studies indicate that the rumbling sounds (borborygmus) and discomfort are more likely to arise from incomplete digestion, delayed passage of foodstuffs, or disorders of intestinal muscular activity than from the quantity of air or gas.

Unconscious air-swallowing, hasty chewing, or gulping effervescent drinks may form a bubble of air at the top of the stomach. As the air is warmed to body temperature, it expands. If not belched for relief, the air passes into the bowel where it can become trapped to cause pain that can be mistaken for a gallbladder or heart attack. Certain foods are known for their gas-producing tendencies and may need to be avoided, but individual reactions differ and much depends on the health of the digestive system. Allergies, emotional upheavals, inadequate nutrients, or relaxing drugs can slow digestion to increase flatulence. Overeating can overwhelm the digestive enzymes, leaving partially digested food to create gas. Many people of African, Mediterranean, or Oriental descent are genetically unable to digest the lactose in sweet milk but can tolerate buttermilk, cottage cheese, hard cheeses, and yogurt, which contain very little of the milk sugar. (A lactose-digestive can be added to regular milk by those who suffer from flatulence due to lactose intolerance.)

Eating slowly at frequent intervals, supplying any needed supplements, and practicing deliberate relaxation (see pages 9-10) often remedy the situation. Of all the symptoms that can arise from bowel disturbances, gas is the least likely to reflect a serious health problem, but medical advice should be obtained if the flatulence persists or is accompanied by severe pain.

Diet and Supplements

No one food produces flatulence for all people at all times. Known for engendering gas are the "windy pulses" (dried beans, cabbage, cauliflower, onions), unripe apples, fresh bread, chocolate, coffee, cucumbers, fried foods, lettuce, meringues, peanuts, radishes, turnips, and whipped cream. Refined carbohydrates such as sugar and white flour, particularly when combined with proteins, can contribute to gassiness. (Sugar, alone, sometimes irritates the lining of the digestive tract to cause flatulence.)

Freedom from gas depends on the proper digestion and absorption of foods by enzymes, hydrochloric acid and bile (see Gallstones), beneficial intestinal flora, and the contractions (motility) of the stomach and intestines. Beginning meals with a raw vegetable salad and ending them with fresh fruit is believed to aid complete digestion. Taking one or two digestive enzyme tablets with each meal may be helpful. (The tablets should contain cellulase, pancreatin, and papain to assist with the digestion of fats, fruits, proteins, starches, and vegetables.) A lack of gastric acid may prevent the absorption of minerals and vitamins needed for intestinal motility and allow partially digested foods to move into the intestines to produce gas. For those with chronic flatulence, but no ulcers, taking nonprescriptive betaine hydrochloride tablets with each meal may provide a solution for bloating and gas.

Foods believed to prevent or relieve flatulence are: beets, endive, garlic, Jerusalem artichokes, olives or olive oil, peaches, sauerkraut, tomatoes, water chestnuts, and yogurt. Both fresh papaya and pineapple contain enzymes that contribute to complete digestion and the avoidance of gas. When fresh papaya is not available, papaya tablets may prove helpful. The old standby, baking soda, is of doubtful value. It may bring up some air from the stomach but can aggravate matters because the gastric juices produce carbon dioxide gas from bicarbonate of soda to create intestinal gas. A daily multi-vitamin-mineral tablet plus experimentation with the following supplements often clears problem flatulence.

> **Acidophilus**—The lactic-acid organisms from acidophilus milk, yogurt, or capsules taken with each meal destroy the gas-forming bacteria in the intestines and reduce odor from any gas that is produced.
>
> **B Complex**—One comprehensive, high-potency tablet daily. B vitamins are necessary for adequate production of stomach acid and regulate the action of the bowels to help eliminate flatulence. An additional 50 to 100 milligrams B-1, B-6, and niacinamide, plus 400 micrograms of folic acid may be helpful. Pantothenic acid is the most vital B vitamin for correction and control of flatulence. Some individuals require up to 20 times the Recommended Daily Allowance of 10 milligrams. Any stress, particularly that of surgery, depletes the body's supply. Hospital tests and clinical studies have shown that taking 250 milligrams of pantothenic acid daily not only relieved post-operative gas pains following abdominal surgery, but that 50 to 100 milligrams of pantothenic acid after each meal prevented intestinal gas and distention for which no physical cause was found.[261] The best food sources of pantothenic acid are brewer's yeast, eggs, kidney, liver, salmon, and wheat germ, but it is difficult to fulfill an elevated requirement for this vitamin without taking supplemental tablets.
>
> **Bee Pollen**—Available in tablets or granules, bee pollen is believed to have the same anti-putrefactive effect as lactic-acid foods such as yogurt.
>
> **Vitamin C**—500 to 3,000 milligrams daily, in divided doses with meals. (Hostile, gas-fomenting microbes cannot survive in an acid environment.[261])
>
> **Charcoal**—Activated charcoal tablets, *not fragments of charcoal briquettes*, may help absorb existing gas.

Case History

Lucille M. had always been troubled with intestinal gas that, in addition to being an embarrassment, caused abdominal cramping. Avoiding flatulent-foods such as beans and cabbage made no appreciable difference. Her doctor could discover no physical reason for the problem, so Lucille munched charcoal tablets.

Her mother packed two of the small black cubes in Lucille's school lunchbox each day, and Lucille relied on this after-the-fact remedy for years. Lucille's little daughter was so accustomed to seeing her mother doubled over with abdominal pain that when she observed a stooped-over ancient on the street her comment was, "Poor man, gas." The hope offered by a series of allergy tests was shortlived; omitting the foods to which she was allergic did not allay the flatulence. Then Lucille attended a nutrition class, read everything she could about dietary supplements—and experimented. She began by taking 500 milligrams of vitamin C with each meal; noticed more improvement after she took bee-pollen tablets between meals; and finally added a third supplement, acidophilus, which combined with the others to effect a permanent "cure." By swallowing two of the acidophilus capsules every time she ate, Lucille found that she no longer needed charcoal tablets—her body no longer produced the abdominally cramping, socially embarassing, gas bubbles.

Potassium—A deficiency of this mineral slows contractions of the intestinal muscles and allows distressing gas pains. Eating generous amounts of fresh fruits and vegetables and using a salt subtitute containing potassium chloride usually provides an adequate proportion of potassium, but supplements may need to be medically prescribed.

Tissue Salts

- **For flatulence with heart discomfort and pain**—Take 3X Calc. Fluor and Kali. Phos. alternately, at frequent intervals while the condition lasts.
- **For flatulence with sharp spasms or cramps**—Take three 6X tablets Mag. Phos. dissolved in a little hot water. If the condition continues, take three tablets of 6X Calc. Phos. Repeat both at frequent intervals until relieved.
- **For flatulence with a sour taste in the mouth**—Take three tablets of 6X Nat. Phos.

Enemas

A two-cup, lukewarm enema of tap water or catnip tea often provides immediate relief from a bout of gas pain and distention.

Exercise

A brisk walk or jog is beneficial for some individuals. Kneading the abdomen may move trapped gas in the colon. Sitting on the floor with the knees drawn up and rocking back and forth may help. Lying on the painful side, drawing up the opposite knee, and rolling from side to side sometimes brings immediate relief.

Folk Remedies

Politely referred to as carminatives, all of these remedies were used to relieve flatulence as well as any griping or windy expulsions.

Apple Cider Vinegar and Honey—Sipping a mixture of two teaspoons each apple cider vinegar and raw honey in a glass of water with each meal is the Vermont folk remedy for improving digestion and preventing the formation of gas.[181]

Garlic—The supreme remedy for thousands of years, Babylonians, Chinese, Egyptians, Greeks, Hindus, and Romans all used garlic to cure flatulence. Whether eaten as raw cloves or taken in capsule form, garlic is believed to stimulate gastric juices, neutralize putrefactive toxins, kill undesirable bacteria, and eliminate gas.

Herbal Teas—Either singly or in combination, these were the favorite carminatives of folk practitioners: bay leaf, camomile, caraway, catnip, cayenne, fennel, parsley, savory, and slippery elm, plus:

- **Anise Water**—Steep one teaspoon anise seeds in one cup boiling water for 10 minutes. Sip as a tea or strain, bottle, and take by the tablespoon as needed.
- **Dill Water**—Made in the same way as anise water, dill water was especially popular as a colic remedy for infants—one-fourth to one-half cup in a nursing bottle was the recommended dosage. Preferred for adults was a combination of one-fourth teaspoon each anise, dill, and fennel, with caraway substituted for the dill on occasion. One cup of the hot tea was to be sipped four times a day. For chronic flatulence, one-fourth teaspoon catnip was added.
- **Fennel and Catnip**—Steep one-half teaspoon each catnip and fennel in one cup boiling water for 10 minutes, then sip a cupful several times each day.

Mustard Seed—Taking two mustard seeds with a glass of water before breakfast, then gradually increasing the number to 12 seeds per day was an old remedy for chronic flatulence. Once the gassiness was under control, the number of seeds could be gradually reduced to one or two daily.

Spices and "Compounds"—Allspice, cardamom, cinnamon, cloves, coriander, ginger, and nutmeg were favored carminatives. One-fourth to one-half teaspoon of the ground spice was steeped in one cup boiling water for 10 minutes, then sipped as a tea or taken by the tablespoonful as needed. One teaspoon whole allspice, cloves, or coriander may be steeped for 30 minutes and used in the same manner.

Compounds to be taken only by the spoonful: one-fourth teaspoon each catnip, cinnamon, fennel, and sage steeped in boiling water for 10 minutes; or, one-fourth teaspoon each ground cardamom, cinnamon, cloves, and nutmeg simmered in two cups wine, strained, and mixed with one cup brown sugar. Either compound may be diluted with warm water, if desired.

Heat

Old-fashioned remedies for flatulence included covering the abdomen with a towel wrung out of a mixture of hot water and brandy with a pinch of salt, or with a poultice of oats simmered in a little vinegar. A modern heating pad or hot water bottle may be as effective in allaying a bout of gas pain.

Nerve Pressure

Press each point for 10 seconds, release for 10 seconds, and repeat three times.

- Press the center of the crown of the head, about 1 inch in front of the "soft spot."
- Press upward on the underside of the center of the skull at the back of the neck.
- Press 1 inch to the left of the center of the chest.
- Using a fist, press the lower corner of the stomach in front of the right hip bone, then move up to the rib cage, across, and down to the left side of the stomach. This is more effective if performed while lying down.

Sources (See Bibliography)

4, 5, 13, 18, 53, 62, 64, 68,75, 76, 78, 84, 89, 92, 98, 99, 101, 106, 121, 142, 152, 156, 168, 173, 174, 180, 181, 184, 190, 206, 211, 215, 226, 228, 229, 245, 252, 254, 259, 261, 284, 288, 305, 318, 319, 325, 330, 334, 335, 353, 354.

FROSTBITE AND CHILBLAINS

Long exposure to severe cold can cause blood in the hands, feet, cheeks, ears, or nose to freeze and ice crystals to form in their tissues. Prolonged immersion in icy water produces the same effect but has been called "trench foot" since World War I when many soldiers suffered from this mishap. These frostbitten areas may turn a violet-reddish color or a greyish or yellowish white, but return to normal when gradually thawed. Chilblains are swollen, inflamed areas of the skin caused by frequent or long-continued exposure to cold which may not have been severe enough to cause frostbite or which was improperly treated. Gradual thawing and warming of the blood vessels and tissues is the key to successful treatment. Vigorous friction, or the archaic practice of rubbing frozen parts with snow, can cause permanent damage and lead to gangrene. Mild frostbite usually clears merely by being in a warm room but more severe cases require some of the natural remedies listed, and may need medical attention.

Prevention

Those living in cold climates or anticipating winter excursions may benefit from taking 50 to 100 milligrams of bioflavonoid rutin tablets daily for several months before exposure to cold. A series of Canadian studies showed that taking large amounts of vitamin C helped prevent frostbite by maintaining body temperature. Body-weight tests indicated that children should take 1,500 milligrams vitamin C daily, beginning in the fall—adults double or triple that dosage.[282]

Dressing appropriately with a waterproof outer layer preserves body heat. Damp clothing should be promptly changed as moisture speeds heat loss. Covering exposed skin with mineral oil or Vaseline helps protect against frostbite and windburn. When frostbite threatens, keeping active increases circulation. Jumping up and down, wiggling toes and fingers, and rotating the arms at the shoulders helps keep the blood flowing. Smoking during exposure is not recommended because tobacco constricts the blood vessels of the skin.

Treatment

Cold clothing should be replaced with a warm garment or blanket. Regardless of what method of warming is used, the temperature should not exceed 100 degrees. Frostbitten parts should not be exposed to a hot stove or fireplace as the frozen tissues may suffer thermal burns at temperatures that would be safe for normal skin. When possible, take a bath in 100-degree water or run lukewarm water over the affected areas for five to 10 minutes. Pat dry without rubbing or breaking any blisters that may have formed. The pain of frostbite is often relieved by covering the frosted area with vitamin E ointment or the oil squeezed from capsules. If fingers or toes are affected, they should be individually wrapped with gauze to prevent them from freezing together. A hot toddy or other warm drink helps stimulate circulation but too much alcohol may cause the chilled blood vessels to expand too rapidly. Exercising the frostbitten parts as soon as they are warmed keeps the blood flowing. Taking a daily B-complex tablet is believed to speed recovery from frostbite.

Folk Remedies

Alum—Dissolve one-quarter ounce to one-quarter pound alum in a basin of hot water. Apply towels wrung out of the mixture to chilblains or frostbitten areas, or soak hands or feet for 20 minutes in the evening, then cover with gloves or bed socks for the rest of the night.

Liquid Applications—Sponge the afflicted areas with diluted boric acid, kerosene, warm slippery elm tea, warm vinegar mixed with salt, or witch hazel. Wheat germ oil may be gently rubbed on the frostbitten parts or they may be sponged with lemon juice and then covered with warmed olive oil. An old before-bed remedy for chilblains was to apply alternate hot and cold compresses for 20 minutes, then rub with turpentine and keep warm overnight.

Rice Bran—An immediate treatment for frostbite is to place the afflicted parts in lukewarm water for a few minutes, then cover with a thick paste of rice bran and water.

Sage Tea—Sipping hot sage tea (one teaspoon sage steeped in one cup boiling water) is thought to help restore circulation.

Vegetables—A Russian remedy for both chilblains and frostbite is to moisten dried cucumber peelings and apply the inner sides directly over the afflicted parts, leaving them overnight for chilblains. Gently rubbing frostbite with freshly cut raw onions or white potatoes is said to relieve the pain. Room-temperature mashed potatoes or turnips can be spread over the frostbitten region. The water in which potatoes have been boiled may be sponged over the area or used as a hand or foot bath for either frostbite or chilblains.

Nerve Massage (Do not massage a frostbitten area.)

- Extend the right arm and use the left hand to massage the triangular hollow between the collarbone and shoulder of the extended arm for 30 seconds. Repeat with the other arm.
- With firm, rapid strokes, rub the area over the kidneys (from the top of the pelvis to the center of the back) for a minute or so to help restore inner warmth.

Nerve Pressure

Press each point for 10 seconds, release for 10 seconds, and repeat three times, but do not apply pressure to a frostbitten area.

- Press a point halfway between the tip of the shoulder blade and the base of the neck. Repeat on the other side.
- Press the hollow behind and slightly below the anklebone on each leg.

Sources (See Bibliography)

3, 19, 28, 53, 62, 88, 98, 113, 139, 142, 156, 168, 176, 226, 227, 282, 288, 312, 315, 319.

GALLSTONES

Gallstones can occur at any age but are more frequent in middle life, develop in four times as many women as men, and appear to run in families. Why they form is not definitively understood, but medical studies indicate many possible causes. Obesity, diabetes, infections, and long periods of inactivity or bed rest are predisposing factors. Women taking oral contraceptives are twice as susceptible as those who are not.[4] Many studies, reinforced by a report in the 1982 *Italian Journal of Gastroenterology*, indict excess sugar and a deficiency of fiber—gallstones are almost unknown among primitive people eating unrefined foods. Extensive medical tests have shown that a "prudent" low-cholesterol diet doubles the chances of developing gallstones.[89] Also associated with increased incidence of gallstones are some of the drugs used to lower body cholesterol. The theory with the most circumstantial evidence is that the stones are precipitated by a decrease in the ratio of lecithin to cholesterol.[261]

Small stones in the gall bladder may lie dormant for years without producing any symptoms. When one of the larger stones obstructs one of the bile ducts, a painful gall-bladder attack results. A blocked duct may cause bile to be distributed throughout the body, producing the yellowish skin of jaundice. Severe or frequent attacks warrant medical evaluation, and may necessitate surgical removal of the gall bladder. Fortunately, after the gall bladder is removed, the bile can pass directly from the liver with no disturbance in function. But prevention and control of gall-bladder difficulties through natural, nonsurgical methods offer preferable options. Especially since nearly 60 percent of the patients in one hospital study suffered a return of their original symptoms after their gall bladders had been removed.[128]

Diet and Supplements

Many authorities feel there is no scientific basis for the long list of dietary taboos formerly attached to gall-bladder diets. The function of the gall bladder is to store and concentrate bile produced by the liver, then release it for the digestion of fats. Little bile is manufactured when the diet is low in protein, or is excessively high in sugar and refined carbohydrates. If the amount of bile is insufficient or the gall bladder is not made to empty itself by the ingestion of fats, the bile becomes super-concentrated, gallstones are more likely to develop, and the fat-soluble vitamins A, D, E, and K cannot be absorbed by the body. The formation of gallstones is encouraged by a diet too low in fat, but studies have confirmed that an over-supply of saturated animal fat increases their incidence. Fried foods or too much fat at one meal can trigger difficulties. Current opinion is that diets for those with gall-bladder problems should contain an evenly distributed one-fourth of the calories in the form of fat. For a rough guide: total daily calories for women are estimated at 2,000—3,000 for men—which would allow 500 to 750 calories from fats.

Food		*Calories of Fat*
1	slice whole-wheat bread, plain	6
1	boiled egg	52
1	ounce natural cheddar cheese	85
1	tablespoon butter, margarine or lard	100
1	tablespoon vegetable oil	120
4	ounces steak	120

Brewer's yeast, liver, powdered skim milk, soy flour, and wheat germ can be used to add protein to the diet without extra fat. The inclusion of at least one teaspoon vegetable oil with each meal stimulates regular emptying of the gall bladder. Adding a few teaspoons of unprocessed bran to the daily diet helps prevent gallstones by clearing out degenerated bile salts and may reduce the size of those already existing.[76] Beet greens have been found to increase the flow of bile and aid in fat metabolism. Pears are believed to have a specific healing effect on the gall bladder. Apple, beet, carrot, celery, cucumber, grape, grapefruit, lemon, pear, and pineapple juices are recommended.

Some folk healers report cures when a glass of equal amounts of lettuce and beet juices was taken daily. Others advise eating or drinking nothing but fresh fruit and vegetable juices for three days. This should be attempted only with medical approval, but, if successful in relieving an attack, may be repeated once each month to prevent a recurrence. Eating small, frequent meals with an ample intake of liquids is believed to aid gall bladder function, especially when supplements are added to the diet.

Vitamin A—10,000 to 25,000 units daily. The vitamin A in fruits and vegetables (carotene) cannot be utilized by the body when the gall bladder is not functioning properly. Both vitamins A and E keep cells from sloughing from the mucous membranes to contribute to the formation of gallstones, and have been known to help dissolve existing ones.

B Complex—One comprehensive, high-potency tablet daily. The B vitamins are essential for efficient fat metabolism. An additional 50 milligrams of B-6 is suggested to assist the body's production of lecithin from unsaturated oils. Adding 25 micrograms biotin and 500 milligrams each choline and inositol often aids the internal handling of fats and cholesterol.

Vitamin C and Bioflavonoids—500 to 1,500 milligrams vitamin C plus 100 to 500 milligrams bioflavonoids. Vitamin C hastens the conversion of cholesterol into bile acids to avoid stone formation. When combined with bioflavonoids, the ducts through which the bile flows are strengthened to improve resistance to accumulated stone-causing wastes. Laboratory tests showed that a lack of vitamin C led to the formation of gallstones.[78]

Vitamin E (see Caution, page 6)—10 IU for each tablespoon of unsaturated oil used, plus 100 to 600 IU daily. Vitamin E is vital for the prevention of oxidation of unsaturated oils within the body. There may be a correlation between vitamin E intake and the increased incidence of gallstones in people on a low-cholesterol diet. In experiments with animals, gallstones have been produced by a deficiency of vitamin E and dissolved by the addition of this vitamin.[75, 89]

Lecithin—One to two tablespoons lecithin granules or 10 to 20 1,200-capsules daily. Studies reported in *The American Journal of Gastroenterology* (vol. 65, 1976) showed that when gallstone patients took lecithin daily, their bile was altered in such a way that stones were less likely to form. Lecithin emulsifies fats, prevents their clumping together to form gallstones, and has been shown to dissolve existing stones as effectively as prescribed medications.[3] (Taking lecithin and vitamin D while adhering to the "prudent polyunsaturated diet" offers protection from both gallstones and heart attacks.) Eating brewer's yeast, nuts, sunflower seeds, and unrefined grains increases the body's production of lecithin.

Magnesium—300 milligrams daily. Magnesium is essential for the assimilation of calcium and helps prevent gallstones.

Tissue Salts—During an attack, take four tablets of 6X Calc. Phos. each two hours.

Folk Remedies

Compresses

- **Castor Oil**—Saturate several thicknesses of cloth with castor oil. Place over the upper right quarter of the abdomen, cover with a towel, then with a heating pad. Keep as hot as is comfortable for an hour or two once each day for three or four days. After removing the compress, rinse the area with a solution of one tablespoon baking soda to two cups water.
- **Milk**—Wring a small towel out of cold milk, place on the upper abdomen, cover with plastic and a wool blanket.
- **Water**—Cover the painful portion of the abdomen with a towel wrung out of hot water (with or without one teaspoon of dry mustard). Replace as soon as it has cooled.

Enemas of catnip tea or strong coffee (not instant or decaffeinated), retained as long as possible, were used to help relieve the pain of an acute attack.

Herbal Teas—Camomile, comfrey, dandelion, fennel, parsley, peppermint, turmeric, or white oak bark teas are recommended to stimulate the flow of bile and help dissolve gallstones.

Lemon Juice—Take three tablespoons of undiluted, unsweetened fresh lemon juice 15 to 30 minutes before breakfast each day for one week. Lemon juice is thought to stimulate, purge, and empty the gall bladder. In the early days, the avaricious bottled lemon juice with a few other ingredients for flavor and sold it as a patent medicine for gall-bladder problems.

Olive Oil is the classic folk remedy for gallstones and gall-bladder pain. The many variations testify to its success through the years.

- Take one teaspoon to two tablespoons olive oil before each meal to trigger the flow of bile. The oil should be followed by one-half cup grapefruit or diluted lemon juice and is said to bring rapid improvement.
- Start with one teaspoon olive oil in grapefruit juice every morning before breakfast and gradually work up to four tablespoons of oil. (One teaspoon apple cider vinegar stirred into one-half cup water may be substituted for the grapefruit juice.) Three weeks of this regimen is reported to dissolve gallstones that had been apparent in x-rays.[53]
- These speedier but more rigorous olive-oil-cures should be undertaken *only* with a physician's approval:
  For three days, eat only steamed vegetables with no fat and drink two quarts of apple juice each day. On the evening of the third day, drink a mixture of one-half cup each olive oil and fresh lemon juice. A variation calls for not eating or drinking anything except apple juice for three days and taking a cup of half-and-half olive oil and apple juice on the evenings of the second and third days. Both versions have resulted in the passage of gallstones on the fourth day.[53,334]
  For even more immediate relief: following a bowel movement or enema several

hours after eating, take one-half to one and one-half cups olive oil (mixed with equal parts citrus juice, if desired) and lie down on the right side for two hours.[13]

Radishes—Either eaten plain or minced and combined with olive oil and lemon juice, radishes were believed to benefit the gall bladder and dissolve gallstones.

Nerve Massage

Massage the outer edge of the right hand just below the pad of the little finger, then massage the outer edge of each foot and the pad under the little toe.

Nerve Pressure

Unless otherwise indicated, press each point for 10 seconds, release for 10 seconds, and repeat three times.

- Press inward and upward under each cheekbone, 1½ inches out from the earlobe toward the nose.
- With the fingers of both hands, press inward and downward on the middle of the upper edge of the collarbones.
- Press 2 inches to the right of the navel, midway between it and the lower ribs.
- Winding rubber bands on the thumbs, first, and second fingers (and on the comparable toes) for five to 15 minutes is believed beneficial for the gall bladder. (The rubber bands should be removed the moment the skin begins to turn blue.)

Sources (See Bibliography)

3, 4, 7, 9, 13, 18, 19, 24, 34, 53, 61, 63, 64, 75, 76, 78, 81, 82, 84, 89, 108, 128, 142, 154, 156, 173, 174, 180, 184, 189, 190, 211, 227, 228, 229, 243, 253, 254, 261, 270, 272, 288, 289, 297, 301, 304, 314, 315, 334, 335, 350, 353.

GLAUCOMA

According to the Cataract Research Institute, more than 2 million Americans have glaucoma and over 300,000 new cases are diagnosed each year. One of the leading causes of blindness, glaucoma is too serious a disorder to attempt self-treatment without the approval and supervision of an ophthalmologist. However, since the medical profession emphasizes that drugs and surgery are merely controls to preserve remaining sight, not cures for glaucoma, most eye doctors do not object to their patients experimenting with some of these natural remedies that have been of help to many people.

There are several types of glaucoma, but all are due to excess fluid in the eye and/ or faulty drainage that results in increased pressure, hardening of the eyeball, and loss of side (peripheral) vision—with the possibility of blindness if left untreated. No one specific cause is known, but heredity plays a role. Screening surveys have shown that in those with a family history of glaucoma, almost one out of every 10 adults had this affliction.[70] It usually occurs after age 40 (although young people with juvenile-onset diabetes are especially susceptible) and may be due to anxiety and stress, allergies or hormonal disorders, infection, or injury.

Early detection and treatment can substantially reduce the incidence of blindness resulting from glaucoma. Most eye specialists agree that emotional upheavals, caffeine-containing beverages, excessive eyestrain from movies, reading, or TV-watching, poor lighting (which causes the iris to "bunch up" to admit more light), and drinking large amounts of liquid at one time should be avoided. Sunglasses should be worn only in bright sunlight. There is enough evidence to indicate that smoking causes harm in cases of glaucoma to warrant limiting the use of tobacco or eliminating it entirely.

Diet and Supplements

While there is no specific diet for glaucoma, ample protein (including organ meats and seafood), leafy greens, colored vegetables, whole-grain products supplemented with brewer's yeast and wheat germ are believed to aid the body in resisting the malady. Eating three carrots boiled in one quart of water and drinking the liquid each day is a folk remedy for regaining sight lost through glaucoma. (Improvement has been noticeable in from two weeks to two months.[3]) Fresh juices from beets and beet greens, carrots, grapefruit, lemons, and oranges are also considered beneficial.

There is controversy over the use of salt for those with glaucoma. Although there is no direct relationship between the high fluid pressure in the eye and high blood pressure, many doctors suggest stringent reduction of salt. Other specialists regard glaucoma as a stress disease resulting from adrenal exhaustion, which causes so much salt to be lost from the body that fluids can pass into the tissues of the eye, and recommend extra amounts of salt until the condition is corrected. Taking a daily multi-vitamin-mineral tablet is usually suggested to avoid deficiencies and assure efficient absorption of nutrients from foods.

In her book, *Let's Get Well*[89], Adelle Davis wrote that an adequate diet plus these supplements taken in divided doses six times daily with "fortified milk" completely cleared glaucoma for the individuals with whom she worked: 3,000 milligrams vitamin C, 600 milligrams pantothenic acid, 12 milligrams each B-2 and B-6. Ms. Davis' original formula required eggs, soy flour, and yogurt but by taking an acidophilus capsule along with the vitamins and utilizing one of the unsweetened protein powders now available, a day's supply of fortified milk can be quickly prepared and stored in the refrigerator. In an electric blender, combine two cups whole or skim milk, one-fourth cup each brewer's yeast, dry milk, and protein powder. If desired, add up to one-half cup frozen, undiluted orange juice, or vanilla and nutmeg for flavor.

Other supplements suggested by nutritional experts:

Vitamin A—25,000 units daily. Vitamin A is essential for eye health.

B Complex—One comprehensive, high-potency tablet daily to alleviate symptoms of anxiety and stress related to a deficiency of B vitamins. A study reported in *Annals of Ophthalmology* [July, 1979] indicated that 100 milligrams of B-1 per day relieved the effects of glaucoma. (Larger doses should be used with caution as they have been known to increase eye pressure.) Other specifics for glaucoma are additional amounts of B-2, B-6, choline, inositol, and pantothenic acid.

Vitamin C—1,000 to 35,000 milligrams daily. As little as 500 milligrams twice a day has lowered pressure in some instances but the *Journal of Holistic Medicine* (Fall/Winter, 1981) reported that mega-doses of vitamin C dramatically reduced intraocular pressure. In one series of tests, the daily amounts used varied from 60 to 250 milligrams of vitamin C per pound of body weight. (An individual weighing 150 pounds might take 7,000 milligrams of vitamin C three to five times per day—preferably at five-hour intervals.) Such massive amounts should be used only with a physician's approval, but no adverse side effects appeared during these tests. Symptoms such as mild stomach discomfort and diarrhea disappeared after a few days and could be mitigated by accompanying each dose of vitamin C with a calcium supplement. All types of glaucoma responded with normal, or near normal, intraocular pressure within 45 days. In some cases the lowered pressure held for several weeks after treatment had stopped.[70] Other studies have shown vitamin C to be even more effective in reducing pressure when 50 to 150 milligrams of bioflavonoids were taken with each dose.

Drugs

Glaucoma victims must be wary of medications not prescribed by their ophthalmologist. Drugs with atropine-like side effects could aggravate glaucoma. These include many medications prescribed for gastritis, peptic ulcer, irritable bowel, or diarrhea.

Glycerine

Drinking 1½ grams of oral glycerine (available in pharmacies) per each kilogram (2.2 pounds) of body weight has been found to ward off glaucoma attacks[168], but should be used only with medical approval.

Nerve Massage

For a few seconds each day, massage the bottom of each foot just below the second and third toes, and the top of the foot where the second and third toes begin.

Nerve Pressure

Place the index fingers under the ends of the jawbone just under each ear and pull forward for 10 seconds, release for 10 seconds, and repeat three times.

Seawater

Using filtered seawater (available in health food stores) as eye drops has reportedly corrected some cases of glaucoma.

Sunlight

Letting bright sunlight filter through closed eyelids while slowly turning the head for two minutes several times each day has been of benefit during the early stages of glaucoma.[76]

Sources (See Bibliography)

3, 6, 7, 13, 19, 34, 64, 70, 71, 72, 75, 76, 81, 82, 84, 88, 89, 168, 189, 236, 254, 261, 297, 309, 315, 316, 350.

GOUT

Once limited to rotund medieval noblemen, gout still afflicts 95 percent more men than women but has become a commonplace malady. Resulting from crystals precipitating out of uric acid, then being deposited in and around joints, gout usually affects the big toe but can occur in the ear, hand, heel, knee, or any other joint in the body. Uric acid is synthesized by the body as well as being derived from the purines (nucleoproteins) contained in foods. Normally it is converted into urea and ammonia, then excreted as urine. Abnormal ingested amounts or increased production of uric acid, or a deficit of the chemicals and nutrients required for its conversion and elimination allow the pain-creating crystals to form.

No single cause of gout has been established, but factors such as improper protein metabolism, injuries, obesity, diuretics or drugs taken for other ailments, emotional strain, or even a change in the weather can provoke an attack. It is hereditary in that a predisposition to high uric acid levels and gout runs in families. Yet not all those with elevated uric acid levels succumb to gout. (Many clinical studies have shown an association between high blood levels of uric acid and high levels of intelligence, without any gouty problems.[13, 261])

Research in England, Italy, and Switzerland has established a correlation between blood-sugar regulation and high uric acid. Australian studies on alcohol consumption and cigarette smoking (both of which have a decided effect on blood-sugar levels) reinforce this theory. Other authorities believe that control of gout depends more on ample intake of fluids and correction of the chemical imbalance causing the crystals to precipitate than on drug or dietary methods of reducing uric acid levels.

Every form of stress has been shown to increase the production of uric acid. Since deficiencies of any nutrient act as a stress on the body, vitamin supplements may be essential—particularly while adhering to a low-purine diet. The symptoms of gout may be similar to those of rheumatoid arthritis, and excess uric acid can produce kidney stones as well as gout, so medical diagnosis and treatment is advisable. But gout is considered the most treatable of all rheumatic maladies. With medical supervision, a wise diet, and supplements, most gout victims today can be kept free from acute attacks.

Diet and Supplements

Cherries are the number-one dietary remedy for gout. While no officially sanctioned tests have established reasons for their curative effects, so many doctors and their patients have achieved good results that the use of cherries to combat gout has moved out of the folk-medicine realm. It is believed that cherries contain an enzyme essential for the conversion and elimination of uric acid to prevent the problem-causing crystallization. As first documented by Dr. Ludwig W. Blau (*Texas Reports on Biology and Medicine,* Vol. 8, No. 3, 1950), eating one cup of fresh cherries on the first day and one-half cup each day thereafter has left many gout-sufferers free from pain. Overnight relief has been obtained by some individuals but others required several days or weeks of "cherry therapy." Fresh, raw cherries are considered the most effective but frozen or canned, unsweetened cherries, even cherry juice, have cleared gout symptoms when they were used every day.

Case History

Willard G. does not believe in vitamins or natural remedies; he thinks they are "quackery." Willard does believe in doctors though, and adhered religiously to the low-purine diet and medication prescribed for the gout in his foot. The pain lessened, then fluctuated with frequent flare-ups. Driving his car was difficult, so Willard moved his accounting office into his living room where he could work with his throbbing toe propped on a pillow. Willard's wife grew impatient with the slowness of his recovery, read about successes with natural remedies, but could not talk Willard into trying any of them. One day she put a bowl of fresh cherries on his work table, raved over their tree-ripened flavor, and commented that they would have to eat a lot of the cherries because she had bought several pounds at a bargain price. The cherries were so delicious that Willard nibbled his way through a large bowlful every day for a week before he questioned the apparently never-ending supply of fresh cherries. By this time his foot was no longer painful, and he had returned to work in his office. His wife admitted that she had purchased more cherries because she wondered if they might have had something to do with his speedy recovery. She suggested that, just for luck, he continue to eat a few every day. Willard still does not believe in vitamins, or in natural remedies; but Willard tells everyone how "lucky" it is to eat cherries when bothered by gout.

From whatever source, adequate amounts of complete proteins should be eaten daily because a deficiency of their amino acids increases the body's production of uric acid. Using generous quantities of fruits and vegetables, and their juices, helps keep the uric acid crystals in solution and facilitates their excretion. Apples, beets and beet greens, blackberries, cabbage, cherries, cauliflower, cucumber, endive, figs, grapes, kale, lettuce, oranges, parsnips, pineapple, strawberries, tomatoes, and turnip greens are considered the most beneficial. Increasing the intake of juices plus milk and water to equal three quarts daily at the first sign of joint discomfort has forestalled gout attacks for many. Parsley eaten along with meat is believed to help eliminate the excessive uric acid produced during the digestion of meat. Brown rice does not cause a rise in uric acid, so its use is advised. Eating acidophilus yogurt daily (or taking acidophilus capsules with each meal) encourages the intestinal bacteria which help dispose of uric acid.

In bygone times, only the gout-afflicted wealthy ate a lot of meat (usually rancid and vitamin-E destructive due to lack of refrigeration) and sweet concoctions, while the gout-free poor subsisted on vegetables, whole grains, and dairy products. (Primitive, underdeveloped nations with high-fiber diets still have no problems with gout.) The traditional low-purine diet for gout is now under scrutiny. Many doctors believe that the biochemic individualities of overproduction and faulty elimination of uric acid have little relation to the amount of anchovies, dried beans, herring, meat broths, organ meats, or other purine-containing foods consumed. Glycine, a substance contained in gelatin, is rapidly transformed into uric acid by those with gout. Avoiding gelatin, along with other high-purine foods, alcoholic beverages, and excessive amounts of sugar or fats during an attack is suggested.

Obesity increases the susceptibility to gout but weight loss should be gradual. Fasts and crash diets should be shunned by those with gout as they increase the concentration of uric acid and prevent the kidneys from properly excreting it. The dietary restrictions imposed during attacks of gout, however, are frequently unnecessary during periods of remission. The use of supplements often extends these remissions permanently.

B Complex—One comprehensive tablet daily, especially when abiding by a low-purine diet which is low in B vitamins. Brewer's yeast is an excellent source of all the B vitamins and has been known to help reverse gout, but is classified with the purines by some experts and, therefore, restricted. Taking an additional 10 to 20 milligrams of B-1 each day has been beneficial for some gout sufferers. Others have achieved complete relief from gout symptoms by taking 400 milligrams B15 each morning and evening for two or three days. Pantothenic acid is of primary importance in preventing and controlling gout—its deficiency has been known to produce the malady. Some individuals have a hereditary need for extremely large amounts of this B vitamin which is necessary for the transformation of uric acid into harmless urea for excretion. From 100 to 600 milligrams of pantothenic acid may be required on a daily basis, with additional amounts taken with 500 milligrams vitamin C plus extra liquids, each two or three hours, during periods of stress or at the first sign of joint pain.

Vitamin C—1,000 milligrams per hour while suffering from a gout attack, then a gradual tapering off to a maintenance dosage of 500 milligrams per day. Vitamin C is as helpful for noninfectious gout as it is for maladies caused bv viruses or bacteria.

Vitamin E (see Caution, page 6)—100 to 1,200 IU daily. A deficiency of vitamin E can cause uric acid to form in excessive amounts and low-purine diets are usually lacking in this vitamin. Soaking a gouty toe in hot water for 30 minutes then rubbing it with vitamin E has helped some cases.

Tissue Salts—To prevent the formation of uric acid crystals, take two tablets 6X Silicea three times each day. During an attack of gout, increase the dosage to three tablets and take an equal amount of 6X Nat. Phos. and Nat. Sulph.

Folk Remedies

Apple Cider Vinegar—Two teaspoons each apple cider vinegar and raw honey stirred in a glass of water and sipped at mealtime was believed to prevent and relieve gout. Liniments made from simmering one tablespoon cayenne pepper in two cups cider vinegar, or heating the vinegar and stirring in all the salt that would dissolve, were rubbed on gout-afflicted joints four times s day to relieve pain. Soaking the painful area in a solution of one-half cup apple cider vinegar and three cups hot water was also thought to alleviate gouty pain.

Apples—Raw, juiced, or cooked into sauce, apples have long been considered a cure for gout. Europeans make a tea from dried apple peels and sweeten it with honey. Vermont folk medicine recommends stirring two teaspoons honey in a glass of apple juice to be sipped with each meal. Other folk practitioners believe that apple cider is the ideal beverage for those with a "gouty constitution."

Baking Soda—One-fourth teaspoon soda dissolved in water and taken three or four times daily was believed to alleviate the pain of gout.

Butter and Wine—An old folk remedy for gout was to heat unsalted butter until it started to boil, add an equal amount of wine, and let it steam until the consistency of an ointment, then rub on the affected area to soothe and heal.

Celery—Eating at least two stalks of raw or cooked celery each day is a gout remedy in both Germany and Japan. American folk medicine suggests celery juice or celery seed tea.

Compresses—Alternating hot and cold compresses over the inflamed joint every two or three hours often brings relief.

Garlic—Eating several cloves of raw garlic each day has been a gout-preventive since the Greco-Roman era. Applying a poultice of cooked garlic is thought to relieve pain in an afflicted joint.

Herbs—Alfalfa, buckthorn, chervil, comfrey, elder flower, ginger, juniper, berry, parsley, plaintain, and sarsaparilla teas were recommended as beverages (four cups per day), or as poultices for gout. Rubbing the affected joint with fresh mint leaves was said to relieve the pain, as was taking a few drops of oil of wintergreen on a sugar cube three times a day.

Pears—Eating a fresh, ripe pear before each meal is a French remedy for keeping uric acid in solution and avoiding gout.

Potatoes—Freshly extracted potato juice (mixed with beet, carrot, or celery juice for palatability) was an old remedy for gout.

Strawberries—The Swedish botanist, Linnaeus, was reportedly cured of gout by eating almost nothing but large quantities of strawberries for several days. Latter-day French herbalists are equally enthusiastic about the "strawberry cure."

Nerve Pressure

Once each day, press each point for 10 seconds, release for 10 seconds, and repeat three times.

- Press inward and upward on the underside of the protuberance at the base of the center back of the skull.
- Press just below the center of the nose toward the upper lip.
- Press between the bone at the ball of the foot and the bottom of the big toe on each foot.

Sources (See Bibliography)

3, 9, 13, 19, 24, 48, 52, 53, 62, 68, 69, 81, 82, 84, 88, 89, 128, 142, 151, 152, 156, 165, 168, 173, 180, 184, 189, 190, 211, 227, 229, 243, 252, 253, 254, 261, 276, 288, 297, 311, 315, 316, 321, 325, 335, 348, 349, 350, 354.

HANGOVER

For thousands of years mortals have been concocting and imbibing alcoholic beverages. For an equal length of time they have been experimenting with remedies for the morning-after-maladies which sometimes follow indulgence in these "drinks of the gods." In the first century A.D., Pliny the Elder suggested that hangover be treated with "the eggs of an owlet and the ashes of a swallow's beak, bruised with myrrh." Hangovers have no respect for race or socioeconomic status. To a hungover Frenchman, it's "la geule de bois"—woody mouth; to a German, it's "katzenjammer"—the wailing of cats. Italians call it "stonato"—out of tune; in Sweden, it's "hont i haret"—pain in the roots of the hair. Thanks to modern research, an understanding of the process involved in the production of hangovers allows them to be prevented or remedied, not just endured as penance.

Alcohol is a mild anesthetic, muscle relaxer, and diuretic. It requires a series of chemical alterations within the liver before it can be excreted from the system. An "average" person can cope with one alcoholic drink per hour, but each individual reacts differently. Body weight has much to do with the rate of absorption. A 240-pound person can handle four or five drinks with no more effect than a 100-pounder gleans from one or two. The alcohol from distilled spirits is absorbed more rapidly than that in beer and wine, which contain nonalcoholic substances to slow absorption. When more than the assimilable amount is imbibed, the brain cells adapt to the anesthetic by becoming supersensitive (hence the sensitivity to light and sound while the cells readjust after the alcohol is no longer present). Relaxed muscles account for the slurred speech and disruption of motor faculties besides allowing blood vessels to expand and create a vascular headache (which see). The diuretic properties of alcohol can cause dehydration as well as increasing urinary losses of nearly all the nutrients needed for good health.

Most happy-hour beverages contain more than pure alcohol. As explained by Dr. Boris Tabakoff, President of the Research Society on Alcoholism, the flavorings and colorings (called congeners) added to everything except vodka, are toxins which further burden the liver and increase the possibility of a hangover. In general, it takes as many hours to recover as the number of drinks that have been consumed. (When the system becomes adapted to functioning with alcohol, it may take up to 12 hours.) Alcohol is readily eliminated from the body but congeners are not. They linger to cause toxic effects the following day. On a scale of 1 to 7, in relation to congener-content and morning-after-aftermath: vodka rates 1; gin, 2; white wine, 2½; beer or Scotch, 3; dark rum and sherry, 5; red wine, 6; brandy or bourbon, 7. These congeners and various other nonalcoholic substances, such as the histamines in red wine, are largely responsible for the stomach irritation and other after-effects of drinking. Hangovers have been produced in volunteers just by giving them nonalcoholic mixtures of congeners.

Another contributory factor is the disturbance of REM (Rapid Eye Movement during dreams) in the sleep that follows an evening of overly generous libations. Without the restorative powers of dream sleep, the morning-after feeling of not having slept at all occurs, and, for confirmed alcoholics, this lack of normal dreaming can have the rebound effect of pink-elephant hallucinations.

Aside from the facetious advice for avoiding hangovers—don't drink or don't stop—there are three stages of hangover elimination: before, during, and after drinking.

Before

An hour or so before a premeditated evening of partying, dine well on high-fat, high-protein foods including some starch and, ideally, some cabbage. Chops or steak, ham, salmon, or a cheese omelet, plus rolls or garlic toast slathered with butter, and an extra spoonful of oil with a green salad or coleslaw will inhibit a too-rapid rate of alcohol absorption. Ancient Greeks and Romans advised eating at least five cabbage leaves dipped in vinegar before and after a lavish banquet to counteract the next day's "wrath of the grapes." Modern scientists have discovered that cabbage is a chelator. It gathers and absorbs the congeners in liquors before they can reach the bloodstream, then carries them out of the system. Taking 500 to 3,000 milligrams of vitamin C, also a chelating agent, will increase the effectiveness of the cabbage in controlling the toxins. Adding one tablet each of a B-complex and a multi-vitamin-mineral formula will fortify the system against anticipated losses due to the diuretic action of the alcohol. Some medical nutritionists recommend the addition of 200 milligrams B-1, 100 milligrams each B-6 and pantothenic acid, 500 milligrams each niacinamide and magnesium, and 15 to 20 milligrams of zinc.

During

Selecting clear alcohols such as vodka, gin, white rum, or white wine, and using natural juices or water as a mixer reduces the complications of congener reactions. (Club soda or seltzer contain no congeners but carbonation speeds the absorption of alcohol.) The evil effects of red wine can be partially avoided by uncorking the bottle and allowing the congeners to evaporate for an hour or so before serving. Nibbling on nuts (almonds are a folk-remedy favorite), cheese, or protein-rich canapes slows the absorption of alcohol. To avoid hangovers, the Russians swear by a bite of black bread along with every sip of vodka. Physical movement, such as dancing, speeds the metabolism of alcohol to lessen possible morning-after misery. Since a "hangover headache" may result merely from an evening spent in a smoke-filled room, going outside for a few deep breaths of fresh air at frequent intervals is wise when drinking with smokers. During a protracted evening of imbibing, taking an additional B-complex tablet is recommended.

After

After the party is over, there are several before-bed options. Drinking one to three cups of tea or coffee (not decaffeinated) while the alcohol is still in the stomach may slow its absorption, help revive the nervous system, and encourage REM sleep when too much alcohol has depressed the system. A bedtime snack of bread and mayonnaise plus peanut butter or cheese, or crackers and honey, plus another vitamin-mineral and B-complex tablet with a glass of milk will assist the assimilation and recovery process during sleep.

Case History

Bill S. was a salesman whose most profitable deals were consummated while dining, and wining, his prospective clients. Bill did not imbibe to excess, yet often found himself miserably uncomfortable and fuzzy-headed at "morning after" meetings. Deciding to experiment with the "if a little is good, more is better" theory, Bill evolved his own hangover preventive and cure. He began taking one of his usual once-a-day-in-the-morning multiple vitamin tablets before going out to dinner with a client, another (with a glass of milk) before going to bed, and an additional multiple vitamin tablet as soon as he awoke. The results were amazingly effective. Even when he did not have time for a fortifying, high-protein breakfast, Bill could greet each day with his normally ebullient spirit and a clear head.

Hangover Remedies

Once it has arrived in full force, the complex anatomy of a hangover precludes its complete cure with any single remedy. A cup of strong tea or coffee (not decaffeinated) and an ice pack on the wrists, back of the neck or head may help constrict the enlarged blood vessels causing the throbbing headache. If a commercial painkiller is used, an acetaminophen (Datril, Tylenol, etc.) is recommended in preference to aspirin which may further inflame an already irritated stomach. An antacid may soothe gastric distress but can do nothing for the other problems. Water will moisten a parched throat and begin to restore the liquid balance of the body but can neither replace lost minerals and vitamins nor eradicate the toxins and unmetabolized alcohol still in the system. Strong spices tidy up the mouth but may contribute to further gastrointestinal upset. The fabled "hair of the dog" will bring on another bite unless taken in very small amounts to allow gradual normalization of the supersensitized brain cells.

The goal is to speed recovery by assisting the body's return to its normal, nonalcoholic state. Individual reactions to hangover remedies are as varied as individual reactions to alcohol. Whatever specifics are selected, replacing lost liquids at the rate of approximately 12 ounces per hour is essential. Dehydration contributes to a hangover—a furry mouth is just one of its symptoms. Gingerale or soda water with a few drops of bitters are less likely to aggravate stomach distress than plain water or strong citrus juices. Beef or chicken broth is usually well tolerated, replaces both lost fluids and minerals, and may help ease nausea.

> **Alcohol**—The phrase, "hair of the dog," was first recorded in 1546 and, throughout history, the majority of hangover cures have included alcoholic spirits in the formula. More than one jigger (three tablespoons) of straight alcohol can prolong the agony by further upsetting the stomach and dilating the already throbbing blood vessels in the head. A small quantity, however, often allows the sensitized cells to ease their way back to normalcy without a painfully disquieting shock to the system. Some of the more famous remedies, such as "Prairie Oyster" with its raw egg to be swallowed whole, are for those with strong, not queasy stomachs. Most of the "bartenders' specials" combine the resuscitating bit of alcohol with ingredients that speed readjustment without being offensive. Almost any appealing combination may be effective, and a touch of any favored spirit may be taken with the nonalcoholic remedies.

- **Beer**—One cup beer mixed with one-fourth cup bitters, or with an equal amount of champagne (Black Velvet) or tomato juice (Shameful Mary).
- **Bloody Bullshot**—One third cup each beef broth and tomato juice blended with three tablespoons each lemon juice and vodka, then poured over ice. One raw egg, a little Worcestershire sauce and a dash of black pepper may be blended in, if desired.
- **Brandy with Peppermint** is the Swiss remedy for a hangover.
- **Las Vegas Flip**—Two-thirds cup tomato juice, one-third cup beer, one raw egg, and two tablespoons heavy cream blended with one ice cube and seasoned with black pepper or nutmeg.
- **Reindeer Milk**—One-half cup milk blended with one-fourth cup each honey, lemon juice, and vodka, plus two ice cubes. Add orange flavoring and nutmeg to taste.
- **Scotch Hare**—Three tablespoons Scotch blended with an ice cube plus one tablespoon each honey and heavy cream.
- **Sherry-Cream Flip**—One-third cup dry sherry, one raw egg, and one tablespoon honey blended with an ice cube, then dusted with nutmeg.
- **Suffern Bawstard**—One tablespoon each brandy, gin, and lime juice, poured over ice in half a glass of gingerale and stirred with a sprig of mint.

Apples—An old remedy for a hangover headache was to eat one or two apples, chewing them thoroughly.

Charcoal—Four to six tablets (not fragments of charcoal briquettes) help absorb any alcohol remaining in the system. An experiment conducted at Columbia University showed that activated charcoal absorbed from 82 to 93 percent of the congeners in alcoholic beverages.[289]

Cream—A glass of heavy cream is the Norwegian remedy for a hangover.

Foods—Ancient Egyptians chewed on cabbage leaves, Russians recommend salted cucumber juice, the Japanese are reported to favor eating persimmons as a hangover cure. For most people, bland foods like poached eggs over toast are more appealing. Proteins do absorb irritating stomach acids and hardy souls may prefer spreading mashed anchovies on rye bread, covering them with onion slices drizzled with olive oil, then heating under the broiler and sprinkling black pepper atop.

Herbal Teas—Camomile, clove, and ginger teas sweetened with honey were old-time favorites. During the 1800s, a combination of one teaspoon thyme plus one-fourth teaspoon each rosemary and spearmint steeped in one cup boiling water was recommended.

Honey and Fructose—The fructose in honey, and to some extent in ripe fruits and tomato juice, accelerates the metabolization of any alcohol remaining in the system. Downing two tablespoons of honey each 20 minutes until a total of six tablespoons have been taken, then eating a soft-cooked egg and taking two more tablespoons of honey has been sworn to as effective by generations of tipplers. Table sugar does not have this effect, but granulated fructose is now available in health food stores and may be substituted for honey in any of the hangover remedies. It should be mixed with lemon juice and water if taken straight. Combining the honey or fructose with a tablespoon of vodka or whiskey is another option.

Juices—Sauerkraut juice, plain or mixed with tomato juice, has been a longstanding hangover remedy. Equal amounts of clam juice and tomato juice, or apple, grape, or orange juice blended with a little honey, provide fructose to speed relief.

Milk and Yogurt—Acidified milks offer easily digested protein. Stirring one cup buttermilk into one tablespoon cornstarch and heating just to simmering with one tablespoon honey, then eating hot or cold as a stomach pacifier is a European remedy. A mixture of equal parts yogurt and tomato juice sparked with lemon juice is another favorite.

Nerve Massage and Nerve Pressure—Massage both thumbs and/or both big toes. (See Headache for hangover-headache massage and pressure points.)

Oxygen and Fresh Air—When a home canister of oxygen is available, eight deep breaths of pure oxygen often trumps a hangover. Breathing nonpolluted, out-of-door-air for 20 minutes is believed to accelerate the process of alcohol metabolism to the same extent.

Primrose Oil—Recent tests by Dr. David Horrobin at the University of Montreal have shown this natural substance to be effective in counteracting the after-effects of alcohol consumption. Also called "Oil of Evening Primrose," it is available from health food stores and should be taken only according to package directions.

Soups—Borscht or chicken soup (both available in cans) is the remedy favored by Russians and Europeans. For a homemade cabbage soup recorded by David Outerbridge in his *Hangover Handbook*[245] and credited with marvelous recuperative powers: shred one fourth of a large head of cabbage into four cups of fat-free beef broth and simmer for 20 minutes. Add one-half cup apple cider, one-fourth teaspoon caraway seeds, and salt to taste. Freeze in one-cup containers in anticipation of future need.

Vitamins and Minerals—Two multi-vitamin-mineral tablets, one high-potency B-complex tablet, and 500 milligrams vitamin C. Take the first thing upon awakening to help compensate for the losses incurred and help the system return to normalcy. Many of the traditional hangover symptoms (aches and pains, bloodshot eyes, irritability, loss of appetite, shakiness, etc.) can be created by vitamin deficiencies alone.

Sources (See Bibliography)

3, 7, 33, 54, 63, 64, 75, 78, 86, 89, 121, 154, 156, 158, 180, 206, 227, 228, 229, 235, 241, 245, 252, 254, 276, 288, 289, 292, 310, 311, 315.

HARDENING AND NARROWING OF THE ARTERIES (ARTERIOSCLEROSIS AND ATHEROSCLEROSIS) AND CHOLESTEROL

Hardening of the arteries (arteriosclerosis) is a thickening of the artery walls accompanied by a loss of flexibility. Atherosclerosis is the clogging or filling up of the arteries by deposits of cholesterol, fat, and/or minerals. As the blood flows through these narrowed channels, tiny particles of chemicals in the blood may begin to cluster on rough spots to form the core of a clot which further blocks the flow of blood. Under certain conditions, one of these clots may break away and be carried through the arteries to cause a heart attack or stroke.

Atherosclerosis is not a new ailment. An Egyptian mummy who had been about 40 years of age at his death 2,100 years ago, had atherosclerosis. But, before 1900 there was very little coronary heart disease. Hardened arteries were considered a normal facet of aging and only during the past few decades has a connection been made between clogged or hardened arteries and heart attacks. Studies have shown many of the elderly to have clear, flexible arteries, so there is controversy regarding the cause of arterial hardening and narrowing.

Continuing research has refuted some earlier-held beliefs about the desirability of avoiding cholesterol-laden foods, and indicated that the type of cholesterol in the blood is the crucial factor. Apparently it is the low-density lipoprotein (LDL) that causes problems, while the high-density lipoprotein (HDL) protects against atherosclerosis and heart disease. Cholesterol is necessary for life, is manufactured by the body, and has many useful functions. Although there is still no official pronouncement, the ratio of "good" HDL to "bad" LDL is now regarded as of more importance than the total serum cholesterol level. As reported in the *Harvard Medical School Health Letter* (November, 1979), the famous Framingham Study has shown that the ratio of total cholesterol to HDL should be no more than 4.5 regardless of age or sex, and that a ratio in the range of 7 to 9 indicates a double risk of heart attack. Numerous other studies have shown little relationship between the amount of cholesterol in the diet and blood cholesterol levels, so the anti-cholesterol crusade is wavering.

Autopsies performed on American soldiers killed in Korea and Viet Nam showed that 77 percent of these healthy young men had arteriosclerosis, while similar studies conducted during World Wars I and II revealed little or no signs of this malady. Since all the soldiers were physically active, ate approximately the same amounts of cholesterol and fat, and were subject to equal stress, an assortment of explanations for this change in arterial health have been offered. Increased sugar consumption along with a deficiency of vitamins B, C, E, chromium, and other minerals and a lack of fiber in modern processed foods are prime suspects. According to Dr. Passwater[249], narrowed arteries are not caused by cholesterol dropping out of the blood but by an accumulation of mutant cells from food additives and pesticides clinging to arterial walls. (He recommends increased amounts of vitamins C and E plus selenium to counteract this.)

Other authorities regard poor blood-sugar control and lack of exercise responsible for the deposits on arterial walls. (It is known that refined sugar and carbohydrates increase the cholesterol level of the blood, and that exercise increases the "good" HDL levels.[208]) *Dr. Reuben's Everything You Always Wanted to Know About Nutrition*[273] reports the theory that polyunsaturated fats and low-cholesterol diets lower blood cholesterol levels only by forcing cholesterol out of the blood and onto the artery walls to create the plaques of atherosclerosis.

Heredity has a role in arterial health because of the inborn thickness of the arterial lining, which varies widely among people of any age group. Clinical studies have shown that identical diets will elevate blood cholesterol for some individuals and lower it for others. Some people have difficulty metabolizing saturated fats while others have a greater problem with refined sugar and alcohol increasing their serum cholesterol.

Until there are more definitive medical conclusions and cures, it seems wise to assume that all the experts are at least partially correct and to experiment with some of the natural remedies which have proven successful for the correction of hardened and narrowed arteries. As stated in *The American Journal of Clinical Nutrition* (November, 1980), "There is increasing evidence that arteriosclerosis is a substantially reversible process."

Diet and Supplements

There is mounting evidence that high cholesterol is an effect, not a cause, and that a "civilized diet" with white flour, white sugar, and processed foods results in hardening of the arteries and atherosclerosis. The recommended diet is one with natural, unprocessed foods predominating—less fat and meat, fewer eggs, more fish and chicken, and more fruits and vegetables.

Blood fats are classified into categories according to their density. The LDLs (low density lipoproteins) of saturated animal fats and hydrogenated vegetable fats are the villains. They pick up the triglycerides (which make up 98 percent of the weight of food fats) and transport them along with about 65 percent of the cholesterol in the blood. The polyunsaturated HDLs (high density lipoproteins) are the heroes. The oils from corn, safflower, sesame, sunflower, or soybeans help reduce the cholesterol in the blood about half as effectively as saturated fats raise it. Monosaturated olive and peanut oils are neutral, they do not seem to affect cholesterol levels. Current research has led most authorities to believe that naturally saturated fats are less likely to encourage hardened arteries than are hydrogenated vegetable fats. (Natural butter or lard in preference to vegetable shortening or partially hydrogenated margarine, and natural rather than processed cheeses.) In light dairy cream, approximately half the fats are saturated, while nondairy creamers contain 75 percent saturated fat from coconut oil, one of the most saturated fats in nature.[120]

International studies of hundreds of thousands of people over periods of from five to 15 years have shown that low-fat diets resulted in lower cholesterol levels than normal or high-fat diets, but that there was no significant difference in the death rates from heart disease. However, current recommendations are that the total percentage of all fats should not exceed one-third of the daily calories (one tablespoon of fat equals approximately 100 calories), with a two-to-one ratio of unsaturated to saturated fats.

Eggs are no longer four-letter words to be shunned. Besides their much-publicized cholesterol, eggs furnish an almost perfect protein plus lecithin and other protective nutrients. Although some authorities still suggest limiting egg consumption to three per week, several clinical studies have shown that after eating over half a dozen eggs every day, healthy people had lower cholesterol than when the tests began. More sophisticated methods of determining cholesterol content have resulted in reduced figures for shellfish. According to the 1982 edition of the Department of Agriculture's *Composition of Foods,* more than 12 oysters or two small lobsters would be required to equal the cholesterol in one egg.

In addition to their beneficial vitamins and minerals, fruits and vegetables are excellent sources of fiber and pectin to speed the progress of cholesterol-containing foods through the system and reduce the amount of cholesterol accumulated in the bloodstream. All fresh fruit and vegetable juices are considered beneficial, with beet, carrot, celery, parsley, pineapple, and spinach heading the list—up to two glasses daily of any combination are recommended.

The high pectin content of apples may account for their reputed ability to keep the doctor away. Pectin (available in other fruits and in supplemental capsules) limits the amount of cholesterol the body absorbs. Eating nothing but cherries for several days is a folk remedy for clearing accumulated debris from the arteries. Lemons and limes are believed to help liquefy fats and prepare them for elimination from the body. Laboratory tests have shown that high-fiber diets reduce the formation of fatty deposits in the arteries and increase the excretion of cholesterol from the body. All whole grains, dried legumes, and root vegetables are rich in fiber, but unprocessed oat or wheat bran is the most concentrated. The amount required for optimum effect varies with individuals and their diets—from one teaspoon for children to as much as three tablespoons three times daily for some adults.

A favorite folk medicine for thousands of years, garlic is now available in capsules which may be more pleasant and breathless than the one-fourth cup of raw garlic used to lower the LDLs and raise the HDL cholesterol levels in scientific tests. However it is taken, garlic dilates blood vessels and reduces cholesterol levels. Eggplant and onions are two other time-proven cholesterol-reducers with modern, scientific backing. Eating grated raw potatoes in salads or cereals is a Russian method of avoiding arteriosclerosis. Hospital tests have shown that yogurt lowers blood cholesterol by as much as 22 points when three cups are eaten daily.[120]

Modern research has also made some changes in the recommendations for beverages. Natural "hard" water helps prevent arteriosclerosis, but both heavily chlorinated and "soft" water have been shown to contribute to its development. Coffee, tea and other caffeine-containing beverages increase the fatty acids in the bloodstream and can be a factor in the development of atherosclerosis, so should be limited if not eliminated. Comfrey, mint, red clover, rosehips, and sage teas are folk-remedy suggestions as substitutes for those with hardening of the arteries.

Skimmed or fat-reduced milk is recommended in preference to whole milk. Questions have been raised regarding the effect of milk fats in relation to heart disease, but taking a folic acid supplement is believed to counteract any possible harm. Milk promotes the body's synthesis of vitamin B-6 to help prevent cholesterol deposits, and combines with fatty acids to increase the excretion of fats. Taking 1,000 to 2,000 milligrams of calcium daily for a year resulted in an average drop of 25 percent in cholesterol for volunteers tested. (*Lipids*, Vol. 7, 1972.)

Many studies have shown that alcoholic beverages, in moderation, lower cholesterol and reduce the risk of heart disease. As shown by recent tests at Baylor College in Texas, three glasses of beer per day raise the "good" HDL cholesterol levels as effectively as regular running or jogging. No more than two or three drinks per day are recommended, however, as more than that amount slows the blood flow and the alcohol not utilized for immediate energy is rapidly transformed into saturated fat.

Tobacco constricts the arteries, reduces HDL levels, and aggravates arteriosclerotic conditions. Pipes and cigars have less effect than cigarettes but it is recommended that all forms of tobacco be limited or avoided, and never accompanied by caffeine-containing beverages which intensify its action.

Whatever the foods selected, dividing the meals into several small ones each day has lowered serum cholesterol levels in a number of experiments, even when considerable amounts of animal fats were incorporated into the diet. Including daily supplements has been shown to prevent or correct hardened or narrowed arteries.

Vitamin A—10,000 to 25,000 units daily, up to 100,000 units for short periods. Clinical studies have shown that large amounts of vitamin A decrease cholesterol levels and increase the proportion of lecithin in the blood. In many of the underdeveloped countries where there is a low incidence of heart disease, the native diet provides large quantities of vitamin A. The tremendous amounts of vitamin A in the livers of fish, seals, and bears may account for the mystery of the fat-eating Eskimos' resistance to heart problems.

B Complex—One comprehensive, high-potency tablet daily. Several nutritionally-oriented physicians recommend adding up to 200 milligrams B-2 plus 500 milligrams each choline, inositol, and pantothenic acid. When taken together, choline and inositol heighten each other's effect. As therapy, 3,000 milligrams choline and 1,500 milligrams inositol may be taken daily, along with extra B-6 and large amounts of vitamin E.[154] As much as 600 milligrams of B-6 is required each day for the proper metabolization of fats by some people. Tests have shown that 100 to 3,000 milligrams niacin (not niacinamide) taken in divided doses every day lowers cholesterol levels. (The brief periods of flushing and tingling are said to diminish with continued use.) Folic acid, especially when taken with vitamins C and E, has been found to be an effective dilator for small arteries. In some cases, B-12 supplements or desiccated liver tablets have decreased serum cholesterol levels.

Brewer's Yeast and Chromium—One to two tablespoons brewer's yeast daily plus an additional 50 to 200 micrograms of GFT chromium. Brewer's yeast not only contains chromium, but intensifies the effectiveness of chromium supplements. As reported in *Journal of the American College of Nutrition* (Vol. 1, 1983), even one tablespoon brewer's yeast per day for eight weeks produced signficantly lower total cholesterol and a higher HDL cholesterol ratio. Other tests using two tablespoons of brewer's yeast plus chromium tablets for six weeks resulted in an average increase in HDL of over 17 percent, and an equal decrease in the "bad" LDL cholesterol.[334]

Vitamin C—500 to 10,000 milligrams daily, taken in divided doses with meals. Some researchers believe vitamin C is the key factor in averting atherosclerosis, which they feel may be a vitamin-C-deficiency disease. Large amounts of vitamin C help keep the artery walls healthy and less susceptible to atherosclerotic lesions, frequently instigate a rapid drop in blood cholesterol, and reduce the potentially dangerous LDL levels. In *Vitamin C, The Common Cold and the Flu*[251], Dr. Pauling reports that tests have shown 1,000 milligrams of vitamin C per day to have the same effect in controlling cholesterol levels as the elimination of five eggs per day from the diet. In another test, 450 milligrams of vitamin C plus 15 grams of citrus pectin lowered LDL as well as total blood cholesterol in six weeks. Dr. Wilfrid Shute[301] has reversed severe cases of atherosclerosis with 5,000 milligrams of C plus 1,200 IU of alpha-tocopherol daily, but large amounts of vitamin E should be taken only with medical supervision.

Cod Liver Oil—One tablespoon (or the equivalent in capsules) daily. As reported in *American Health* (May/June, 1982), studies have shown that cod liver oil reduced cholesterol by 15 percent and triglycerides by up to 85 percent. Biochemists have discovered that fish liver oils contain a substance with qualities similar to aspirin that may avert strokes by making blood platelets less sticky and possibly less likely to clot, without any of aspirin's side effects.

Vitamin E (see Caution, page 6)—400 to 1,200 IU daily. Vitamin E reportedly increases HDL levels while reducing total serum cholesterol, elevates blood lecithin, and helps dissolve arterial scars so that atherosclerotic deposits will not form. It also protects the essential fatty acids from being destroyed within the body and is of particular importance for those using unsaturated oils because they can deplete the body of vitamin E even though they contain the vitamin.

Kelp—Up to one teaspoon (or five tablets) of this dried, powdered seaweed is often recommended as a daily supplement for those with a sluggish thyroid. Kelp is a rich source of iodine which stimulates the thyroid and may help lower cholesterol.

Lecithin—One to five tablespoons lecithin granules daily. In worldwide studies, lecithin has proven effective for maintaining low cholesterol levels with a normal diet, lowering LDL levels and total cholesterol, and increasing the ratio of HDL cholesterol. In addition to emulsifying fats in the blood to prevent atherosclerosis, lecithin is believed to break up existing deposits on arterial walls.

Dr. Rinse utilized lecithin in his famous Breakfast Formula for preventing or correcting hardened and narrowed arteries. For an instant version: combine one tablespoon each lecithin granules, brewer's yeast, and wheat germ. Add cereal or yogurt, one teaspoon powdered bone meal, then sweeten to taste with brown sugar or honey.

Magnesium—200 to 400 milligrams daily when blood cholesterol levels are elevated as this condition is believed to increase the need for magnesium.

Seleniun—150 to 300 micrograms daily. Selenium works with vitamins C and E to prevent degeneration of the arteries and protect against arterial deposits.

Tissue Salts—Three or four tablets of the following 6X-potency tissue salts may be taken three or four times a day for reduced circulation caused by hardened or clogged arteries.

- Calc. Phos. if the hands and feet are always cold.
- Silicea for internal chilliness. If accompanied by cold extremities, add Nat. Mur.

Zinc—10 to 50 milligrams daily. Adequate amounts of zinc reduce the chances of cholesterol deposits clinging to the arteries. Recent tests have shown blood-fat levels to decrease as blood-zinc levels rose, and zinc supplementation has improved the condition of patients already suffering from hardened arteries.[256]

Exercise

Considerable evidence indicates that a sedentary lifestyle contributes to hardening of the arteries. Physical exercise stimulates circulation and strengthens heart muscles. The long-recognized protective effect of exercise may be due to its increasing HDL cholesterol levels. Any strenuous exercise program should be undertaken only with medical approval. Exercise alone is not the solution—athletes and blacksmiths develop arteriosclerosis. Exercise plus vitamins C, E, and lecithin is the combination favored by many medical nutritionists.

Nerve Pressure

Press inward and upward against the hinge of the jawbone, just in front of the ears. Press for 10 seconds, release for 10 seconds, and repeat three times once or twice each day.

Relaxation

As reported in *Your Good Health* (May, 1983), stress instigates a constant production of hormones, causing artery cells to mutate and form plaques. Devoting a few minutes each day to deliberate relaxation (see pages 9-10) may help counteract this effect.

Sources (See Bibliography)

3, 5, 12, 13, 24, 25, 37, 62, 68, 78, 81, 84, 89, 119, 120, 128, 136, 154, 159, 163, 165, 166, 173, 175, 189, 194, 203, 208, 227, 228, 229, 238, 243, 249, 250, 251, 252, 256, 261, 264, 270, 273, 274, 280, 282, 296, 297, 299, 301, 303, 319, 325, 331, 332, 335, 344, 348, 349, 350, 353, 354.

HAY FEVER AND SINUS PROBLEMS (See Also Allergy)

Known as a "catarrhal affection" for hundreds of years, the name "hay fever" was first used in the 1820s to describe indispositions occurring during the haying season in England. Allergic rhinitis is the medical term for seasonal hay fever. Perennial allergic rhinitis refers to the type that lasts throughout the year. Irritated sinus passages frequently accompany bouts of hay fever but "sinusitis" is a bacterial infection (see Infections) initiated by an allergy or cold that causes swollen tissue to plug up the opening of the sinuses. Blotting rather than forcefully blowing the nose may help avoid such infections.

Hereditary "chinks in the armor" may weaken the body enough to allow an allergen to gain a foothold. Individuals whose parents are allergy-free are less likely to be troubled by hay fever than those from families with allergy problems. When instigated by the inhalation of pollen, hay fever is usually seasonal but a conglomeration of nonpollen dusts may cause it to last all year. Air conditioners and home humidifiers are often helpful for this type of hay fever. (Humidifiers must be cleaned at frequent intervals to prevent the growth of molds which might cause additional allergic-respiratory distress.) Food allergies may be related to either type of allergic rhinitis, but the customary misery of itchy eyes, sneezing, and drippy or stuffy nose is nearly always caused by inhaled substances—although there are instances of emotion-triggered or psychosomatic hay fever.

Deficiencies of vitamins, protein, or almost any nutrient can increase the permeability of the cells so that harmful substances enter them more readily. When foreign irritants reach the blood, the body forms histamines. In most normal persons, the liver destroys any excess histamine. Those with allergies are often unable to produce sufficient amounts of the histamine-destroying enzyme, either from inherited tendencies or from liver toxicity (possibly engendered by the overuse of antihistamine drugs). Some commercial antihistamines may thicken the mucus lining the nasal passages and sinus cavities, blocking them to create pain and infection. Thinning the mucus to keep it flowing by using a humidifier, or avoiding the formation of excess mucus by taking vitamins C, B-6, and pantothenic acid may be safer solutions. Natural remedies and the antihistamine action produced by the body do not provoke the drowsiness or other possibly harmful side effects that may result from over-the-counter or prescription medications.

Diet and Supplements

The relationship between diet and hay fever is still not clear but it seems that alcohol, coffee, fried foods, salt, sugar, and tobacco can contribute to allergic conditions. Doctors have found that mild, dormant food allergies can be aroused as a result of the additional stress put on the body during hay fever season. In their book, *The Complete Allergy Guide*[267], Howard Rapaport and Shirley Linde cite strong evidence to show that chocolate candy is a major cause of allergic rhinitis, particularly in children, and that eating chocolate can intensify the effects of other mild allergies already present. Drinking pasteurized-homogenized milk has been found responsible for hay fever in some adults as well as children. (This can be home-tested by avoiding milk for two or three weeks.) Some authorities believe that hay fever is due to an excess of fats and concentrated carbohydrates in the diet, and can be corrected by the same treatment used for controlling low blood sugar (which see).

Much body fluid is lost through coughing, sneezing, and nasal discharge, so the intake of liquids should be increased. The enzymes in raw juices are believed to neutralize the sensitivity-causing histamines that trigger hay fever symptoms. One or two daily glasses of equal amounts of cabbage, carrot, cucumber, and tomato juice, or any combination of beet, carrot, celery, cucumber, parsley, and spinach juices, have been found helpful. Alternating one day of regular meals with one day of nothing but fresh raw fruits and vegetables and their juices has brought relief for some seasonal-hay fever sufferers.[334] Eating acidophilus yogurt every day (or taking acidophilus capsules with meals) is also beneficial because the acidophilus destroys certain histamine-liberating bacteria in the intestinal tract.[89]

Individual reactions are so varied that no one remedy can be expected to help everyone uniformly, but the most universally successful is a three-vitamin combo taken each four or five hours when beset by hay fever, sinus problems, or post-nasal drip.

> 500 milligrams vitamin C + 500 milligrams bioflavonoids (available in combination tablets)
> 100 milligrams pantothenic acid
> 50 milligrams B-6

If no relief is discernible after 30 minutes, a second round of all three can be taken. Some individuals may need to increase the amounts to 1,000 milligrams each vitamin C and pantothenic acid and 500 milligrams B-6 before their symptoms disappear. Since these vitamins are water soluble, any excess is merely excreted, but, if continual use is required for more than a few days, it is wise to take a comprehensive B-complex tablet daily to avoid the possibility of creating a deficiency of the other B vitamins.

Case History

Before Gayle D. began teaching school she simply endured her annual bout of hay fever by hibernating inside her house for three weeks each spring. Knowing that she must find another solution this year, Gayle got a prescription for antihistamines from her doctor, and tried first one and then another over-the-counter remedy—all with discouraging results. If they worked at all they made her either too drowsy or too nervous to cope with her second-grade students, so she took the medication only in the evenings and suffered through the days in bleary-eyed, sniffly misery. A fellow teacher, observing her discomfort, described the Vitamin C-Pantothenic Acid-B-6 remedy (see above) that several of her friends had found effective. Gayle stopped at a health food store on her way home from school, took the combination as directed, and noticed some relief within a few minutes. After experimenting with the doubled amounts, Gayle found that taking the regular dosage every two hours worked better for her—worked so well in fact that she thoroughly enjoyed their class trip to the zoo on a breezy spring day.

A more complex hay fever cure is recorded by Rex Adams in *Miracle Medicine Foods*[3]: to the C, pantothenic acid, and B-6 combination, add one vitamin A and D supplement, 600 IU vitamin E, six tablets each bone meal and kelp, three capsules each unsaturated fatty acids and lecithin, two garlic perles, and one tablespoon brewer's yeast each day.

Since allergic reactions lower the body's resistance, many nutritionally-oriented physicians advise giving it a boost with a daily multi-vitamin-mineral tablet in addition to any supplements taken therapeutically.

Vitamin A—25,000 to 100,000 units daily for one to four months, then 10,000 to 25,000 units per day for maintenance. Vitamin A protects the mucous membranes against air pollution, decreases the permeability of the cells, thins mucus, and reduces susceptibility to infection. A deficiency can harden the membranes to prevent the mucus from moving normally. Vitamin E is required for proper utilization of vitamin A. Adding 10 to 50 milligrams of zinc each day aids the mobilization of vitamin A and is believed to help prevent sinusitis.

B Complex—One comprehensive, high-potency tablet daily, to compensate for the stress created by allergic reactions. Additional amounts of B-6 and pantothenic acid have an antihistamine, antimucus effect and are particularly effective when taken with vitamin C and bioflavonoids (see above).

Vitamin C—1,000 to 10,000 milligrams daily to detoxify foreign substances entering the body, decrease cell permeability, and inhibit the production of histamines. Tests in Yugoslavia established that 500 milligrams of vitamin C were more effective than a prescription bronchodilator in increasing breathing capacity for people working in environments polluted with dust.[261] Because vitamin C is used up during the detoxifying process, the quantity required is in proportion to the amount of toxic material entering the body. Small amounts of vitamin C do not have an antihistamine effect, but taking as little as 250 milligrams at three-hour intervals has been advantageous in some cases. Severe hay fever symptoms have responded in minutes after 2,000 milligrams of vitamin C were taken.[89] Continuing to take 1,000 milligrams each hour frequently abates an attack that resisted the first dosage.[305] When taking vitamin C for hay fever, the benefits are intensified if bioflavonoids are included. Separate tablets of bioflavonoids are available, as are combinations with vitamin C. Best results have been obtained with the addition of the B vitamins listed above.

Calcium—Up to 2,000 milligrams per day, depending on the amount of dairy products used. A lack of calcium is considered one of the main factors in allergies of all kinds.

Vitamin E (see Caution, page 6)—100 to 600 IU daily. Although vitamin E is not usually recognized as having antihistamine properties, tests conducted in Japan have shown that vitamin E suppresses hay fever symptoms, particularly when taken before the irritation occurs.[3]

Tissue Salts

- **For acute hay fever**—Take 3X Ferr. Phos. and Nat. Mur. in alternate doses each half hour until relieved.
- **For chronic, year-round hay fever**—Take 12X Kali. Phos., Nat. Mur., and Silicea each two hours in alternation for two days, then twice daily.
- **For sneezing**—Take three tablets of 6X Silicea. (Often stops a violent sneezing-fit in mid-sneeze.)

Case History

Linda C. developed a peculiar complication during her pregnancy. She had never been troubled by either allergies or hay fever, but now she went into a paroxysm of sneezing at the touch of a cool breeze or a draft of cold air. Linda tried to stand behind the refrigerator door when she opened it, but the sneezes usually began before she could place anything on a shelf. With advancing pregnancy the prolonged bouts of sneezing became more than a nuisance, they were discomforting. She did present a comical sight, however, as she attempted to cover her nose and mouth while holding her abdomen with both hands. A friend who had not been able to resist laughing at Linda's maneuvers pulled out a purse pillbox and told Linda to place three of the tiny white pellets under her tongue. Before the friend could explain that the pellets were a tissue salt, silicea, Linda's sneezes had ceased. For the remainder of her pregnancy Linda kept a container of 6X Silicea within reach so that she could halt each incipient bout of sneezing after the first sneeze or two.

- **For a stuffy nose**—Take 3X Kali. Mur. four times during the day or night.

- **For ulcerations inside the nose from constant irritation**—Use Calc. Phos. in the 3X potency three times daily for children. For adults, use 12X Silicea three times a day.

Exercise

Vigorous exercise such as rope skipping or stationary bike riding produces a constricting effect in the small blood vessels which sometimes improves hay fever symptoms in less than five minutes.[52]

Folk Remedies

During the years between 1600 and 1800 a diet of foxes' lungs and the application of leeches to draw out evil humors were recommended for the miseries of a catarrhal affection. Some of the less exotic folk remedies, however, are still being used with success.

Apple Cider Vinegar—For an acute nasal drip: three times a day for four days, drink a glass of water containing five tablespoons of apple cider vinegar. Reduce to three tablespoons vinegar twice a day for one month, then to once a day. When the condition has cleared, one glass of the mixture each two weeks is suggested for preventive maintenance.

Castor Oil—Stir five drops of castor oil into a glass of juice or water and drink before breakfast each morning to help sinusitis and nasal congestions.

Citrus Peel, which contains bioflavonoids, has been used in numerous ways:

- **For a runny nose**—Dry 1-inch squares of tangerine peel at room temperature for one week. Store in an air-tight container, then chew and swallow one square to squelch a drippy nose.
- **For seasonal hay fever**—Take one teaspoon grated lemon or orange peel, plain or sweetened with honey, each morning and night.
- **To prevent sleep-disturbing clogged nasal passages**—Soak small strips of orange peel in apple cider vinegar for several hours. Drain, add honey to the peel and cook until thick, then eat several strips at bedtime.

Cod Liver Oil—For sinus congestion and pain, take one tablespoon cod liver oil each morning.

Coffee and Chocolate—Although either can trigger or intensify hay fever for some individuals, drinking several cups of strong black coffee has relieved sneezing and itching in some cases. An old English folk remedy was drinking three or four cups of a mixture of coffee and hot chocolate each day.

Comfrey Tea is believed to reduce sensitivity to pollens and have a positive effect on allergy coughs. For hay fever, drink one cup of comfrey tea at noon and one at night. When disturbed by coughing, take one-half cup strong comfrey tea with one teaspoon honey.

Fenugreek Tea—Drinking one cup of fenugreek tea each day for a month or two before and during hay-fever season has been successful in alleviating the symptoms for many people.

Garlic—Eat raw garlic (or take two garlic perles) every four hours to relieve congestion caused by hay fever. Garlic is believed to destroy the offending bacteria in the intestinal tract that are responsible for forming histamines.

Honey and Bee Pollen—Raw, unfiltered honey with its natural pollen content has long been used to build up immunity to hay fever and to relieve its symptoms. For best results, the honey should be made by bees in the areas near where the hay fever occurs.

- Take two tablespoons raw honey each day, starting one month before the hay-fever season. Supplementing the honey with bee pollen granules or tablets may increase the benefits. In the South, an equal amount of whiskey is used to enhance the effectiveness of the honey.
- Chewing honey-comb cappings once each day for a month before the hay-fever season has either prevented or reduced symptoms. If an attack does occur, chewing one teaspoon of honey comb is believed helpful.
- Taking a 1,000-milligram bee-pollen tablet three times a day for one month has quelled chronic post-nasal drip for some individuals.

Horseradish—To help clear the sinus passages without damage to the mucous membranes, take one-half teaspoon prepared horseradish plus a few drops of lemon juice each morning and evening. When fresh horseradish is available, grate ¼ pound and mix with the juice of one lemon. Store in the refrigerator, then take one teaspoon twice each day. (Horseradish acts as a solvent and cleanser of abnormal mucus.)

Mustard—To open sinus passages, folk healers mix one teaspoon dry mustard with two tablespoons vegetable oil, then massage into the forehead.

Onion—Another favorite folk remedy for unclogging nasal passages and helping restore free breathing:

- Cover a sliced, raw onion with one cup water and let stand for one minute. Remove the onion and sip the water. Repeat with a fresh onion several times each day.
- Grate half a raw onion into two cups scalded milk and drink. Repeat morning and evening.
- Inhale the vapors of a fresh-cut onion several times a day and place a bowl of sliced onions by the bedside at night.

Potato—To relieve congested sinuses: quarter one large potato and boil in two cups water until tender. Remove the potato and inhale the steam.

Rose Petals and Pekoe Tea—To relieve sore, irritated eyes: steep one teaspoon dried rose petals in one cup hot water. Filter and apply the liquid to the eyes four or five times each day. If desired, one teaspoon prepared pekoe tea may be used in place of or in addition to the rose petals.

Nerve Massage

- Briskly rub both ears to relieve a stuffy nose.

- Massage the thumbs, index and middle fingers, and the webs between them, on both hands.
- Rub the front tip of each toe, just below the toenail.
- Massage a spot on the bottom of each foot about an inch toward the toes from the heel pad and a little toward the outer edge of the foot.

Nerve Pressure

For sneezing—Press the hollow directly above the center of the upper lip for 10 seconds and repeat three times.

For general symptoms of hay fever (unless otherwise indicated, apply pressure for 10 seconds, wait 10 seconds, then repeat for a total of 30 seconds pressure.)

- Use the index fingers to press in an upward direction on both sides of the nostrils.
- Wrap the thumbs, first, and second fingers of both hands with rubber bands. Leave in place for 10 to 15 minutes—less, if the fingers begin to turn blue.
- Press a point in the center of the chest.
- Press 1½ inches directly below the navel.
- For up to 20 minutes' relief from sinus pain, pinch the skin between the eyebrows three times for 10 seconds each; or apply 10 seconds of pressure to each of these spots in succession for two or three rotations: the top of the head at the center of the skull...the hairline directly above the nose...the center of the forehead...both sides of the nose just below the bridge...both sides of the nostrils ...both sides of the jawline, directly beneath the corners of the mouth.

Sources (See Bibliography)

3, 7, 9, 13, 22, 48, 52, 53, 62, 63, 64, 67, 68, 76, 78, 85, 86, 89, 94, 98, 116, 142, 152, 153, 156, 160, 165, 168, 173, 180, 181, 189, 226, 229, 243, 254, 261, 288, 293, 297, 305, 315, 318, 325, 327, 328, 330, 333, 334, 335, 350.

HEADACHE—TENSION, VASCULAR, AND MIGRAINE

Humanity's oldest and most common malady, headaches are never fatal but some of the attempted remedies have been. Prehistoric skeletons bear testimony to a crude form of trephination—holes chiseled in skulls to allow the escape of pain-provoking demons. During the Middle Ages, pseudo-physicians cut into the skulls of headache sufferers and pretended to remove "head stones," explaining that stones caused head pain in the same manner as stones in the kidneys. Ancient Greeks attributed headaches to an excess of body fluid, or humor, which they drained by using heated cups to draw blood from cuts in the scalp or temples.

During the past few decades, scientific studies have analyzed the interrelationship between the blood vessels of the circulatory (vascular) system, the nerves, and specialized muscles within the confines of the head. From the bewildering variety of causes and kinds of headaches, two principal categories emerge. Tension headaches resulting from involuntary contraction of neck, scalp, and forehead muscles in response to stressful situations, and "vascular"—such as migraine, hunger, and high-altitude headaches—caused by dilation of the blood vessels. Dr. Harold Wolff, a pioneer in the study of headaches, describes them all as "biologic reprimands"—warnings that the body is out of balance. Identifying which type of headache is present makes it possible to apply proper treatment for prompt relief. Remedies for miscellaneous or combination headaches follow the segments on Tension, Vascular, and Migraine headaches.

Tension Headaches

By far the most common, tension headaches are controllable and are not dangerous, just miserable. When certain muscles are subjected to prolonged tension (from slumping over a desk, hunching one shoulder to hold a telephone, straining to see in poor light, driving in traffic, or from psychological stresses of anxiety, excitement, resentment, or repressed anger), they contract. This restricts the flow of blood and temporarily damages muscle cells which then transmit warning signals of pain to the brain. The painful sensation tends to be a dull ache, usually more intense across the forehead and temples. When the tension is relaxed and normal blood-flow resumed, the pain fades away. A feeling of tightness in the neck muscles is an early-warning sign of tension headache. Shifting position, taking a walk, or moving as many parts of the body as possible, and breathing deeply while putting the immediate emotional pressure into perspective, often forestalls the headache.

> **Beverages**—One glass of wine or other alcoholic drink may encourage muscle relaxation and help dilate the constricted blood vessels. Coffee, however, should be avoided during a tension headache as caffeine has a constricting action on the blood vessels. Its excessive use has been linked to some cases of recurrent tension headaches.
>
> **Exercise and Massage**—Pressing the fingertips in the center of the forehead and drawing them gently toward the ears is particularly beneficial for tension headaches. Squeezing and releasing the tense neck muscles often helps, as does locking the fingers behind the back of the neck and tilting the head back as far as possible. This should be followed by drooping the head forward and slowly rolling it in the widest possible circle while pressing the base of the skull with the fingertips.

Case History

Marlys L. had a headache every workday afternoon. She went to an ophthalmologist who declared that her eyes were fine. Neither her doctor nor her dentist could discover a physical explanation for her headaches. Marlys tried pain pills but they upset her stomach, befuddled her mind, or made her nervous—and did little to alleviate the headaches. When she complained to her husband, he told her to quit her job—it was too stressful. When she mentioned her daily headaches to her employer, he offered to hire a part-time assistant for her; but she refused because there was not enough work to warrant another employee. Marlys enjoyed her position as office manager and could not believe that merely being busy at something she did well could be the cause of her headaches. She did, however, sign up for a class on stress management, and learned that stress could be physical as well as mental. By practicing the relaxing "neck roll" (described above) at least once each hour, and nestling the telephone on her right shoulder instead of the left when she was not writing down what was being said, Marlys "cured" her persistent headaches by forestalling their arrival.

Garlic—Taking one minced clove of garlic in one teaspoon raw honey is a remedy credited to the American Indians. (Scientists have demonstrated that garlic dilates the small veins and arteries.)

Heat increases the blood supply to taut muscles, making them more pliable and carrying away the pain-inducing toxins that accumulate in strained tissue. Standing under a hot shower with the water pulsating on the back of the neck, or soaking in a comfortably hot tub for 15 minutes, is most effective but a hot towel, hot water bottle, or heating pad placed at the back of the neck may suffice.

Nerve Massage—To relax neck tension, massage one big toe and rotate it round and round, then repeat with the other foot. When toe-massage is not feasible, massaging the thumbs of both hands may bring relief.

Nerve Pressure

- **For headache from eyestrain or sinus pressure**—Use the tips of the thumbs to press upward under the beginning of the eyebrows next to the nose. Exert pressure for 10 seconds, release for 10 seconds, and repeat three times.
- **For headache due to nervous strain or neuralgia**—Press the thumb against the roof of the mouth and maintain pressure for from three to five minutes. If the headache is extensive, shift the pressure to cover the rest of the roof of the mouth.

Pillows—Feather-stuffed bed pillows may be a cause of allergic headaches for some individuals, but switching to foam rubber pillows may result in tension headaches for others. (The springy action of foam pillows causes a gradual tightening of the neck and upper back muscles in an attempt to hold the head still—causing compression on the spinal cord.[53])

Tissue Salts

- **For a frontal headache**—Take three tablets each 6X Kali. Phos. and Mag. Phos. each half hour while acute, then less often.
- **For a heavy headache**—Take three tablets 6X Kali. Sulph. each half hour until the pain lessens.

Vitamins and Minerals—An extra 10,000 to 25,000 units of vitamin A each day may correct recurring tension headaches due to overuse of the eyes. Niacin (not niacinamide) dilates the capillaries and blood vessels. Taking 50 milligrams at the onset of a tension headache may produce a flush and prickling sensation, but often relieves the congestion. Up to 1,000 milligrams of niacin, in divided doses during the day, has been used to bring relief in severe cases but such massive doses should have medical approval. Two to four dolomite tablets (containing calcium and magnesium) aid muscle relaxation and act as tranquilizers.

Vascular Headaches

This category encompasses the wide range of throbbing, pulsating headaches resulting from blood surging through swollen, stretched blood vessels. The enlarged veins and arteries irritate adjacent nerve endings which send pain messages to the brain. Vascular headaches are often designated as "toxic" because they signal an imbalance in the body caused by some toxic substance. These headaches can be triggered by inhalants (cigarette smoke, motor exhaust or paint fumes, smog, high-altitude air, etc.) or sleeping in a poorly ventilated room or with the head under the covers. Any reduction of the concentration of oxygen in the blood requires dilation of the blood vessels to provide sufficient oxygen for the brain.

Individual reactions to certain foods, or lack of proper food, are believed responsible for most vascular headaches. Research regarding the causes of migraine headaches has shown that many "ordinary" headaches also are triggered by serotonin (a pain inducer) and/or the amino acid, tyramine, present in aged cheeses, avocados, bananas, beer, canned figs, chicken livers, chocolate, cola drinks, pickled herring, red wine, and spinach. Allergists add cane sugar, citrus fruits, corn, eggs, fish, milk, nuts, plums, pork, and wheat to the list of possible instigating factors.

Monosodium Glutamate (MSG), the flavor-enhancer so prevalent in Oriental foods, TV dinners, and other commercially prepared foods, enlarges the blood vessels. The nitrates and nitrites employed as perservatives in bacon, corned beef, frankfurters, hams, and lunch meats relax the muscles that control the size of the blood vessels, allowing them to stretch enough to bring on headaches for many people. (Nitro-glycerine, used in the treatment of angina, is a nitrate compound.)

To self-test for reactive foods, eliminate all questionable items from the diet for one week. Then reintroduce them one at a time, eating the same food twice in one day. When a headache does result, postpone further testing for at least four days. A second test of each offending substance may be wise. Once the testing is complete, the incriminated foods and future headaches may be avoided. A study reported in the *Canadian Journal of Neurological Sciences* (May, 1981) indicated that food allergies caused 75 percent of the vascular headaches for 250 volunteers tested.

Hunger headaches occur when the blood-sugar levels drop so low that more blood must be pumped through the head to maintain an adequate supply for the brain. Excitement, emotional pressure, or extreme physical exertion cause the body to consume sugar at a faster rate, thus lowering the glucose levels even when regular meals have been eaten. (Adverse reactions to certain foods can produce the same effect.) Since the end result of eating sugar is a depletion of sugar in the blood (see Low Blood Sugar), a glass of milk or a handful of peanuts is a better remedy than a candy bar. Sugar "binges" of birthday cake or Christmas goodies trigger headaches for some individuals. If headaches appear with regularity, reducing the amount of sugary foods and eating a protein-rich snack between meals may prevent them.

Too much heat from the sun dilates blood vessels as well as depleting the body's mineral supplies through perspiration. Anything that upsets the hormonal balance—

anger, extreme exertion, even sexual orgasm—may trigger a vascular headache in members of either sex. The menstrual cycle, oral contraceptives, and estrogen supplements help account for the preponderance of these headaches among women. Frequent vascular headaches that do not respond to natural remedies, or those accompanied by fever, warrant medical examination as they may accompany high blood pressure or other maladies.

Beverages—Drinking a glass of fresh cabbage, celery, lettuce, or other green vegetable juice may neutralize the reaction of food chemicals in the system to bring quick relief. Recurrent headaches may be thwarted by limiting one meal every other day to nothing but raw juices. Coffee has a constricting effect on blood vessels. Those who are not accustomed to drinking much coffee may derive immediate relief from a cup of it taken strong and black. However, people who regularly consume large amounts of caffeine in coffee, tea, or soft drinks adapt to this vascular constriction and may suffer a headache when deprived of their customary quantity. Alcohol dilates blood vessels (see Hangover) so should be shunned while a vascular headache is in progress. The Vermont remedy, publicized by Dr. Jarvis[181], was a mixture of one tablespoon each apple cider vinegar and raw honey in a glass of water. This was to be repeated in 30 minutes, if necessary. Drinking ginger tea while heating the feet with a mustard plaster (or in hot water with dry mustard) was a favorite folk remedy for this type of headache.

Foot Baths—Soaking the feet in hot water for 15 to 20 minutes draws blood away from the head to bring relief from a throbbing headache. Adding a spoonful or so of dry mustard to the water is a folk-medicine tip for intensifying the effect. When an appropriate basin is not available, half-fill a bathtub with hot water and sit on the edge to soak the feet and ankles.

Ice Packs—Cold helps contract swollen vessels and reduce the pulsating flow of blood. Place the ice pack on the forehead, on top of the head, or around the neck. Cold packs are especially effective when combined with a hot footbath.

Nerve Pressure—Press each point for 10 seconds, release for 10 seconds, and repeat three times.

- Press the soft spot on the front part of the top of the head.
- Hook the thumbs under each side of the jawbone while applying pressure to the temples with the fingers.
- Gently press the carotid arteries on both sides of the Adam's Apple.

Tissue Salts

- **For pain primarily in the back of the head**—Take three tablets each 6X Ferr. Phos., Kali. Mur., and Kali. Sulph. each half hour for an acute condition, then less often.
- **For a frontal headache with nausea**—Take three tablets of 6X Calc. Sulph. three times daily.
- **For a sick headache focused on top of the head**—Take 6X Nat. Phos. frequently until relieved.

- **For a sick headache accompanied by neuralgia**—Take 6X Nat. Sulph at frequent intervals.
- **For sharp or shooting headache pain**—Take 6X Mag. Phos. at 15-minute intervals until relieved.

Vitamins and Minerals—B vitamins are necessary for normal body metabolism and the control of blood-vessel dilation. Headaches resulting from a lack of these vitamins may be due to poor absorption rather than an insufficiency in the diet. Eating acidophilus yogurt daily (or taking the capsules with meals) may re-establish the bacteria, sometimes destroyed by antibiotics, which help the body absorb and synthesize B vitamins. Immediate relief has been obtained by taking the following vitamin-mineral combination to normalize circulation, combat toxicity, and relax the nerves:

1 high-potency B-complex tablet
50 milligrams B-6
100 milligrams pantothenic acid
1,000 to 2,000 milligrams vitamin C
2 dolomite (calcium + magnesium) tablets

MIGRAINE AND CLUSTER (OR HISTAMINE) HEADACHES

The name, migraine, is derived from the Greek word used by Galen to describe this disorder in 200 A.D. Six-thousand-year-old Sumarian writings refer to the ravages of migraine headaches, and the tomb of Pharoah Ahkenaton contained formulas to be prepared from hippopotamus hide and poppy seeds for their treatment. Before headaches were clinically classified, migraines were known as "sick headaches." Now they fall under the vascular heading but are subdivided into "classic" or "common" migraines, and "cluster" headaches. Migraines are discriminatory by nature—10 times more men than women have cluster headaches, while classic and common migraines occur in four times more women than men.[24] No one who is subject to any of them requires a descriptive analysis of the symptoms, but understanding the anatomy of a migraine may aid in coping with its immediate problems and preventing future attacks.

Classic migraines are preceded by a 15-to 30-minute "prodrome" or "aura"—a set of symptoms including visual disturbances, flashes or zigzags of light, nausea, distorted perception, and other extraordinary sensations. Some of the religious visions of the Middle Ages are attributed to the visual effects and distortions of the prodrome—Lewis Carroll immortalized his in *Alice in Wonderland*. In the common migraine, the prodrome symptoms may last for several hours or several days but are generalized into feelings of unease or excitement, with only slight disturbances of perception. Cluster headaches tend to recur in rapid succession over a period of weeks or months, then disappear for several months before returning in another cluster of headaches. They lack the prodrome symptoms, usually affect only one side of the head, are even more painful than other migraines, but rarely last longer than an hour or so.

Migraine headaches progress through a sequence of blood-vessel narrowing followed by blood-vessel widening. (Prodrome sensations are a result of the constriction. Pain is produced by the dilation and irritation from chemical substances in the blood or around the swollen blood vessels.) A hereditary, genetic instability of the system of nerves controlling the constriction and dilation of arteries is considered responsible for the migraine syndrome. Some authorities believe that migraine and Meniere's Disease (which see) are related to the same metabolic imbalance.

Any of the "triggers" listed under vascular headaches can bring on a migraine for a susceptible individual. Diets rich in animal fats provoke some migraines, a sudden increase in salt intake may cause problems as may changes in barometric pressure, and the connection between hormonal estrogens and migraine in women has been firmly established. In 95 percent of migraine victims, eating ice cream or other extremely cold foods without allowing them to warm in the mouth stimulates nerve endings which can instigate a migraine headache.[235] Breathing pure oxygen for 15 minutes shrinks the dilated blood vessels and usually cures a cluster headache. Alcohol should be avoided as it further dilates blood vessels and even a few sips can precipitate another attack during a cluster episode.

Several experts, including Dr. Miles Atkinson (an otologist on the faculty of New York University) consider migraines to be a matter of nutrition rather than being of emotional or psychosomatic origin. Much publicity has been given recent research regarding tyramine-containing foods, and self-testing frequently brings good results (see Vascular Headaches, above). But years of recorded medical reports show that over 80 percent of migraine sufferers have abnormal glucose tolerance levels (see Low Blood Sugar). The value of B vitamins in maintaining normal vascular control has been well-established. A B-complex tablet taken with vitamin C plus extra B-6 and pantothenic acid has an antihistamine, anti-toxic effect that counteracts inhaled and ingested substances that might otherwise bring on a migraine attack (see Hay Fever).

Headache clinics across the country are reporting success rates of 95 to 98 percent by helping their patients identify their own particular "triggers" so they can be avoided, adjusting their diets to prevent fluctuations in blood-sugar levels, increasing vitamin intake, and encouraging the use of self-relaxation techniques (see pages 9-10).

The control of migraine headaches is an individual matter. For do-it-yourself therapy, a statistically sound program would entail adhering to a low blood sugar diet, reinforcing it with vitamins B and C, and testing for known migraine-causing foods while relieving mental tensions through physical exercise and positive thinking. Less involved than it sounds, this regimen has permanently prevented migraines for many people and is worth the effort to avoid even one day of migraine suffering. Any of the vascular or miscellaneous remedies may be helpful once a migraine is in full force but, when counterattacked on the onset, some migraines have been bested by the following natural remedies.

Apple Cider Vinegar—To prevent migraine headaches, take two teaspoons apple cider vinegar in a glass of water with each meal. When the pain of a migraine has started: combine equal amounts of apple cider vinegar and water in a saucepan, bring to boiling, and inhale the vapors for 75 breaths.[168]

Coffee—Drinking one cup of strong black coffee (not decaffeinated) with or without the juice of half a lemon, at the first stage of the prodrome, may prevent a migraine from developing.

Exercise—A few minutes of vigorous exercise when the pressure first begins to build up has stopped all varieties of migraines for many people. Aerobic exercise is believed to suppress some trigger mechanism related to migraines. According to *Medicine and Science in Sports and Exercise* (Vol. 13, No. 2, 1981), migraine sufferers had significantly fewer headaches during a 15-week program of walking and running for 30 minutes a day three days each week.

Hair Dryer—When used at the first sign of a migraine, the humming sound and heat from a stand-type hair dryer banished pain for two-thirds of the volunteers in scientific tests.[52,315]

Honey—At the onset of a headache, take one tablespoon raw honey, then take another in 20 minutes with two or three glasses of water.

Hot and Cold Applications—During the first-stage symptoms, applying heat to the neck and head may relieve the constriction. Once the blood vessels have dilated, ice packs can be used to decrease their size and reduce both circulation and the sensitivity of the painful nerve endings.

Nerve Massage

- Place the thumbs behind the earlobes and firmly massage the bottom of the lobes with the fingers.
- Using oil to lessen friction, vigorously rub the second joint of each thumb.

Case History

As a practicing psychiatarist, Dr. Tad V. found his increasingly frequent migraine headaches more than a discomforting nuisance; they were a menace to his professional future. When his college roommate, now a medical doctor who had studied reflexology, arrived for a visit during one of Tad's headaches, Tad was more than willing to experiment with anything that might relieve his misery. The visiting doctor began by massaging the ball of Tad's right foot, worked his way up to the pad behind the nail on Tad's big toe, and smiled with relief when Tad winced with pain. They had located the pressure point. Then he told Tad to take over and gently, but persistently, rub the toe until the pressure was no longer painful. Surprisingly, the pain in Tad's head was also fading. Even more amazing, by massaging his toe at the first indication of an approaching headache, Dr. Tad has never suffered from another migraine—and it has been over 20 years since that first demonstration of nerve massage.

Nerve Pressure—Press the thumb of one hand into the palm of the other as firmly as possible, then repeat with the other hand.

Tissue Salts—At the onset of a migraine headache, take three tablets of 6X Nat. Mur. Repeat in four hours, if needed.

Vitamins and Minerals—Deficiencies of any vitamin or mineral can trigger migraines for some individuals, particularly under stress conditions. A daily, preventive combination recommended by Dr. Van Fleet[325] is: 30,000 units vitamin A, 6,000 milligrams vitamin C, 1,000 IU vitamin D, and 30 milligrams zinc. Either singly or in various combinations, other dietary supplements have reduced the frequency and intensity of migraines for many people and completely abolished them for others.

- **B Complex**—One comprehensive tablet plus two tablespoons brewer's yeast daily has brought complete relief to some migraine sufferers. Others, particularly women taking oral contraceptives and individuals who drink much alcohol, have found that adding 100 milligrams of B-6 solves the problem. Some have received the most help by taking 50 milligrams of B-6 plus 1,000 milligrams of calcium each day between headaches. Taking 50 milligrams of niacin (not niacinamide) at the first symptom of a migraine may abort it. If no flushing is experienced, the dosage should be repeated in 10 minutes. (The flushing and prickling indicate that the capillaries are being dilated to relieve the pressure.)
- **Vitamin E** (see Caution, page 6)—Taking 1,200 IU of vitamin E in four divided doses each day has prevented migraines for some individuals.
- **Lecithin**—The moment a migraine threatens, take one tablespoon lecithin granules or 10 1,200-milligram lecithin capsules. Another option is to blend one teaspoon each lecithin granules and brewer's yeast with one tablespoon wheat germ and one glass of fresh vegetable juice, apple juice, or milk. (Myalin sheaths, composed largely of lecithin, insulate the nerve endings of blood vessels against outside influences.[331]) Taking one tablespoon of lecithin granules every day has been known to reduce the frequency and duration of migraines, and has prevented recurrence in some cases.
- **Tryptophan**—According to *Dr. Atkins' Nutrition Breakthrough*[24], taking two grams of this amino acid each day between headaches, four grams when a migraine does strike, has proven effective for half the migraine patients he treats.
- **Zinc**—15 to 50 milligrams daily. Studies have shown migraine headaches to decrease in incidence and severity when zinc supplements accompanied an adequate diet.

Miscellaneous Headaches

Many headaches are a garden-variety combination of tension plus vascular dysfunction. Very few are caused by serious conditions such as brain tumors or cerebral hemorrhages. However, perpetual or severe headaches that do not respond to natural remedies should be investigated by a physician. They may be the result of an imbalance of the bite (temporomandibular joint syndrome) or spinal maladjustment. True "sinus headaches" are rare but when they do occur, professional draining may be required.

Experts warn that drugs of any sort are not sufficient for those with extremely painful headaches. Over-the-counter painkillers such as aspirin and acetaminophin (Datril, Tylenol, etc.) are generally too mild to help migraine sufferers. The intensity of pain has been scientifically measured by "dols" on a scale of 1 to 10. Most headaches range between 2 and 4 dols, but some have registered as high as 8 or 9. Since pain relievers like aspirin act primarily by increasing the amount of nerve stimulation needed to produce pain, a headache that is producing a 2-dol pain may disappear when two aspirin are taken, but a 4-dol headache will not be reduced to 2-dols by the two aspirin, and increasing the dosage does not help. Aspirin is an acid that irritates the stomach lining and may trigger an ulcer attack in susceptible people. Acetaminophens achieve similar pain relief without upsetting the stomach, but prolonged or excessive use of either can harm the kidneys or liver. The more-potent painkillers available by prescription may prove counterproductive and lead to addiction.[314] Tracking down the provoking factors in order to prevent repeated episodes of pain is the goal. Meanwhile, all-purpose headache remedies abound.

Diet and Supplements

The *Medical Tribune* (March 31, 1982) reports that holistic doctors have cured more than 90 percent of all chronic teenage headaches within two weeks by simply deleting refined carbohydrates and caffeine from their diets. Eating generous amounts of beets, and/or drinking 16 ounces daily of 8 ounces carrot juice plus any combination of apple, beet, celery, cucumber, lettuce, or watermelon juice, is believed to help relieve excess nerve pressure in the head.

Clinical studies have shown that persistent headaches can result from iron deficiency, with or without anemia, or from a lack of vitamins B-6 or pantothenic acid. Taking vitamins B-1, B-2, and B-12 have also proven beneficial. The headaches preceding or accompanying menstruation are usually relieved by supplements of calcium and vitamin D. Vitamin C deactivates many toxins—2,000 to 4,000 milligrams of this vitamin taken at the onset of occasional headaches has a reported success-rate of 50 percent.[24] For headaches associated with either low blood pressure or low blood sugar, Adelle Davis[89] suggested taking one-half each teaspoon baking soda and salt in a little water. *Earl Mindell's Vitamin Bible* recommends the following daily combination for chronic headaches:

> One 100-milligram B-complex stress tablet
> 100 milligrams three times daily of niacin or niacinamide
> 2 to 4 dolomite (calcium and magnesium) tablets

Dr. Van Fleet's *Extraordinary Healing Secrets from a Doctor's Private Files*[325] reports both preventive and curative results from filling a humidifier with a solution of vitamins A, C, D, and crushed zinc tablets in boiled water, then inhaling the mist for 10 minutes every hour. After the headache has cleared, taking the same vitamins orally and using the mist several times a day has prevented recurrence.

Exercise

A few minutes of vigorous exercise at the onset of a headache may prevent its development by delivering more oxygen to the body.

Folk Remedies

Folklore holds that gathering all the clippings from a haircut and burying them under a rock will prevent headaches. One of the more appealing remedies is an old French cure recorded by M.F.K. Fisher in *A Cordiall Water.*[121] Thin slices of boiled ham, fluted pickles, crisp zwieback, or fresh bread and butter were to be attractively arranged on a tray, then eaten in bed in a quiet room with a glass of wine as an accompaniment.

Apple Cider Vinegar—Combine three tablespoons apple cider vinegar with one tablespoon raw honey and take at the onset of a headache. Or, follow the advice from Mother Goose and soak a piece of brown paper in vinegar, fold several times, then place on the forehead.

Herbs—Inserting marjoram in the nostrils and then inhaling deeply was a headache cure in 16th-Century Italy, but a cup of strong herbal tea followed by an hour's bed rest has been the standard headache remedy for hundreds of years. Basil, camomile, catnip, fennel, peppermint, rosemary, sage, and thyme were the favorites. Some herbalists have found combinations of herbs to be more effective. Any of these mixtures should be steeped in one cup boiling water, then slowly sipped: one-half teaspoon each catnip, marjoram, peppermint, and sage; or peppermint and scullcap plus sage; or one-half teaspoon scullcap plus one-fourth teaspoon each camomile, catnip, and celery seed; or one-fourth teaspoon each marjoram, rosemary, and celery seed.

Lemon—Peel a fresh lemon and rub the inside of the skin on the temples. Or, add the juice of one lemon to a glass of warm water, stir in one teaspoon baking soda, and drink slowly. Or, stir the juice of one lemon into one pint hot pekoe tea. Drink one cupful, then cool and drink the second cup in two hours.

Poultices—Bind wilted beet or mint leaves or slices of raw potatoes on the forehead. Or, combine beef tallow and turpentine, spread on a bandage, and tie tightly around the head. Or, place moistened baking soda, bruised garlic, shredded horseradish, or onion between pieces of gauze and apply to the back of the neck and/or the bend of both arms and legs for half an hour.

Strawberries—Eat a large bowl of fresh strawberries (or those frozen without sugar). Strawberries are believed to contain organic salicylates similar to the active ingredients in aspirin.

Nerve Massage

- Place the fingers of both hands in the hollows at the base of the skull and massage firmly for three minutes.
- Squeeze and massage the thumb and first two fingers, plus the webs between them, on both hands.
- Massage the first three toes plus the connecting skin between the big toe and the one next to it, on both feet.

Nerve Pressure

The well-publicized acupressure technique of applying pressure to the head at half-inch intervals is reportedly successful, but time consuming. Stimulating any (or all) of the following individual pressure points has proven equally successful for many. Unless otherwise indicated, each point is to be pressed for 10 seconds, released for 10 seconds, and repeated for a total of 30 seconds pressure.

- Press just above the top of the nose where the eyebrows would come together. Then press the tiny hollow at the outer edge of each eyebrow, about ½ inch toward the ear.
- Press inward and upward against the bone midway between the center base of the skull and the bony ridge behind each ear. Then cup the palms of the hands over the ears and push for two minutes. Follow by gently pressing the hollow of the temples while rotating the head.
- With the fist tightly clenched, press the mound between the thumb and the index finger. Repeat with the other hand. Then press the top of each hand, 1½ inches below the web between the little finger and the one next to it.
- Tightly wrap rubber bands around each finger just below the fingernail. Leave in place for 10 minutes, or until the fingers begin to turn blue.
- Press the crease on the inner wrists, in line with the little fingers.
- Press the top of each foot, three-quarters of an inch from the web separating the first and second toes.
- Squeeze the toenails of the second and fourth toes on both feet for 10 seconds each, then pull each toe for another 10 seconds.
- Press just below the ball of the foot in line with the third toe. Repeat with the other foot.

Relaxation

Stress, whether from emotional pressure, physical exertion, inhaled or ingested toxins, or nutritional deficiencies is another term for the "imbalance" many doctors consider responsible for headaches. Going beyond resting with a cool cloth on the forehead to deliberately relaxing both mind and body often dissipates a headache. Practice is necessary for perfection, but for immediate relief during a headache, the basic outline given in the Introduction (pages 9-10) may serve the purpose if concluded with the positive thought that the entire body will feel refreshed and pain-free following the period of relaxation.

Sources (See Bibliography)

3, 4, 5, 6, 9, 23, 34, 40, 42, 52, 53, 62, 63, 64, 68, 69, 73, 75, 78, 88, 89, 98, 107, 121, 134, 142, 143, 151, 152, 153, 156, 165, 167, 168, 171, 173, 174, 178, 180, 181, 184, 190, 212, 214, 226, 227, 228, 235, 236, 243, 254, 257, 261, 262, 263, 270, 288, 289, 291, 293, 297, 314, 315, 316, 323, 325, 333, 334, 345, 354.

HEARING LOSS AND TINNITUS

Hearing deterioration begins at the age of 10, presumably a protective action as the body senses that loud noises are potentially damaging and adjusts the volume.

Hearing loss may be so slight that it never becomes a handicap but can often be prevented, slowed, or even reversed by natural means.

Noise deafness (a form of nerve deafness) is caused by prolonged exposure to noise levels greater than the ear can tolerate without damage. It is, therefore, preventable. A decibel measures the smallest amount of sound the average human ear can distinguish. Normal conversation registers 60 decibels; a heavy truck rumbling by, 100 decibels; and amplified dance bands have been charted between 120 and 140 decibels. The American Medical Association recommends the use of ear plugs or shields when continuing sounds are more than 90 decibels. Ears can recover from brief exposure to loud noise, but chronic exposure wears down the hearing nerve endings to cause hearing impairment that is temporary at first but can become permanent. Even an accumulation of low-level sounds from air conditioners, appliances, background music, etc. can reach the danger point. No scientific instruments are required to assure ear safety: If it is necessary to shout in order to carry on a conversation with someone a few feet away, turn down the sound, don a protective device, or move out of range.

Conduction deafness may be due to wax in the ear canal. Normally, earwax preserves hearing by protecting the inner ear from bacteria, dust, and other foreign objects. When it becomes sufficiently laden with these impurities, it works itself out of the ear with the motion of the jaw in eating, talking, and yawning. Increased air pollution can overburden the earwax to create a troublesome substance that is not easily expelled. Modern diets, with their few really chewy foods, offer little challenge to the jaw muscles and can contribute to the buildup of earwax and gradual hearing impairment.

Lack of essential fatty acids can be responsible for excessive earwax. Adding one tablespoon cold-pressed, polyunsaturated oil such as safflower or sunflower to a daily salad may be beneficial. Using a hairpin or cotton-tipped swab in an attempt to remove earwax can lead to infection or perforation of the eardrum, and further hearing loss. Any wax that can be removed by such means was already working itself out of the ear, and the wax that remains is packed in more tightly. The safest treatment is to eat foods that require hearty chewing. Inserting a piece of cotton dipped in olive oil may help reduce earwax. A few drops of hydrogen peroxide has proven helpful for some individuals. The peroxide should be allowed to remain in the ear until it has stopped fizzing, then be shaken out. Some over-the-counter preparations contain only glycerine and antiseptic, so may be used for the same purpose by those who are sensitive to hydrogen peroxide. In severe cases, medical intervention may be necessary— conduction deafness can result from injury to the eardrum or middle ear and require surgical correction.

Tinnitus (ringing, roaring, or hissing sounds in the ear) may be the result of excess earwax, may be caused by infections in other parts of the body, by deterioration of the delicate sensors within the ear from too much noise, or by reactions to certain medications. Aspirin has been known to produce congestion in both the middle ear and the labyrinth. Large doses of other drugs—barbiturates, quinine, the "miacins," cocaine, and other narcotics—can instigate tinnitus. It can also result from too much caffeine or from exposure to chemicals such as carbon monoxide or the benzene used by dry cleaners.

Reflex tinnitus is a reaction to stress, is often considered psychosomatic, is usually temporary, and can be brought about by anything from an emotional upset to tight shoes. Some people can train their minds and bodies to relax on command (see pages 9-10), quieting tension-caused sounds in their heads. If the nonexistent noise cannot be turned off, it can often be overridden by the pleasant sound of soft music.

Transient deafness can be occasioned by a nagging partner or parent, or other mental disturbance, and usually disappears when the "trigger" is removed. Temporary "airplane deafness" (caused by the pressure from altitude changes) can be prevented or relieved by chewing gum or yawning and swallowing in rapid succession. Blowing to puff out the cheeks while both nose and mouth are closed is also helpful (see Earache).

Diet and Supplements

Diet as well as quiet can contribute to hearing health. Clinical studies have shown that over 50 percent of those with hearing loss and/or ringing in the ears also had elevated serum cholesterol.[159] Reducing the cholesterol level (see Hardening of the Arteries) has reversed hearing losses of 50 to 60 percent and restored normal hearing acuity.[154] In another study, 87 percent of 444 patients with impaired hearing had abnormal glucose tolerance indicative of hypoglycemia, diabetes, or a pre-diabetic condition.[52] Emphasizing protein and complex carbohydrates in the diet while restricting sugars and saturated fats often brings improvement (see Diabetes and Low Blood Sugar). A glass or two of fresh fruit and vegetable juice each day is believed to invigorate the sensory receptor cells. In his book, *Helping Yourself with New Enzyme Catalyst Health Secrets*[334], Carlson Wade recommends a "Hearing Health Shake" composed of mixed vegetable juice, one-half cup fresh citrus juice, and one teaspoon each brewer's yeast, lecithin granules, and wheat germ to improve hearing. Other authorities believe a decline in sensory perception may be due, at least in part, to free-radical damage to the brain and suggest generous daily amounts of the antioxidants listed on page 3.

> **Vitamin A**—10,000 to 25,000 units daily. Vitamin A is an ear as well as an eye vitamin. When taken with lecithin, it aids the cilia cells vital to hearing. Otosclerosis (a conductive-type hearing impairment in the elderly) can often be slowed or improved with supplements of vitamin A plus vitamin E (see Caution, page 6).

> **B Complex**—One comprehensive tablet daily. There is considerable evidence that a lack of (or an increased need for) B vitamins may contribute to both nerve deafness and tinnitus. Taking an additional 50 milligrams of B-6 three times a day has solved the problem in some cases by its action as a natural diuretic to stabilize inner ear fluids. Two or three daily doses of 100 milligrams niacinamide and one to three tablespoons brewer's yeast each day has improved hearing for some individuals.

Vitamin C—1,000 to 10,000 milligrams daily, depending on individual tolerance levels. Taking large amounts of vitamin C in addition to the B vitamins has resulted in improved hearing acuity, particularly for the high tones. Adding supplements of vitamin E and selenium are believed to increase the amount of oxygen reaching the cells for further improvement.

Minerals—Manganese deficiency can be a cause of deafness in infants, ear noises, or hearing impairment in adults. Beets, egg yolks, green leafy vegetables, nuts, peas, and wheat germ are good dietary sources; and manganese is available in 50-milligram tablets. Extra potassium from bananas, fresh vegetables, sunflower seeds, or supplementary tablets, has reduced ear noises for many individuals. Tissue salts are credited with improving hearing in a number of cases:

- **For hearing loss with tinnitus which is worse at night**—Take three tablets of 12X Kali. Sulph. each two hours during the evening.
- **For chronic deafness not caused by bone changes**—Take two three-tablet daily doses, alternately, of each Kali. Mur., Kali. Phos., Kali. Sulph., and Silicea, plus supplements of vitamins A and C with each meal.

Case History

Della W.'s job with a travel agency necessitated many intercontinental trips. When she first noticed the hissing sounds in her right ear she attributed them to jet-lag aftermath or to a reaction from the medication she had been given for an infection she had developed in Europe—and assumed the problem was only temporary. Rather than fade away, however, the hissing increased in volume. A medical checkup disclosed that her blood pressure and cholesterol were normal, and even a lavage treatment to wash out any accumulation of ear wax failed to abolish the irritating sounds. While chatting with a fellow passenger on her next flight, Della mentioned her discomforting ear noises. Her seatmate, a health-nutrition writer who had been doing some research on natural remedies for tinnitus, shared his notes with her. At their next stop, Della bought B-complex tablets and a bottle of multiple-minerals, took one of each, and asked the stewardess for a banana in place of the chocolate cake offered for dessert. The pharmacy in her destination city provided 100-milligram niacinamide tablets, and by the time she got home Della could tell that the hissing sounds were decreasing. Stirring brewer's yeast into her morning tomato juice helped even more, and, although forgoing her stimulating coffee breaks was a sacrifice, eliminating caffeine from her diet was well worth the blissful silence that ensued.

Exercise

Regular walking, jogging, or other exercise has improved hearing by providing more oxygen and glucose to the ears.

Folk Remedies

Almond Oil and Turpentine—The nightly insertion of a piece of cotton saturated with equal parts almond oil and turpentine was believed to correct hearing loss caused by an abnormally dry condition of the ear passages.

Apple Cider Vinegar and Honey—Mixing two teaspoons each apple cider vinegar and raw honey in a glass of water and sipping with each meal is a folk-medicine prescription for preserving good hearing and reversing many types of hearing loss.

Cabbage and Wine—Equal parts fresh cabbage juice and wine, used as ear drops, was believed to improve hearing.

Cotton—To correct ringing in the ears and impaired hearing, place a wad of cotton in the space between the last tooth and the angle of the jaw. Then bite down hard for several minutes two or three times each day.

Garlic—Combine 1 ounce minced garlic (one large bulb) with one cup almond oil and let stand for one week. Strain, bottle, and place a drop or two in the ear to correct temporary deafness. Another option is to dip a large clove of peeled garlic in honey and stuff it in the ear overnight.

Onion Juice—To correct poor hearing and ringing in the ears, place a drop of onion juice in the ear every other day. Reduce the frequency as the condition improves, eventually using only one drop every 10 days for maintenance.

Nerve Massage

For general relief of ear problems—Massage the area on the bottom of the feet between the third, fourth, and little toes.

To relieve ringing in the ears and hearing loss due to thickening of the ear membrane—Massage the joints of the little finger and the one next to it, as well as the little toe and the one next to it, on both hands and feet.

Nerve Pressure

For hearing loss with tinnitus

- Using a pencil eraser, press on the gums behind the wisdom teeth.
- Using the index fingers, press 1 inch to both the right and left of the center of the chest where the breast muscle joins the breastbone. Press for 10 seconds, release for 10 seconds, and repeat three times once each day.
- Several times each day, wind rubber bands around the tips of the fourth fingers and leave in place until the fingers start to turn blue.

To reverse hearing loss

- Press the teeth of an aluminum comb against the tips of the fingers for five minutes at a time. Follow with finger-pressure against the floor of the mouth for an equal period, then brief pressure against the roof of the mouth and the back of the tongue.
- Forcibly lift the end of the third fingernail of the right hand with the third fingernail of the left hand for a few minutes at a time. Repeat the same

procedure with the fourth fingers. The same pressure may be applied to the middle and fourth toenails of both feet by using the fingernail of the index finger to do the lifting.

Sources (See Bibliography)

3, 6, 33, 52, 62, 63, 68, 71, 84, 89, 98, 142, 154, 156, 159, 165, 173, 174, 180, 226, 227, 229, 236, 239, 247, 252, 261, 270, 288, 315, 316, 334, 353.

HEARTBURN AND HIATAL HERNIA

Considered a symptom distinct from indigestion, heartburn is defined as a burning sensation beginning in the lower chest and traveling upward toward the neck. Technically known as pyrosis or gastroesophageal reflux, heartburn is caused by stomach acid backing up through the muscular ring (sphincter) at the junction of the esophagus and stomach. Most heartburn is the result of "operator error" rather than physical abnormality. A combination of aging, emotional tensions, genetic tendencies, and over-indulgence in alcohol, chocolate, citrus juices, coffee, fat, and tobacco can reduce sphincter tension so that pressure in the stomach forces a portion of it to protrude into the esophagus as a "hiatal hernia." When necessary, hiatal hernias can be surgically corrected, but, although more than half the population over 50 is believed to have some form of hiatal hernia[18], few experience any discomfort and the majority of heartburn sufferers are not herniated.

Eating when exhausted or emotionally upset increases the flow of stomach acids. Eating too much too rapidly, or swallowing air, so overloads the stomach that a backup (acid reflux) is almost inevitable. Chronic constipation with straining for evacuation can push the stomach upward to lead to heartburn. Obesity, a tight belt, or other constricting clothing can interfere with normal abdominal distention after a meal and trigger heartburn. Besides the obvious preventives of relaxing before dining and slowly eating small, frequent meals instead of one or two large ones, there are several other suggestions for avoiding heartburn.

Sipping cold drinks through a straw; restricting the amount of air-filled foods such as souffles, milk shakes, or carbonated beverages; and refraining from chewing gum reduces swallowed air which can form a bubble at the top of the stomach. When the air in this bubble is warmed to body temperature, it expands and may be belched with sufficient force to carry stomach acid into the esophagus. Not drinking any liquids for 30 minutes before or after, or during, meals may allow the digestive enzymes to perform at full strength and prevent heartburn. Sugar is a source of irritation to the delicate membranes of the esophagus, particularly when taken in the form of candy or soft drinks on an empty stomach. Certain foods may trigger heartburn due to an allergy-type reaction and should be avoided through trial-and-error experimentation as for other allergies. Smoking can instigate heartburn for some people. Bending over or lying down within an hour or so after eating can remove the downward pull of gravity on stomach contents and encourage heartburn. Chronic sufferers may benefit from elevating their beds by placing 4- to 6-inch blocks under the legs at the head of the bed.

Case History

Grace E., a vivacious widow in her seventies, decided the time had come to do something about her chronic heartburn. After a thorough medical examination which resulted in a diagnosis of hiatal hernia, Grace opted for experimenting with home remedies before resorting to surgery. Reading the pamphlet the doctor had given her convinced Grace that she must change her eating habits. As an artist with a picture always in progress she frequently went right to work with nothing more than a glass of fruit juice for breakfast, sipped tea or soft drinks throughout the day, and ate a large meal in the evening. By adjusting her schedule to include some food with her morning juice, taking a few minutes for a sandwich plus soup or a salad at noon, and reducing the size of her dinner, Grace avoided her daytime heartburn. Eliminating fatty foods, such as pork chops, from her evening meal made her life even more comfortable. She was still experiencing some nighttime discomfort and, rather than hire someone to put blocks under the head of her bed, tried stuffing pillows under the head-end of the mattress. Success! No more being awakened by burning sensations in her chest—and no surgery required.

When heartburn does occur, natural remedies are preferred over commercial antacids or bicarbonate of soda. Soda creates carbon dioxide gas which brings apparent relief by belching. But the belch would not be necessary if the soda were not taken in the first place, and may force leftover stomach acid into the esophagus to create more heartburn. Antacid tablets or alkalizers are not considered beneficial for heartburn sufferers. Although they offer temporary relief by neutralizing stomach acids, they destroy vitamins and minerals and interfere with digestion. The stomach reacts by secreting more acid to finish its job, thus creating a vicious cycle. Their continued use can lead to deficiencies which cause more serious problems.[89,261] A glass of milk has been shown to have the same effect as an antacid preparation and, while it may have a slight acid rebound, does not have the other undesirable side effects of commercial preparations. Betaine hydrochloride or papaya enzyme digestive tablets often assist complete digestion so food does not remain in the stomach in an undigested state to necessitate the release of additional stomach acids.

Folk Remedies

Apple Cider Vinegar—Stir one or two teaspoons apple cider vinegar in a glass of water and sip with each meal. If desired, two teaspoons raw honey may be added to the mixture.

Buckwheat or Oatmeal—Eating a bowl of cooked buckwheat groats or oatmeal each morning is believed to relieve persistent heartburn.

Carrot or Celery—Thoroughly chewing and swallowing a small stick of raw carrot or celery often relieves heartburn.

Garlic—For chronic heartburn, eat a clove of garlic with each meal (or take two garlic perles).

Horehound—Sip horehound tea or eat a piece of horehound candy.

Lemon—Stir one teaspoon fresh lemon juice in one-half glass water and sip to relieve heartburn.

Milk—A glass of cool milk before or after meals is the standard folk remedy for heartburn. Drinking several cups of goat's milk throughout the day is said to provide relief from chronic heartburn.

Onion—Eating one half of a thinly sliced raw onion with a slice of bread was believed to take care of heartburn.

Peas—Eating half a cup of fresh green peas each day, or soaking dried peas overnight and chewing them the next morning, were folk-medicine preventives.

Peppermint—An infusion made from one-half cup peppermint steeped in two cups boiling water, strained and taken by the tablespoonful was the remedy for heartburn in 1850.

Salt—Dissolve one teaspoon salt in one-fourth cup water and drink to alleviate heartburn.

Sugar—Eating one or two teaspoons of white or brown sugar was an old remedy for quickly relieving heartburn.

Nerve Pressure

Press a point 1 inch to the left of the center of the chest for 10 seconds, release for 10 seconds, and repeat three times.

Tissue Salts

For all heartburn, but especially when the pain goes through to the back, take frequent doses of three tablets each Ferr. Phos. and Nat. Mur. in the 6X potency.

Sources (See Bibliography)

18, 19, 53, 68, 88, 89, 131, 142, 153, 156, 158, 165, 168, 173, 175, 180, 190, 226, 227, 237, 254, 261, 269, 270, 288, 293, 297, 315, 320, 325, 328, 333, 334, 335, 354.

HEMORRHOIDS (PILES)

These discomforting varicosed veins in and around the rectal opening are a malady attributed largely to a civilized diet and a sedentary lifestyle. Hemorrhoids are practically unheard of in primitive, underdeveloped nations, yet in the United States their incidence has increased from an estimated 49 percent of those over 40 in 1970 to more than half of those over 30 in 1981.[314]

"Straining at stool" or constipation (which see), prolonged sitting or standing, tension, and emotional stress are considered the principal causes. Hemorrhoids that develop during pregnancy usually disappear with delivery. Obesity, an attack of diarrhea, or the strain of coughing, sneezing, or lifting can aggravate an existing condition. Breathing freely while lifting or during bowel movements is believed to reduce abdominal pressure on the homorrhoidal veins. If blood clots form within the distended veins, causing them to become "thrombosed," the thin skin covering them may rupture to cause bleeding. If these clots do not dissolve with natural methods, they can be "evacuated" surgically—a procedure usually performed in the doctor's office rather than a hospital.

The American Pharmaceutical Association has stated that ordinary Vaseline is as effective as the products sold as protectants, and has approved of Witch Hazel as an astringent.[314] Products containing local anesthetics or vasoconstrictors to shrink blood vessels bring temporary relief but may eventually oversensitize the affected tissues to cause itching or bleeding. Most hemorrhoids respond to natural treatment within a week or two, but those that are persistent should receive medical attention. Although few hemorrhoids ever become cancerous, they may occur as a side effect of other diseases.

Diet and Supplements

The bland, low-residue diet once advised for hemorrhoid sufferers has been found to be a contributing factor rather than a cure. A high-fiber diet including fresh fruits, vegetables, ample fluids, and one to three tablespoons unprocessed bran daily is now recommended to relieve pressure on the stretched veins, help prevent bleeding, avoid the necessity for stool softeners or harsh laxatives, and forestall the formation of new hemorrhoids. Sugar and refined foods made of white flour should be limited or avoided, as should chocolate, cocoa, coffee, and cola drinks which promote anal itching. During an attack it is usually advisable to eliminate scratchy foods such as nuts and coarsely ground or cracked grains in cereals or breadstuffs. (Some folk healers recommend eating three or four almonds daily, along with generous amounts of ripe papayas and grated raw carrots.) Other foods reputedly helpful for hemorrhoids are: bananas, parsnips, persimmons, plums, prunes, pumpkin, sweet potatoes, and winter squash. Eating yogurt or taking acidophilus capsules with meals also contributes to the health of the bowel. Carrot juice and okra juice lubricate and coat the intestinal tract and are believed to promote healing. Juices of apples, beets, celery, cucumber, grapefruit, lemon, orange, papaya, pineapple, and spinach are also considered helpful.

Vitamin A—10,000 to 25,000 units daily for prevention of infection and healing. An ointment containing vitamins A and D may be helpful for lubrication and relief of pain.

B Complex—One comprehensive tablet daily plus 10 to 25 milligrams B-6 after each meal. Bleeding hemorrhoids have been produced in volunteers deficient in B-6 and corrected when the vitamin was supplied. An adequate diet plus B-6 supplements brought a "miraculous recovery" to every hemorrhoid sufferer with whom nutritionist Adelle Davis[89] worked. Taking one to two tablespoons of brewer's yeast each day has been credited with speeding the relief.

Bioflavonoids—100 milligrams four times daily for one week, then two or three times a day for a month has reportedly cured thousands of hemorrhoid cases in European clinics. Another group of medical nutritionists corrected hemorrhoids with oral supplements of 60 to 600 milligrams of the bioflavonoid, rutin, taken in divided doses daily. Rutin is nontoxic. As much as 3,000 milligrams has been used for a day or so to relieve hemorrhoids. Other cases have cleared in 48 hours when 1,200 milligrams citrus bioflavonoids plus 600 milligrams each hesperidin bioflavonoids and rutin were taken in divided doses each day.[52,261]

Vitamin C—1,000 to 6,000 milligrams daily. Vitamin C strengthens the walls of the veins near the anus to reduce the possibility of clotting, aids healing, and assures proper assimilation of the bioflavonoids. Regular intake of large amounts of vitamin C has been found to help maintain soft stools without the side effects of commercial stool softeners.

Vitamin E (see Caution, page 6)—400 to 600 IU daily. Vitamin E promotes healing, improves circulation, and has demonstrated a remarkable ability for preventing or dissolving blood clots. In addition to the oral supplements, vitamin E ointment, the oil squeezed from capsules, or liquid lecithin or wheat-germ oil (both contain vitamin E) can be applied directly to the hemorrhoids. Pierced capsules of vitamin E, lecithin, or wheat-germ oil may be used as suppositories to alleviate discomfort. For painful internal hemorrhoids, an ounce of vitamin E ointment or wheat-germ oil can be injected into the rectal area with a baby syringe.

Tissue Salts—Unless otherwise indicated, take half-hourly or hourly doses for an acute condition, three or four doses daily for chronic hemorrhoids.

- **For pain from inflamed hemorrhoids or those bleeding bright red blood**—Take two tablets of 6X Ferr. Phos. each 10 minutes until the condition improves, then every hour or two. Dissolve three tablets in one-half cup warm water and apply externally as well. For bleeding hemorrhoids with dark, clotted blood, take 6X Kali. Mur. each 30 minutes for several hours.
- **With low back pain, constipation and itching**—Take 12X Calc. Fluor. internally and dissolve three tablets in one-half cup warm water to use as an external lotion.
- **With sharp, darting pains**—Take 6X Mag. Phos.
- **When accompanied by a feeling of heat**—Take 12X Nat. Sulph.

Exercise

A brisk daily walk plus a few minutes of calisthenics is considered preventive medicine for hemorrhoids—the "sitting man's disease."

Folk Remedies

Despite the healthful physical activity and preponderance of natural foods ascribed to our ancestors' lifestyles, the plentitude of folk-cures for "piles" indicate that hemorrhoids have been a problem for hundreds of years.

Aloe Vera—Apply aloe vera gel (available in health food stores) to external hemorrhoids. To relieve bleeding hemorrhoids: make a suppository from a leaf of an aloe plant by cutting a section ¾-inch wide and 2½ inches long, then peeling and folding it in half.

Apple Cider Vinegar—The Vermont folk remedy for chronic hemorrhoids is to stir two teaspoons each apple cider vinegar and raw honey in a glass of water to sip with each meal. A variation said to stop any itching and make the piles vanish in three weeks is to stir one teaspoon of the vinegar in the glass of water to drink with each meal and to use another glass of the same mixture for daily external applications.[293] Annoying itching may be relieved by saturating a cotton ball with apple cider vinegar and inserting it overnight.

Cranberries—Wrap one tablespoon finely chopped raw cranberries in a square of cheesecloth and insert in the painful area. Repeat in one hour.

Enemas—An enema of plain warm water, strained white oak bark tea, or a mixture of one tablespoon cornstarch and two cups water (cooked and cooled, if desired) often brings temporary relief from piles and, some believe, has a long-term curative effect.

Herbs—Cayenne tea, taken internally is thought to relieve hemorrhoids by stimulating circulation. Flax seed, rose hips, slippery elm, uva ursi or white oak bark teas can be sipped every four hours, applied externally, or injected two tablespoons at a time with a baby syringe.

Ice—A Eurasian remedy for hemorrhoids is to insert a piece of ice for 30 seconds once each day and gradually increase the time to 90 seconds. When the hemorrhoids have eased, cold compresses may be used.

Ointments—Castor oil, cocoa butter, cod liver oil, or petroleum jelly can be used to provide a coating over inflamed tissues and reduce swelling. Sunflower seeds, simmered in cream and thoroughly pulverized, were believed helpful. Some folk practitioners advised a mixture of strong white oak bark tea strained and boiled until thick, then combined with an equal amount of bacon grease. Another option was one-fourth cup butter simmered with two tablespoons smoking tobacco, strained, then applied three or four times daily.

Onions and Leeks—Eating one large, boiled leek each day was a remedy for piles in the 1870s. Eating fried onions or onion soup daily has reportedly stopped persistent hemorrhoidal bleeding. A poultice said to relieve hemorrhoids in two days can be made by cooking a mixture of chopped green onions and wheat flour in bacon grease, spreading it on a cloth and applying just before bedtime.

Potato or Garlic—One of the favorite remedies was to whittle a raw potato into a suppository and insert it overnight. Both soothing and astringent, the potato is believed to speed healing. A peeled garlic clove may be used in the same manner.

Talcum Powder—Dust over the anal area to ensure dryness and prevent moist crevices from encouraging the growth of bacteria and fungi which could cause infection.

Witch Hazel—Applying this herbal liquid after bathing helps shrink hemorrhoids. Small squares of soft cloth can be saturated with a mixture of Witch Hazel and glycerine for use in place of toilet paper.

Nerve Massage

This combination of hand and foot massage is said to relieve pain in a few minutes and bleeding hemorrhoids in two or three days.

- Massage around the outer edges of the palms of both hands with a press-and-roll motion. Then use the thumbs to massage the center of the arms about one-third of the way to the elbow.
- Massage all around the heels on both feet, pressing in toward the bone and down toward the heel pad, using the thumb for one side and the index finger for the other. Then massage the cord on the back of the leg from just above the heel to the calf of the leg. Massage a few moments with the heel extended, then stretch the foot down and rub the cord again.

Nerve Pressure

Using the handle of a tablespoon, press down on the center of the tongue as far back as possible without gagging; maintain pressure for at least two minutes. Then pull down on top of the bone forming the depression at the hollow of the throat and push up on the tip of the coccyx (tail bone), repeating each pressure three times for 10 seconds each.

Sitz Baths

Sitting in warm water is undoubtedly the oldest of all remedies for hemorrhoids. Soaking in 6 inches of water for 20 minutes three or four times a day can be both soothing and healing. These sitz baths have been found even more effective when camomile or white oak bark tea was used as the liquid, or when one cup of cornstarch or one-fourth cup Witch Hazel was added to the tub. When sitz baths are impractical, a towel wrung out of hot water and applied for 20 minutes several times a day may bring relief.

A "water treatment" described by David Carroll in *The Complete Book of Natural Medicines*[62] calls for sitting in hot water for 10 minutes, draining the tub, running 6 inches of cold water and immersing the lower torso for 30 to 60 seconds. This should be followed by rubbing the entire body with a towel wrung out of ice water, then normal drying. The treatment should be repeated five times a week for a month, or until the hemorrhoids have cleared.

Sources (See Bibliography)

3, 13, 18, 23, 34, 52, 53, 62, 63, 64, 66, 68, 76, 81, 82, 84, 89, 106, 142, 145, 152, 156, 168, 174, 176, 180, 181, 184, 189, 190, 214, 226, 229, 253, 254, 261, 269, 272, 274, 289, 293, 297, 301, 303, 312, 314, 316, 318, 325, 333, 335.

HEPATITIS AND CIRRHOSIS OF THE LIVER

Hepatitis is an inflammation of the liver. The most common form, viral hepatitis A (infectious or epidemic hepatitis, formerly called catarrhal jaundice) is passed directly from person to person, contracted by inhaling airborne germs from infected individuals, or by ingesting contaminated food or drink. It has an incubation period of from two to six weeks. Viral Hepatitis B (serum hepatitis or serum jaundice) is chiefly spread through contaminated blood transfusions or inadequately sterilized hypodermic needles or ear-piercing equipment. It requires a six-week to six-month incubation period. Serum hepatitis is not considered contagious but recent evidence indicates that it can be spread through sexual contact.

Toxic hepatitis is liver inflammation caused by chemicals or drugs. Some antibiotics, dry-cleaning chemicals, insecticides, sleeping pills, sulfa drugs, tranquilizers, etc. can cause liver damage in people who are sensitive to them, but the disease cannot be transmitted to others. One of the functions of the liver is to cleanse the system of toxic chemicals and wastes. When it becomes overloaded with harmful material there is a cumulative deterioration and hardening of liver cells resulting in faulty functioning and the chronic disease, cirrhosis. Once called gin-drinker's liver or hardening of the liver, cirrhosis may result from hepatitis, malnutrition, or an overabundance of sugar and saturated fats in the diet, as well as from too much alcohol. The classic role of alcohol in producing cirrhosis of the liver is now considered to be very indirect—only an estimated 10 percent of alcoholics develop cirrhosis. Alcoholic cirrhosis is believed to be primarily the result of nutritional deficiencies, particularly of B vitamins.

All these liver maladies begin with similar flu-like symptoms, may cause a jaundiced yellowing of eyes and skin, and require bed rest plus a nutritious low-fat diet with total abstinence from alcohol. All should be monitored by a physician. Many doctors advise injections of gamma globulin (a substance derived from human blood that carries hepatitis antibodies) for individuals who have been exposed to the infectious virus. Infectious hepatitis requires isolation plus special care of linens and eating utensils.

The usual duration of hepatitis is two to six weeks but total biochemical recovery and the correction of cirrhosis requires at least six months. The indispensable liver serves at least 500 functions in the operation of the human body. When allowed a respite from some of these chores and furnished the proper nutrients, the liver can almost entirely regenerate itself. Seemingly hopeless cirrhotics have recovered with a regimen of diet and supplements plus adequate rest.

Diet and Supplements

Optimal nutrition is the key to liver regeneration. Small, frequent meals with a daily total of from 2,500 to 3,000 calories are recommended. The diet should be low in saturated fat, high in protein, fruits, vegetables, and natural grains. Apples, artichokes, beets, carrots, citrus fruits, cucumbers, garlic, leafy greens, ripe papayas, sesame seeds, summer squash, and walnuts are considered especially beneficial. Distilled water, herbal teas, milk, and natural juices should be substituted for coffee, tea, and soft drinks. In his book, *New Enzyme Catalyst Health Secrets*[334], Carlson Wade reports many successes with a daily glass of "Liver Tonic." This is made by combining one-half cup each fresh orange and grapefruit juice with one teaspoon desiccated liver and one-half teaspoon each brewer's yeast and honey. If jaundice is present, a combination of 8 ounces carrot juice plus 8 ounces of any mixture of apple, beet, celery, citrus, cucumber, grape, parsley, or watercress juice daily is suggested by Gary and Steve Null in their *Complete Handbook of Nutrition*.[243]

Clams and oysters should be well-cooked to inactivate concentrations of hepatitis virus they may have picked up from contaminated waters. Beef liver, long acclaimed as the best food for liver repair, is now under scrutiny because of the amount of toxins assimilated by the animals. Processed foods containing chemical additives or preservatives should be avoided and the use of salt limited. Honey and blackstrap molasses may be used, but sugar has been shown to have the same toxic effect on the liver as alcohol—which is absolutely forbidden during liver inflammation and for at least six months after recovery.

Since liver functions are so varied, a deficiency of almost any nutrient can contribute to its degeneration. In addition to the therapeutic use of the following supplements, a daily multi-vitamin-mineral tablet is usually recommended.

Vitamin A—50,000 to 100,000 units daily for one or two weeks, then 25,000 units per day as a maintenance dosage. Tests have shown that persons with liver damage (particularly when the damage is not caused by alcohol) have difficulty converting the carotene from foods to an assimilable form of vitamin A and are often deficient in this vitamin.

B Complex—One comprehensive tablet daily to combat the stress of illness, plus optional, individual supplements.

- According to the *Scandinavian Journal of Gastroenterology* (Vol. 13, 1978), taking 200 milligrams B-1 each day for one week brought improvement for patients with chronic liver disease.
- Vitamin B-6 and niacin (50 to 100 milligrams of each, daily) have proven beneficial in many cases, but massive amounts of niacin may produce positive liver tests even when the condition is improving.
- Choline is essential to prevent fatty degeneration of the liver. Daily doses most often used are 500 to 1,000 milligrams, but up to 10,000 milligrams a day for two weeks has brought rapid improvement in some cases.
- As reported in the December 20, 1952 issue of the *Journal of the American Medical Association,* 30 to 50 micrograms of B-12 daily speeded recovery from liver infections in a series of hospital tests. Fifteen years ago the hospital death rate from advanced infection of the liver was 48 percent. Today, with larger doses of B vitamins, the death rate has been reduced to 15 percent. 100 to 1,000 micrograms of B-12 per day have been effective in maintaining normal blood and marrow in patients with liver damage (*Pathways to Living,* Vol. 16, 1982).

- Taking 50 to 150 milligrams of B-15 each day for several months is credited with preventing fat-infiltration damage when the liver is overly burdened with toxins.
- Nutritionist Adelle Davis recommended that large amounts of B-6, pantothenic acid, and vitamin C be taken as a preventive measure before and several days following a blood transfusion. Her treatment for the acute stage of hepatitis was to take at least 2 milligrams each B-2 and B-6, 100 milligrams pantothenic acid, and 500 milligrams vitamin C with and between each meal and every three hours during the night, if awake. The vitamins were to be taken with the "fortified milk" described in *Let's Get Well.*[89] (For modernized variations of fortified milk, see Index.) A less complex, but effective, regimen is to take one high-potency B-complex tablet, 100 milligrams pantothenic acid, and 1,000 milligrams vitamin C three times a day with one glass of milk into which one tablespoon sugar-free protein powder has been stirred.

Case History

Janice K. was so accustomed to her dual occupations as music teacher and real-estate saleslady that a week of isolated inactivity following her physician's diagnosis of infectious hepatitis left her feeling bored as well as miserable—and the prognosis was for another five weeks of the same! With the hope of shortening her recovery period, Janice telephoned a nutritionist-friend to see if there were any natural remedies that might speed the process. Janice had been taking a daily multiple vitamin, and she had some dietary supplements on hand, so they evolved a supplemental regimen utilizing what was available. Once each day Janice added one-fourth cup each brewer's yeast and protein powder to a quart of whole milk, whirred it in her electric blender, and stored it in the refrigerator. She drank a glass of the mixture with her breakfast, lunch, and dinner—and accompanied each glass with 100 milligrams of pantothenic acid and 1,000 milligrams of vitamin C. Before bed she drank the final glass of fortified milk with a B-complex tablet and another 1,000 milligrams of vitamin C. Within a few days Janice felt the lethargy receding; and by the end of three weeks after his diagnosis, astounded her physician by being totally "clear" and ready to return to work.

Brewer's Yeast—3 to 5 tablespoons daily. This nutritional yeast is a rich source of high-grade protein and B vitamins, and assists the liver in its detoxification function.

Vitamin C—3,000 to 10,000 milligrams (or tolerance level) in divided doses daily. Many reports have been published regarding the effectiveness of 20,000 to 50,000 milligrams of vitamin C in clearing hepatitis in a matter of days. When taken on exposure to hepatitis, this vitamin acts as a preventive. Vitamin C is nontoxic, even in massive amounts, and the possible stomach irritation or diarrhea may be mitigated by accompanying it with milk or calcium supplements. The dosage should gradually be reduced, then maintained at 2,000 to 6,000 milligrams per day for six months after the symptoms have cleared.

Vitamin E and Selenium—100 to 400 IU vitamin E daily (see Caution, page 6). An antioxidant that hastens regeneration and helps prevent dangerous scarring from liver damage, vitamin E is especially important if jaundice is present. Taking 100 to 200 micrograms of selenium daily increases the effectiveness of vitamin E and aids the liver's detoxification process.

Lecithin—One or two tablespoons granules or the equivalent in capsules each day. Lecithin contains choline, helps prevent fatty degeneration, neutralizes some toxins, and is believed to improve liver function.

Folk Remedies

A temporary diet of nothing but lean meat, skinned chicken breasts, and grape juice was an old-fashioned cure for liver disorders and jaundice. European folk healers encouraged drinking a daily glass of fresh beet or cabbage juice, or equal amounts of liquefied dill pickles and raw carrots or tomatoes. Grated or juiced red or white radishes were also believed beneficial to the liver.

Apple Cider Vinegar and Honey—Sipping a glass of water in which two teaspoons each apple cider vinegar and raw honey have been stirred has long been believed to help regain and maintain liver health. The liquid should be taken three times a day, either with or between meals.

Dandelion and Apples—A folk-medicine favorite for liver ailments was a combination of cooked dandelion leaves and grated raw apples, to be eaten in generous amounts each day.

Garlic—One teaspoon minced raw garlic mixed with one tablespoon olive oil and taken before bed each night was believed to rejuvenate the liver.

Herbal Teas—Cornsilk, dandelion, goldenseal, licorice root, parsley, sage, sarsaparilla, and turmeric teas were considered specifics for liver problems. A highly recommended mixture was one teaspoon dandelion, one-fourth teaspoon each anise, fennel, and flaxseed simmered for 15 minutes in one cup water. The dosage was one cupful each morning and evening.

Horseradish—Believed to help the digestion of fats and stimulate liver action, a large horseradish was grated into a cup of scalded milk, allowed to stand for 10 minutes, then strained and sipped. (Grated fresh horseradish is used in Russia to treat epidemic hepatitis.[335])

Lemon—A favorite folk-formula for improving liver function was to stir the juice of half a lemon into a cup of hot water. One cupful was to be taken each morning and night. For the yellowing of jaundice, the remedy was to take a mixture of one teaspoon each lemon juice and honey blended with an egg yolk for each of three consecutive mornings.

Nerve Massage

Once each day use a firm, rolling motion to massage the outer edge of each hand near the base of the little finger and the pad under the little toe of the right foot.

Nerve Pressure

Press each point for 10 seconds, release for 10 seconds, and repeat three times once each day.

- Use the tips of the thumbs to press inward and upward on the bony notch beneath each eyebrow just above the corner of each eye.
- Press 1 inch below and to the right of the center of the chest.
- In a line with the center of the chest, press against the rib directly under the right arm.

Sources (See Bibliography)

3, 7, 9, 12, 13, 18, 19, 25, 28, 37, 43, 49, 63, 81, 84, 88, 89, 99, 142, 151, 152, 156, 171, 173, 174, 175, 176, 180, 181, 189, 214, 226, 227, 228, 229, 243, 249, 251, 252, 253, 254, 257, 261, 270, 288, 289, 293, 297, 315, 318, 333, 334, 335, 353, 354.

HICCUPS

Medically described as involuntary spasmodic contractions of the diaphragm along with sudden closure of the glottis (the upper opening of the larynx), hiccups (singultus) are usually caused by irritation of either the vagus or phrenic nerve. The characteristic sound comes from an attempt to breathe in while the air passage is closed. Hiccups can arise from nervous tension, a fit of laughter, eating too much or too rapidly, too much alcohol, or swallowing irritating substances. Persistent hiccupping may indicate underlying disease and should have medical attention, but most hiccups are merely temporarily annoying or embarrassing mishaps. The options for ending the spasms and annihilating the hiccups are many and varied.

Asphyxiate Them

Breathe into a paper bag (never a plastic one) for two minutes.
Hold the breath as long as possible.
Inhale and hold the breath for a count of 25. Exhale and bend over, allowing the arms to dangle, for a count of 25. Straighten up and repeat the sequence.

Drown Them

Slowly sip, or drink without stopping: a glass of cold beer, pineapple juice, or water, or hot dill tea. Keeping the eyes closed and using earplugs during the process is said to be helpful.
Place a metal knife, fork, or spoon in a glass of water. Sip the water while holding the upper part of the utensil against the temple with the lower part remaining in the water.
Attempt to drink a glass of water from the far side of the glass or while holding a pencil clenched in the teeth.

Stir one teaspoon apple cider vinegar in a glass of water and drink it down.

Bring one cup dried apples to a boil in one cup water. Strain and drink the hot liquid.

Place one teaspoon caraway seeds, dill, ginger, mint, dry mustard, or baking soda in a cup. Fill with boiling water and sip.

Swallow one teaspoon honey, onion juice, or vinegar.

Sip a small glass of orange juice, sugar water, or vermouth.

Sip one tablespoon fresh lemon juice with a few drops of bitters or grains of sugar mixed in.

Gargle with hot or cold water for at least one minute.

Feed Them

Eat small pieces of dry bread or soda cracker, chewing each bite at least 10 times.

Chew charcoal tablets. In extreme cases, continue until relieved.

Chew dill seed or fresh mint leaves.

Eat a slice of fresh orange, one teaspoon peanut butter, or one or two pickled peppers.

Eat a teaspoonful of white sugar. (This has worked for patients who had been hospitalized with hiccups for as long as six weeks.[52]) A variation is to moisten one teaspoon brown sugar with vinegar and eat it.

Dissolve three tablets of the tissue salt, Mag. Phos., under the tongue.

Pulverize or chew a ¼-inch section of white chalk and swallow it.

Push or Pull Them Away

Place the heels of the hands on the closed eyes and gently push for at least 30 seconds.

Push in and up under the cheekbones adjoining the nose. Maintain pressure for 10 seconds, release, and repeat three times.

Push in on the center of the upper lip for 30 seconds.

Thrust the tongue out of the mouth for as long as possible. Or, grasp the tongue with the fingers and gently pull to keep it extended for two or three minutes.

Push down on the middle of the tongue with a tongue depressor.

Place the palms of the hands along the sides of the neck and push in for at least one minute.

Interlock the fingers behind the back of the neck and, while tipping the head back, push in with the thumbs under the edge of the jawbone.

Place the palms on the collarbones and push in for 30 seconds. Release and repeat for another 30 seconds.

Push in on the center of the small depression in the breastbone about 2 inches below the hollow of the throat. Release after 10 seconds and repeat three times.

Interlock the fingers and exert as much pressure as possible.

Use the right thumbnail to press firmly against the largest knuckle of the left middle finger on the side toward the index finger. Release after 10 seconds and repeat three times.

Apply clothespins to the tips of the thumbs and fingers. Remove the moment the skin begins to change color.

Push in on the abdomen 1½ inches directly below the navel. Release after 10 seconds and repeat three times. Then, bend over and touch the toes. Remain in this position for two minutes.

Lean backward with the head hanging down over a bed or sofa.

Rub Them Out

Gently rub both closed eyes with the index fingers. Then massage the hollow at the back of the neck for 30 seconds.

Rub the soft pad at the base of the thumb on each hand. Then massage the thumbs and the next two fingers on both hands for two minutes, giving special attention to the webs of skin between them.

With the palm of the hand, rub the solar plexus area for 30 seconds. Or, use the heel of the hand to massage upward from the navel to the solar plexus, making slow, deep, circular movements and allowing one minute to move from the navel to the bottom of the breastbone.

Rub the center portion of the sole of the foot between the ball of the foot and the arch. Push in firmly with the thumb and fingers while massaging for several minutes. Repeat with the other foot.

Startle Them

Take a hot bath. Or, place a towel wrung out of hot water over the diaphragm.

Make a poultice of one-half teaspoon cayenne pepper to one cup vinegar thickened with cornmeal and/or whole-wheat flour, then apply to the diaphragm.

Shout or sing as loudly as possible.

Force sneezing by inhaling a drift of black pepper, tickling the nose with a feather, or taking a pinch of snuff.

Swallow small bits of crushed ice, with or without holding the nose. Or, place an ice cube just below the Adams Apple for one minute.

Splash cold water on the back of the neck or hold an ice cube there for one or two minutes. Or, wrap ice cubes in a towel and place them over the solar plexus for three minutes.

Throw Them Up

If all else fails, induce vomiting by holding a finger down the throat.

Sources (See Bibliography)

3, 34, 52, 53, 62, 63, 67, 68, 81, 142, 156, 159, 168, 173, 190, 226, 277, 288, 293, 297, 315, 318, 319, 329, 335, 345.

INDIGESTION—GASTRITIS (See Also Flatulence, Heartburn, Nausea, and Ulcers)

Defined as any sense of stomach discomfort or pain generally related to meals, the term "indigestion" covers assorted maladies such as biliousness, dyspepsia, gastritis, and sour stomach.

Simple indigestion (upset stomach) is usually brought on by overindulgence in food or drink, too rapid eating with insufficient chewing, or eating when emotionally upset, exhausted, or constipated. The discomfort occurs only occasionally and disappears in a few hours. Dyspepsia refers to frequent or chronic indigestion. In addition to any of the same causes as occasional indigestion, nutritional deficiencies, lack of digestive juices, allergy-type reactions to certain foods, antibiotics, or other medications, or continual stress may be responsible for chronic indigestion.

Gastritis is an inflammation of the stomach lining resulting from allergies, too much alcohol or tobacco, over-use of aspirin, fatty or spicy foods, food poisoning, or infectious diseases. Sometimes violent in onset and accompanied by vomiting, the symptoms usually fade away within a day or two. (The mucous membrane lining the stomach is replaced every 36 hours[156] and food wends its way through the 30-foot digestive tract in approximately 48 hours.[18]). If the inflammation reaches the intestines, intestinal flu (gastroenteritis) can result. Chronic indigestion or gastritis which does not respond to natural remedies should receive medical attention as it might be a symptom of serious disease.

Diet and Supplements

Since each individual reacts differently to specific foods and beverages, the traditional bland diet plus antacids is now being forsaken in favor of a more personalized holistic approach. By supplying the nutrients needed for proper digestion and eliminating individual "triggers," digestive problems can usually be cured rather than merely soothed.

Which food does not seem as important as how and when it is eaten. When the body is adequately supplied with proteins, vitamins, and minerals, not deliberately abused or tied in tension knots, the digestive system impartially processes whatever comes its way. Eating smaller meals at more frequent intervals and chewing them thoroughly gives the stomach a better chance to do its job before sending the partially digested foods on to the intestines.

Many people of African, Mediterranean, or Oriental ancestry are genetically unable to digest cow's milk but have no problem with yogurt or other fermented milk products. Fatty foods, particularly when deep fried, take longer to digest and require extra gastric juices which may back up into the esophagus to cause heartburn, or remain in the stomach to cause irritation. An overabundance of refined carbohydrates can disturb the normal digestive pattern—sugar, alone, is a gastric irritant for some. Cooked, dried legumes such as baked beans contain a substance that creates gas as it is broken down for absorption. Allergies, alcohol, caffeine-containing beverages, and a long list of "strong" or spicy foods may create problems for certain individuals. Some nutritional experts believe that combining too many kinds of foods at the same meal is responsible for indigestion. They suggest eating only one food group (cereal, protein, fruit, etc.) at a time. By making positive use of beneficial foods and supplements and eating a well-balanced diet with enough roughage to prevent constipation, most people can improve their digestive well-being to the point that a normal diet can be eaten without difficulty and occasional dietary indiscretions tolerated.

Acidophilus—Eating acidophilus yogurt, drinking acidophilus milk, or taking acidophilus capsules with each meal encourages the growth of friendly bacteria and the synthesis of B vitamins in the intestines. When not controlled by these lactobacillus acidophilus bacteria, the putrefactive bacteria flourish and multiply to produce a histamine that releases gases which can pass into the blood to cause allergic reactions, indigestion, and nausea.

Antacids provide fast, temporary relief from the symptoms of occasional indigestion but do nothing to correct the cause of dyspepsia. Combination antacid-aspirin products add to the problem by further irritating the stomach. Commercial antacids, baking soda, even milk—anything that neutralizes stomach secretions—can cause "acid rebound." After being temporarily reduced, the gastric acids bounce back to even greater levels.[18] Some doctors feel the sale of antacids should be banned because their continued use can impair protein digestion and vitamin C absorption, allow B vitamins to be destroyed, and bring about an imbalance in body chemistry that can result in constipation, diarrhea, and/or muscle weakness and cramps.

Hydrochloric Acid—Medical analyses have shown that a deficiency of stomach acid, rather than over-acidity, is the most common cause of indigestion. Hydrochloric acid is essential for the digestion of protein and the absorption of vitamins and minerals. A diminished supply may be compensated for by beginning meals with protein foods rather than a salad, and by not drinking while eating. Increasing the intake of protein, garlic, and lactic-acid foods (sauerkraut, sourdough bread, and soured-milk products) is believed to stimulate the flow of gastric juices and assist digestion. Many people, particularly the elderly (but not those with ulcers), have found that taking one or two tablets each of betaine or glutamic-acid hydrochloride (available in health food stores) and dolomite (calcium plus magnesium) with each meal has corrected chronic indigestion.

Papaya—Ripe papaya fruit has long been used as a digestive aid in Hawaii, India, and Pakistan. An extract of papaya (papain) is the principal ingredient of most meat tenderizers. Research has shown that papaya contains enzymes which help break down all foods, not just proteins, in the stomach. Eating a piece of fresh papaya before meals or drinking the crushed pulp thinned with orange juice often prevents distress from foods that otherwise cause problems. When fresh papaya is not available, two papaya enzyme tablets may be taken with each meal.

Vitamins and Minerals are necessary for proper digestion. One multi-vitamin-mineral tablet once or twice daily may help correct digestive problems, but additional supplements may be required.

- **Vitamin A**—For the stomach inflammation of gastritis, up to 25,000 units taken three times daily for five days is recommended.
- **B Complex**—One comprehensive, high-potency tablet each morning and evening. Many studies have shown that a shortage of B vitamins reduces hydrochloric-acid production and slows the contractions which move food along the digestive tract. Additional daily supplements of 50 to 100 milligrams each niacinamide and pantothenic acid may benefit all types of digestive problems.
- **Magnesium**—One or two magnesium (or dolomite) tablets taken after meals often helps counteract stomach acidity.
- **Potassium** deficiency slows the intestinal contractions necessary for the digestion and absorption of food. Eating leafy green vegetables and fresh fruits plus using a salt substitute containing potassium chloride usually assures an adequate supply of this mineral. Potassium supplements are available without prescription but large amounts should be taken only with medical approval.

Tissue Salts

- **For occasional indigestion**—Take 3X Kali. Sulph. each 10 minutes for half an hour, then each 25 minutes for an hour or so.
- **For discomfort after eating fats or starches**—Take three doses (three tablets each) 6X Kali. Mur. at hourly intervals.
- **For bilious conditions or a bitter taste after eating**—Take 6X Nat. Sulph. at hourly intervals. If nausea is present, adding alternate doses of 6X Nat. Mur. and Silicea may be beneficial.
- **For indigestion with vomiting**—Take 6X Ferr. Phos. at half-hourly intervals with sips of cold water.
- **For chronic indigestion that is worse in the evening**—Take 12X Kali. Sulph. in the afternoon and again in the early evening.
- **For gastritis**—Take 6X Ferr. Phos. and Kali. Mur. alternately each half hour and, if accompanied by nervous exhaustion, take 6X Kali. Phos. at two-hour intervals.

Folk Remedies

Apple Cider Vinegar—Thanks to Dr. Jarvis' book on Vermont folk medicine[181], apple cider vinegar (with or without natural honey) is the best known of all folk remedies for digestive ailments. Two teaspoons of the vinegar in a glass of water taken before a meal is said to prevent possible food poisoning. With a teaspoon of honey added, the mixture is believed to stimulate and improve digestion.

Apples—Slowly eating the grated mush of peeled and cored green apples is said to cool the burning sensations of gastritis and speed the healing process. For ordinary indigestion, shred cored ripe apples, sweeten with honey, and season with cinnamon or sesame seeds, then eat slowly before or between meals to soothe the "butterflies" and facilitate assimilation of food. Simmering apple parings in milk for 15 minutes, then straining and drinking one cup of the warm liquid each hour until relief is felt is a Polynesian remedy for indigestion.

Bananas are rich in potassium and usually well-tolerated. Oriental practitioners believed bananas re-established the yin-yang balance in the digestive system but directed that they never be eaten with acid fruits, starches, or proteins.

Blackberries—Drinking a little blackberry juice, or blackberry wine, was a standard remedy for dyspepsia.

Blueberries—Mashed raw (or frozen unsweetened) blueberries sweetened with honey were an old tonic for rejuvenating the digestive tract.

Bran and Oat Water—For chronic indigestion: stir one-fourth cup each unprocessed bran and rolled oats in one quart water. Cover and let stand for a day, then strain and drink one cup of the liquid before each meal.

Cod Liver Oil—For dyspepsia: stir four teaspoons cod liver oil in a glass of tomato juice and drink before every meal. One-fourth teaspoon kelp granules may be added, if desired.

Garlic—When taken regularly, garlic (either fresh or in capsule form), is believed to improve digestion and cleanse the digestive tract. Externally, garlic may be used in poultices or foot baths to relieve stomach upsets.

Herbs and Spices—The most widely used "digestive teas" are anise, catnip, dill, fennel, and peppermint. Also thought to aid digestion when sipped at the close of a meal are: camomile, caraway, cayenne, cinnamon, ginseng, golden seal, horehound, horseradish, nutmeg, parsley, red clover, sage, savory, slippery elm, thyme, white oak bark.

Anise Water (one teaspoon of the seeds steeped for 10 minutes in one cup boiling water), or one-half teaspoon each catnip, anise, and fennel prepared in the same manner was used as an antacid.

Peppermint was the favored digestive remedy of the American Indians and ancient Egyptians. A strong infusion of peppermint tea can be bottled to take by the spoonful for stomach upsets. Or, a combination of one teaspoon peppermint plus one-half teaspoon each caraway and fennel seeds can be steeped in one cup boiling water for 10 minutes, then sipped after meals.

For chronic indigestion: steep one-half teaspoon mustard seed in one cup hot water and take 20 minutes before eating. Or, prepare this herbal mixture and store in an airtight container, then steep half a tablespoonful in one cup of hot water for five minutes to drink before each meal. Crush or grind one tablespoon each anise, caraway, and fennel seeds. Mix with three tablespoons dried thyme, two tablespoons camomile, and one tablespoon peppermint.

Following gastritis, fenugreek or tarragon tea is believed to promote healing of the digestive tract.

Hot Water—The oldest and easiest of preventives and remedies, sipping a small cup of scalding water before breakfast, or before every meal, was credited with preventing and correcting dyspepsia. For an occasional attack of indigestion, taking extremely hot water by the teaspoonful may suffice. If desired, one-fourth teaspoon salt may be added to each cup of water.

Juices—Carrot, celery, coconut, cranberry, papaya, pear, pineapple, spinach, and tomato juices are believed to help digestion, as are combinations of juices such as carrot-cucumber-lettuce-parsley. A remedy for chronic dyspepsia was to chop one whole, unpeeled grapefruit into two cups boiling water, let stand overnight, then strain and drink the liquid before breakfast. Because of their high alkalinity, raw vegetable juices are thought to be particularly helpful in cases of chronic gastritis, but the liquid from cooked sauerkraut was recommended in the folklore-collection, *The Foxfire Book*.[345]

Lemon—For chronic indigestion: stir the juice of one lemon in a cup of hot water and drink before every meal.

Milk—Scientific tests have shown one glass of milk to be as effective as commercial antacid preparations for relieving the immediate distress of "acid indigestion," and almost as likely to trigger an acid rebound. Some doctors discourage its use but most feel that its soothing effect and nutritional benefits are to be preferred over non-nutritional products with other possible side effects. Soured milks such as buttermilk, kefir, and yogurt are definite digestive aids. The Swiss swear by their "Essig-Milch" made by stirring one tablespoon vinegar in one-half cup buttermilk.

Mustard and Molasses—For chronic conditions: combine one tablespoon whole mustard seed with one-fourth cup dark molasses and take one or two tablespoons each day.

Olive Oil—For chronic gastritis with an irritated stomach: take one teaspoon to one tablespoon olive oil every morning.

Pineapple—Beginning and ending meals with fresh pineapple is a Polynesian folk-favorite for insuring good digestion.

Vegetables

- **For acid indigestion**—Folk healers recommend eating alfalfa sprouts, one large radish, grated turnip, or sipping freshly juiced raw cabbage or potato.
- **For simple indigestion**—Thoroughly chewing a couple sprigs of fresh parsley or a few bites of raw celery, then drinking a glass of water is said to correct the problem.
- **For immediate relief from a sour stomach**—Thoroughly chew and swallow a bite or two of raw potato.
- **For dyspepsia and indigestion**—Tomatoes were considered a "sovereign remedy." According to Mrs. Beeton's *Book of Household Management*[27], published in 1861, important medicinal properties were ascribed to this "fruit" even though many persons found its flavor offensive.

Nerve Massage

- Massage the area between the thumb and index finger on the inside of the left hand.
- Massage the area directly under and around both armpits.
- Massage completely around both kneecaps.
- Massage and pull the middle toe on each foot for at least one minute.
- Massage the area between the ball of the foot and the center of the arch on both feet. If a tender spot is discovered, rub for five minutes twice a day to improve chronic indigestion.

Nerve Pressure

Unless otherwise indicated, press each point for 10 seconds, release for 10 seconds, and repeat three times.

- Press a point in the center of the crown of the head, about 1 inch in front of the "soft spot."
- Press inward and upward on the underside of the center back of the skull.
- Press inward on the corners of the mouth.
- Press the outer side of the upper bone of each arm, midway between the elbow and the shoulder.
- Press (or wrap with rubber bands) the four fingers of the left hand.
- Press 1 inch to the left of the center of the chest.
- While lying with the knees bent, use the fist to press in front of the right hipbone. Then move up to the ribcage, across to the left side and down to a point in front of the left hipbone, using eight or 10 separate pressures of 10 seconds each. Repeat the sequence three times.
- Press all four corners of an imaginary square around the outer edge of the navel.

Smoking

Smokers troubled by indigestion are advised to abstain until the close of a meal rather than smoking immediately before or during a meal. Smoking suppresses the contractions of the stomach walls, may delay stomach emptying, and slow the peristaltic action.

Stress

Any type of stress, mental or physical, can slow stomach activity to such an extent that food may be left as a partially digested lump or rushed on through the digestive tract to cause diarrhea and/or nausea. Not only obvious emotional upsets or physical fatigue but anxiety, grief, happy excitement, or pain can have the same effect. For this type of indigestion, a few minutes of deliberate relaxation (see pages 9-10), concluding with the mental statement, "My stomach is relaxed and comfortable," has been beneficial in many instances.

Sources (See Bibliography)

3, 5, 7, 8, 12, 13, 18, 27, 34, 53, 62, 63, 68, 71, 75, 76, 81, 84, 85, 89, 121, 131, 142, 152, 154, 156, 168, 174, 180, 181, 184, 189, 190, 211, 215, 226, 227, 229, 243, 253, 254, 261, 270, 276, 288, 289, 297, 314, 315, 319, 325, 328, 333, 334, 335, 344, 345, 354.

INFECTIONS (See Also Fever and Specific Maladies)

Everyone harbors millions of germs at all times and acquires more with everything ingested, inhaled, or touched. Fortunately, human cells resent the presence of these invaders. The body's defensive forces wage constant warfare against this horde of potentially harmful microbes. When resistance is weakened by stress (physical or mental) or by nutritional deficiencies, these organisms flourish and multiply to cause any of numerous infections such as colds, dental abscesses, influenza, kidney or bladder infections, "strep" throat, tonsillitis, etc. which may require medical assistance for control. A high degree of immunity is acquired through one attack of some maladies, like measles, but most other infectious diseases provide no barrier to subsequent infection. Scrupulous cleanliness aids in preventing both spreading and acquiring germs, and proper handling of foodstuffs prevents the growth of bacteria that cause food poisoning.

Germs are exceedingly small—viruses are even smaller than bacteria—and have strange habits. Some are immediately obvious, as with food poisoning. Others remain dormant while awaiting either reinforcements or the fertile environment supplied when antibodies are scarce. Occasionally they settle down in one location to create a mild, chronic infection which never quite clears up and may be the basis for allergic reactions. Allergies to foods and inhalants are a frequent cause of childhood infections. These perpetual infections, as well as those in the nose or on the face, should receive medical attention before the germs infiltrate the blood transport system and spread throughout the body.

Antibiotics offered hope for a world free from infection, but they proved to be a mixed blessing. While miraculously effective in certain conditions, antibiotics do not affect viruses like those of the common cold. They destroy many of the beneficial bacteria necessary for normal body metabolism and disease resistance, may trigger unpleasant side effects for some individuals, and, in addition, encourage the survival-of-the-fittest syndrome—strains of hardy, antibiotic-resistant germs. Whenever antibiotics are prescribed, eating acidophilus yogurt daily or taking acidophilus capsules with each meal can help combat the damage to friendly bacteria in the digestive tract.

Regardless of other treatments used, hydrotherapy (alternate applications of hot and cold water or packs) is often recommended to improve circulation in the affected area and help the body throw off the infection. Hands, arms, feet, or legs can be soaked first in hot water, then in cold for three minutes and the alternations repeated three times. For other parts of the body, separate towels wrung out of hot and cold water can be applied.

For fungus infections on the skin, applying a paste made from brewer's yeast and vitamin E oil twice each day is often effective. For vaginal yeast-infections, possibly triggered by past antibiotic treatments, a local application of acidophilus may be necessary to prevent recurrence following a temporary cure by an anti-yeast medication. According to *Dr. Wright's Book of Nutritional Therapy*[353], combining one-half cup plain acidophilus yogurt with two tablespoons acidophilus culture (available in health food stores or by shaking out the contents of acidophilus capsules) and inserting two teaspoons of the mixture into the vagina on each of five successive nights will replace the helpful bacteria. A cleansing douche each morning with two tablespoons vinegar in one quart warm water is recommended. This vinegar douche, used once or twice a week, may also correct vaginal inflammation and discharge caused by Trichomonias, but, if the affliction continues for more than a week or so, medical help should be obtained.

While it is possible that some infections may be psychosomatic in origin, it is the opinion of most nutritionally oriented physicians that proper diet plus supplements is the best defense against infections and can often either abort an incipient illness or shorten its duration.

Diet and Supplements

Adequate protein is needed for good resistance. The body's defensive forces (antibodies, lymph cells, and white blood cells) are made of protein. (Clinical studies have shown that antibodies decrease to one-tenth that of normal after only one week on a low-protein diet.[92]) When infection does strike, increasing the amount of protein obtained daily from meats, eggs, milk, brewer's yeast, soy flour, and wheat germ has proven most effective in increasing antibody production.

Garlic is so well-known for its value in treating infections that it has been dubbed "Russian Penicillin." A daily intake of six garlic cloves (minced and swallowed, added to green salads, or mixed with butter and spread on toast) or the equivalent in garlic perles, is the suggested amount. Onions, whether raw or cooked, have many of the same beneficial properties of garlic because of their high sulphur content. One 8-ounce cup of plain acidophilus yogurt is reported to have an antibiotic value equal to 14 penicillin units.[188] Labels are required reading when shopping for yogurt. Not all commercial brands contain acidophilus and, even when included, the bacterial benefits are reduced by long storage or the addition of sugared fruits.

Fresh pineapple contains an enzyme believed to destroy many kinds of infectious germs. Tomatoes are a natural antiseptic and protect against infection. The juices of beets, carrots, lemons, oranges, and tomatoes are especially beneficial but too much citrus may make body fluids so alkaline that they promote the growth of bacteria. Folk medicine recommends drinking either a cup of hot water into which one-fourth cup apple cider vinegar and two tablespoons raw honey have been stirred, or comfrey tea which is believed capable of drawing infection from the body. Folk practitioners also advise the proverbial two teaspoons each apple cider vinegar and honey stirred in a glass of water and sipped with each meal to increase resistance by creating an acid medium in which germs do not multiply.

Refined sugar should be avoided or stringently limited as it depresses the immune system, impairing its ability to fight infections.[353] Many authorities believe abnormal blood-sugar levels encourage susceptibility to infection. However, taking small amounts of natural carbohydrates (fresh or cooked fruit, or eggnog made with honey) every hour or two can often forestall or halt the headache and nausea accompanying an infection. This modified version of the "fortified milk" recommended by Adelle Davis in Let's Get Well[89] is an eggnog that can be whirred in a blender, refrigerated, and taken in half-cup amounts every few hours. It provides protein and carbohydrates plus other nutrients. When used as the liquid for taking vitamin supplements, it acts as both a buffer and an enhancer. (See Index for more simplified variations.)

2 cups skim or whole milk
2 whole eggs or 2 egg yolks
1/2 cup frozen, undiluted orange juice and/or one small banana

1/4 cup each brewer's yeast, powdered milk, and soy flour
1/4 cup acidophilus yogurt or the contents of two acidophilus capsules
1 tablespoon lecithin granules
1/2 teaspoon each dolomite and bone-meal powder (optional)
Nutmeg and/or vanilla for flavoring, if desired

In addition to a daily multi-vitamin-mineral tablet, the following supplements have been found beneficial:

Vitamin A—25,000 to 50,000 units per day for one month. 100,000 to 200,000 units daily for three or four days during measles, infections of the skin or mucous membranes (colitis or infections of the bladder, kidneys, lungs, sinuses, or throat). Infections create an increased need for vitamin A in order to resist germ invasion and allow the body to produce antibodies and white blood cells. Large amounts of this vitamin have been found successful in counteracting the side effects of cortisone and related drugs that block the immune response, slow healing, and increase the susceptibility to infection.[6]

B Complex—One comprehensive, high-potency tablet with meals three times a day for at least one month. Infections create body stress that increases the need for B vitamins. Even a mild deficiency of vitamins B-1, B-2, B-6, biotin, choline, folic acid, niacin, or pantothenic acid reduces the amount of antibodies produced, lowers resistance, and prevents the body's defenses from being stimulated when antitoxins or other forms of immunization are given. Some people require far more B-6 and pantothenic acid than others. As much as 600 milligrams B-6 and 4,000 milligrams pantothenic acid daily, besides the B-complex tablets, may be needed to increase antibody production. Lecithin contains choline and is believed to help fight infection by increasing the gamma globulin in the blood, but, when using large amounts, both calcium and magnesium should be increased to balance its high phosphorus content.

Vitamin C—100 to 1,000 milligrams each hour or two while the infection is severe, then 500 to 5,000 milligrams per day for maintenance. Vitamin C is a potent therapeutic agent that works almost as antibodies do in destroying harmful bacteria and viruses, and has an antibiotic effect. Massive amounts (up to 40,000 milligrams per day) have been found nontoxic, so as much vitamin C as can be tolerated without the development of diarrhea is recommended. Taking bioflavonoids and calcium with vitamin C enhance its effectiveness and decrease the possibility of side effects. A combination that frequently halts an infection if taken at the onset is: 2,000 milligrams vitamin C, 200 milligrams pantothenic acid, and 20 milligrams B-6. During the first day, half these amounts should be taken every two or three hours with the fortified milk described above.[89]

Vitamin E (see Caution, page 6)—100 to 600 IU daily. Without ample vitamin E, vitamin A is destroyed by oxygen within the body so that what may appear to be a deficiency of vitamin A is actually a lack of vitamin E. The alpha tocopherol form of vitamin E also repairs capillary damage to help repulse further infections, and prevents the formation of internal scar tissue which often follows nephritis, rheumatic fever, etc.[300]

Selenium—150 to 200 micrograms daily. Especially when taken with vitamin E, selenium increases the body's production of antibodies. When the combination is used along with vaccinations, their protective effect is increased as much as 20 times.[249]

Sodium is lost from the body during most infections. This causes fluid to accumulate in the inflamed area, creating swelling and pain. The folk remedy of drinking a cup of hot water containing one-half teaspoon each baking soda and salt often gives prompt relief from a localized inflammation with swelling.

Zinc—30 to 150 milligrams daily. An undersupply of zinc causes low resistance to infections. Extra amounts are particularly helpful in combating those of bacterial origin, and, when taken in combination with B-6 supplements, zinc helps open swollen air passages and tissues to aid in the control of infection.

Exercise

Good muscle tone improves defense mechanisms against infection. "Sit-ups" in particular increase the circulation of blood through the liver to assist the antibodies in their battle with infections.

Nerve Massage

Massaging the top of each foot, from one side of the anklebone to the other, is believed to improve the condition of the lymph glands and encourage antibody production.

Nerve Pressure

Press in and up on the lower edge of the cheekbones, about 2 inches in front of the ears. Then press the tips of the two floating ribs on the left side of the back, just above the waistline. Press each point for 10 seconds, release for 10 seconds, and repeat three times.

Sources (See Bibliography)

3, 6, 7, 12, 13, 19, 30, 34, 53, 78, 88, 89, 92, 99, 153, 154, 156, 173, 174, 175, 180, 181, 184, 188, 228, 229, 249, 250, 252, 253, 254, 256, 257, 260, 288, 293, 297, 300, 301, 305, 312, 328, 331, 350, 353, 354.

INSECT BITES AND STINGS

The bites and stings of ants, bees, mosquitoes, spiders, wasps, etc. are usually merely painful or itchy mishaps. In the United States only black widow and brown recluse spiders are poisonous, and dangerous scorpions are limited to the Southwestern deserts. But a few people are allergically sensitive to common venoms. (Egyptian hieroglyphics from 2641 B.C. indicate that King Menes died from the sting of a hornet.) Those who have known allergies such as hay fever or drug sensitivity should watch for severe reactions that may be delayed for as long as two weeks following a bite or sting. When there is a previously established allergy, a poisonous bite or sting, or one in the eye, mouth, or throat, the area should be chilled immediately. If possible, a tourniquet should be applied between the heart and the site of the sting to impede venom absorption while enroute to the nearest doctor.

After over a hundred years of controversy regarding the acid-vs-alkaline properties of various insect venoms it has now been discovered that they are a complex mixture of both and that the same natural remedies may be used for all.[241] Preventive measures are also similar. Insects confuse people with flowers when brightly colored clothing or cosmetic scents are worn. Bees are thought to be attracted by colors and drawn to coarse materials as well as flower-like scents. Mosquitoes prefer men to women, dirty to clean, like to bite those wearing wet clothing, and are particularly attracted to the color blue.

The stinger left by a bee, hornet, or wasp should be removed by scraping rather than pinching to avoid squeezing in any more venom. If a tick attaches itself to the skin it is important to remove rather than mash it. Covering the tick with any heavy oil or grease may close its breathing pores and force it to release its hold. Gasoline, kerosene, or turpentine may have the same effect. If none of these is available, a lighted match or cigarette can be held to the tick's back. Once the tick is removed, the area should be washed and disinfected, as should a wasp sting since wasps are carnivorous creatures who may have had their feet in contaminated materials.

Diet and Supplements

The daily consumption of large amounts of brewer's yeast or garlic is said to repel insects. According to William Dufty in *Sugar Blues*[105], sweetness is what appeals to insects and they are no longer interested in people who have been on a sugar-free diet for a year or so.

B Vitamins—Taking 100 milligrams B-1 before and each three or four hours during exposure is said to produce a skin odor repellent to bees, fleas, flies, and mosquitoes. Taking 100 milligrams pantothenic acid plus 500 milligrams vitamin C immediately after the attack helps detoxify the poisons from all stings or bites. When 50 milligrams of B-6 are added, allergic reactions are often alleviated.

Vitamin C—1,000 to 2,000 milligrams as soon as bitten or stung. Repeat in an hour or so if discomfort is still present. Massive amounts of vitamin C (up to 4,000 milligrams) have been known to detoxify even black widow spider bites when taken every few hours for several days. Bioflavonoids enhance the action of vitamin C. Continual use of vitamin C and bioflavonoid supplements strengthens cell permeability to help immunize the body from allergic reactions to insect bites or stings. Taking calcium with the vitamin C decreases both sensitivity to pain and the likelihood of stomach irritation. Moistened vitamin C powder applied directly to the area often brings immediate relief from itching and burning.

Vitamin E—Local applications of vitamin E ointment, or the oil squeezed from capsules, often reduces the pain from a sting or bite. Taking oral doses of 200 milligrams vitamin E every three or four hours has increased the effectiveness (see Caution, page 6).

Tissue Salts—For severe bites or stings: take 6X Kali. Phos., Nat. Mur., and Silicea every 10 minutes for one hour. For subsequent swelling, substitute Kali. Mur. for Nat. Mur. and take three or four doses per day. For immediate relief, make a paste of these tablets with water or saliva and apply locally.

Folk Remedies

Prevention—Sponging the face and other exposed areas with camomile tea or vinegar, or rubbing them with fresh parsley, is believed to repel flying and crawling pests. Rubbing olive oil on the face and hands before going to bed is said to prevent gnats and mosquitoes from biting during the night.

Treatment—

Ice is a multi-purpose remedy for all types of bites and stings. Chilling the area keeps the venom localized and has an anesthetic effect on both pain and itching. Soaking an affected hand or foot in a basin filled with ice cubes, water, and half a cup of baking soda is most effective. For swelling, dissolve one tablespoon epsom salts in a little hot water and use in place of the baking soda. For swelling around the eyes, cover the area with cloths squeezed out of a mixture of one teaspoon baking soda and one cup ice-cold water. An ice compress can be placed over a paste of baking soda, or used with any of the other remedies.

Liquids and Lotions—Dab for five minutes, or cover with cloth saturated in any of these liquids: rubbing alcohol, ammonia diluted with water, baking soda and water (plus salt, if desired), the liquid from crushed chrysanthemum leaves, cinnamon tea (eat the cinnamon sticks from which the tea was brewed), cod liver oil, kerosene, lemon juice or vinegar (or a mixture of the two), olive oil, hot salt water, tobacco juice, or turpentine.

An old-fashioned aromatic lotion that was kept on hand for relieving bites and stings can be made by combining one teaspoon each cinnamon, cloves, ginger, lemon peel, orange peel, and sassafras with one cup vinegar and allowing it to stand, covered, for 10 days. It should be stirred or shaken occasionally, then strained and bottled.

Honey was believed especially helpful for bee stings but was used on all bites and stings. Other options are to cover the affected area with vitamin E squeezed from a capsule, castor oil, or wheat germ oil and either plunge it into ice water or cover with an ice pack.

Pastes and Poultices—Commercial meat tenderizer is the modern folk-remedy for bee and wasp stings. Sprinkle the tenderizer on a moistened gauze pad, or make into a paste with water, then apply for 20 minutes to one hour. Activated charcoal (available in health food stores) combined with water to make a paste and applied to the sting also draws out the poison and reduces both pain and swelling. Older remedies are: a paste of baking soda and water or ammonia allowed to dry and harden for an hour, a mixture of butter and salt, fresh cow manure wrapped in cloth and left in place overnight, moist clay or plain mud, raw meat (especially beef), wet salt, snuff, damp tea leaves, a spoonful of moistened tobacco, or a covering of toothpaste. Another option believed to relieve pain and swelling was to rub any four different kinds of fresh leaves together, then apply to the sting.

Vegetables—Mashed or juiced fresh garlic (or the oil from capsules) has been used for all venomous bites and stings, even those of scorpions, since the time of Mohammed. The crushed leaves of cabbage or blades of leeks, fresh grated horseradish wrapped in cheesecloth, onion juice, sliced onions, or raw potato slices were used to relieve the pain of insect bites and stings.

Case History

Casey K. was wearing his new Hawaiian shirt and having a wonderful time playing hide-and-seek with his older sisters in his grandmother's backyard. Then the bee stung. The little boy's howls of pain sent the girls in search of their grandmother. She quickly scraped out the stinger, gave him an ice cube to hold over the spot to deaden the pain, and consoled him with the explanation that the bee had mistaken his brightly colored shirt for a pollen-containing flower. She took Casey with her to the kitchen while she sliced an onion, bandaged one of the slices over the raised red spot on his arm, and told him about the way bees carried pollen to help trees and plants produce delicious fruits and beautiful flowers. By the time Casey's parents arrived to pick up the children, the swelling had gone down. The only evidence of the insect sting was the excited tale, related by the girls, of their assistance in procuring help for him, and Casey's insistence in describing the process whereby bees help make food and flowers for people to enjoy—and use their stingers only when confused or frightened.

Relief of Itching (see also Eczema)—Apply after-shave lotion, rubbing alcohol, ammonia, a paste of baking powder and ammonia, a poultice of cornstarch moistened with lemon juice and Witch Hazel, mashed garlic, lemon or lime juice, mud, the juice of parsley leaves, suntan lotion containing PABA, a mixture of ethyl alcohol and crushed PABA tablets, moistened tobacco, vinegar, or wet soap.

Sources

3, 7, 13, 27, 52, 53, 62, 68, 73, 76, 81, 89, 98, 105, 111, 123, 142, 152, 153, 156, 168, 177, 184, 215, 226, 227, 229, 241, 288, 297, 305, 315, 318, 319, 325, 328, 345.

INSOMNIA

Defined as stressful wakefulness that leaves the victim uncomfortable and unable to function efficiently the following day, insomnia can refer to difficulty in falling asleep, frequent awakening, or being wide awake after a few hours sleep. Many sleeping problems are self-induced by an attempt to get more sleep than the system can accommodate. A recent survey revealed the national sleep average to be seven and one-half hours per night for adults under 40, with a drop to six hours by age 65.[292] The eight-hour myth is just that—individual sleep requirements are determined by an internal clock that may be pre-set for anywhere from three to 11 hours out of each 24. Rapidly growing children need more sleep than adults, and the slowing of reparative processes during extreme old age may require an increase in sleeptime.

Electronic tracings of brain waves show there are four stages of sleep. Normally operating in 60- to 90-minute cycles, they begin with a light sleep during which conscious thought processes may continue. In stages two and three, breathing deepens and heart rate and body temperature declines. From the deep sleep of stage four there is a return to stage two and the rapid eye movements (REM) of dream sleep for 10 to 15 minutes, then down again as the cycle repeats. All the stages are necessary for physical and mental well-being. Insomniacs often feel they have not slept at all because a preponderance of their sleeping time has been spent between stages one and two.

Insomnia can result from environmental disturbances such as too much light or sound, a poor mattress, mental stress, nutritional deficiencies, or the physical disorders of asthma, diarrhea, low blood sugar, etc. A few nights of wakefulness are merely discomforting but prolonged insomnia can endanger health and require medical attention. Once the obvious causes have been controlled, most authorities on sleep suggest the following rules for correcting and avoiding insomnia.

- Take daytime naps only as an intentional portion of sleeptime. Even almost-dozing before the fire or television reduces the amount of sleep required at night. When the schedule permits napping, 15 minutes sleep in the middle of a work day provides more efficiency than five times as much late, light sleeping in the morning.[270]
- Limit liquids during the evening and avoid caffeine-containing beverages or medications.
- Develop a pre-sleep ritual of at least six things to do in the same order each night before going to bed.
- Do not take sleeping pills unless under doctor's orders, and then for no more than 10 consecutive nights. Besides losing their effectiveness and becoming addictive, sleep-inducing medications reduce or prevent the dream-stage of sleep necessary for good mental health.
- Do nothing in bed except sleep—no reading, television watching, etc. (Sexual activity is the one permitted exception to this rule)
- Never remain in bed longer than 30 minutes if awake. Get up and do something boring until sleepy. Do not encourage future wakefulness by reading a novel or eating. If awakened by a bad dream, sit in a chair for five minutes and, during that time, stroke the right forearm from wrist to elbow for 30-seconds to break the neural pattern and prevent continuing the dream when sleep returns.

Diet and Supplements

Eating a heavy meal just before retiring is never recommended but going to bed hungry can cause restless sleep as the drop in blood sugar sets off a release of adrenalin.

Certain foods aid sleep because they are high in the amino acid, tryptophan, which the body converts to a chemical (serotonin) essential to sleep. Carbohydrates plus small amounts of fat assist in the utilization of tryptophan. A chocolate bar, fruit and cheese, or a chicken sandwich with a glass of milk often instigates drowsiness. Other foods high in tryptophan are egg yolks, all milk products, nuts, poultry, and meats. Two other amino acids, arginine and ornithine, are sleep-inducers. Chicken has a relatively large concentration of both. These amino acids are available as supplements, but if used should be taken on an empty stomach just at bedtime.

The type of insomnia determines when the major portion of the day's high-carbohydrate foods should be eaten. If the problem is an inability to fall asleep, the high-carbohydrate foods should be eaten two to four hours before bedtime; if it is light sleep or frequent awakenings, the foods should be eaten immediately before bed.

When nervous tension seems to be the cause of sleeping difficulties, drinking carrot juice combined with an equal amount of apple, celery, grape, pear, spinach, or watermelon juice may be of help. A glass of wine or other alcoholic beverage aids relaxation but overindulgence can disturb the natural sleep pattern, interfere with the dream cycle, and cause restless or short sleep. Salty foods should be avoided before bedtime as salt stimulates the adrenal glands just as caffeine does.

Sleep problems caused by nutritional deficiencies can be remedied with natural supplements which work differently from pharmaceutical sleep-inducers in that their dosage can gradually be reduced and eventually eliminated. Rather than altering sleep patterns and creating a dependence on drugs, the supplements lead to normal sleep.

B Complex—One comprehensive tablet daily. Deficiencies of almost any of the B vitamins can cause insomnia. Additional amounts of specific B vitamins aid sleep and encourage pleasant dreams when taken an hour before bedtime.

- 100 to 2,000 milligrams of niacinamide reduces nervousness and enhances the action of tryptophan.
- 50 to 400 milligrams of B-6 has a tranquilizing effect—being able to recall several dreams each week indicates a sufficient dosage.
- 1,000 to 10,000 milligrams of inositol has been found to produce sedation as effectively as a tranquilizer, especially when accompanied by niacinamide, but massive amounts should not be taken on an every-night basis.
- 100 to 2,000 milligrams of pantothenic acid calms overstimulation and has a tranquilizing effect.

Brewer's Yeast—One to three tablespoons stirred into warm broth or milk and taken before bedtime provides protein and B vitamins to promote sleep. Honey or blackstrap molasses may be added to increase drowsiness.

Vitamin C—500 to 2,000 milligrams daily. Vitamin C acts as an anti-anxiety agent. Its effect lasts approximately six hours when used as a relaxant and is especially effective when taken with B vitamins, calcium, and/or tryptophan.

Calcium—At least 1,000 milligrams daily in addition to the calcium obtained from foods and milk. Known as the sleep mineral, calcium is essential to healthy nerves and sound sleep. Its absorption is dependent on vitamin D, magnesium, and phosphorus, and decreases with age. Taking 500 to 1,000 milligrams of calcium lactate (or a combination of bone meal and dolomite) with a glass of warm milk just before bed frequently eradicates sleep problems. Adding supplements of B-6 and pantothenic acid practically guarantees a restful night.

Tissue Salts—

For occasional sleeplessness from excitement, worry, or working late: take three or four tablets of 6X Ferr. Phos. an hour before retiring. Ten minutes later, take three or four tablets of 6X Kali. Phos. If needed, repeat the dosage in an hour.

If stomach acidity or heartburn accompanies insomnia: take three or four tablets of 6X Nat. Phos. an hour before bedtime and repeat in 30 minutes, if necessary.

If sleeplessness is accompanied by a pounding heart: take one tablet each 12X Calc. Fluor., Kali. Phos., and Nat. Mur. at bedtime and in the morning until the condition has improved.

When insomnia is accompanied by itching: take three tablets of 6X Nat. Phos. Repeat in an hour, if needed.

Tryptophan—1,000 to 3,000 milligrams an hour before retiring. For small children who have difficulty sleeping, a 500-milligram tablet can be crushed and stirred into a before-bed glass of milk. Some authorities recommend taking no more than 10 milligrams of B-6 with the tryptophan as it may cause the tryptophan to break down before it can be utilized by the brain for inducing sleep. However, in their book, *Life Extension*[252], Durk Pearson and Sandy Shaw suggest 100 milligrams B-6 and 1,000 milligrams vitamin C as accompaniments for 2,000 milligrams tryptophan. Numerous scientific tests have shown this amino acid (usually available as L-tryptophan) to be effective in relieving all forms of insomnia without becoming habit-forming, but it is not recommended on a daily basis. Taking up to 500 milligrams of niacinamide increases its sleep-promoting effect. Eating foods high in tryptophan can contribute to normal sleep, particularly when taken in the evening, but the therapeutic effect requires a tremendous disproportion of tryptophan in relation to the other amino acids.

Exercise

Adequate physical exercise is necessary for normal sleep. Thirty minutes of vigorous exercise each day, preferably before 4 p.m., is recommended. Excessive fatigue can be a cause of insomnia but a short walk or a few minutes of these isometric exercises before going to bed may induce sleep.

- Stand with the hands on the rib cage and exert pressure for one minute.
- Put the palms together in front of the chest and press one against the other for a minute or so. Or, interlock the fingers and squeeze. Or, push the fingertips of one hand against those of the other.
- Stand beside a wall with the right shoulder touching it. With the right wrist

and hand, push against the wall as hard as possible for one minute. Repeat with the left shoulder and hand.

Folk Remedies

Too much blood in the brain was considered a cause of insomnia. Raising the head of the bed and using a thick pillow was advised, as was eating just before retiring so the work of digestion would draw blood from the brain.

Apple—Slowly eating an unpeeled apple shortly before retiring is an old folk remedy for insomnia that has been scientifically substantiated by tests at the University of Michigan.[227]

Bread—Butter a thin slice of bread, sprinkle with cayenne pepper, and eat slowly just before going to bed.

Cold Compress—Squeeze a cloth out of ice-cold water and place on the back of the neck to soothe the brain.

Garlic—Crushed garlic stirred into warm milk, or a bowl of garlic soup made with chicken broth, is thought to induce sleep. When children wake in the night with bad dreams, rubbing garlic on their feet is said to bring a return of peaceful sleep.

Herbs—Camomile tea, long recognized by herbalists as a harmless sedative, showed striking sleep-inducing action in tests reported in the *Journal of Clinical Pharmacology* (January 10, 1974). Camomile was also used to quiet nightmares in both children and adults. Other teas advocated by folk healers are: anise, basil, catnip, dill, ginger, lettuce seed, licorice root, marjoram, peppermint, rosemary, sage, and scullcap. A favorite combination was one teaspoon peppermint, one-half teaspoon rosemary, and one-fourth teaspoon sage steeped in one cup boiling water, then strained and sweetened with honey. In the 1840's, washing the hair in strained dill tea was thought to promote sleep.

Honey—A quickly assimilated carbohydrate that reaches the bloodstream 20 minutes after ingestion, honey has long been used as a sleep-inducer. Folk remedies call for stirring one teaspoon to two tablespoons honey in herb teas, warm milk, or hot water with a few teaspoons of lemon juice. A variation is one-fourth cup honey, one tablespoon apple cider vinegar, and two teaspoons bee pollen granules stirred into a cup of freshly boiled water and sipped at bedtime. Dr. Jarvis'[181] formula for insomnia was three tablespoons apple cider vinegar blended with one cup honey and kept in a jar by the bedside. Two teaspoons of the mixture was to be taken upon retiring and another two teaspoons each half hour while wakeful. Taking two teaspoons each honey and vinegar in a glass of water with each meal is advised as maintenance for normal sleep.

Case History

Colleen F. could teach anything to anybody. During the school year she taught in a departmentalized program for seventh and eighth grade students; during the summer she taught the alphabet to pre-schoolers, and conversational Spanish or typing to adults. But, even Colleen could not teach when she was half asleep. She attributed her sleepless nights to enthusiasm over her work, and refused to succumb to sleeping pills. However, she had to get some rest—and stop dozing at her desk. A colleague's mention of Dr. Jarvis' book led to the solution of her problem. At bedtime each night, Colleen stirred two tablespoons of honey into a glass of warm milk, added a tablespoon of apple cider vinegar, and drank the mixture before the milk could curdle. The results were fantastic. Colleen slept the night through and awakened refreshed, ready to enjoy helping her students learn whatever the subject might be.

Hot Water—Either taken by the cupful internally or used as a foot bath (with or without the addition of dry mustard) hot water was believed to produce drowsiness.

Leaf Lettuce (not Iceberg head lettuce) was a favored sedative. The leaves may be eaten raw, chopped and simmered in broth for a soup, or minced and steeped in boiling water for five minutes before straining to sip as a before-bed tea.

Milk is the perennial solution for sleeplessness. In addition to its emotionally soothing effect, a glass of warm milk temporarily neutralizes stomach acids, contains generous amounts of calcium and tryptophan, and is a mild, natural sedative. During the 1800s, hot milk with honey and freshly grated nutmeg (plus a pinch of red pepper, if desired) was the standard remedy for insomnia. Some folk practitioners preferred a mixture of one cup buttermilk, two tablespoons honey, and the juice of one lemon. Those who have difficulty with cow's milk may find goat's milk more easily digestible. Blending one tablespoon carob powder and two teaspoons honey with a cup of goat's milk provides a pleasant change-of-taste.

Onions—Believed to have great soporific powers, onions were eaten raw or cooked. Those who could down two large raw onions before bedtime reported magical results. Others may prefer an onion soup made by cooking the two onions in broth, adding the juice of one lemon, and one teaspoon butter.

Nerve Massage

- Stroke the forearms with the fingernails for five or ten minutes.
- Massage each foot for three minutes. Start with the toes, pulling each one for 10 seconds. Then massage the sole, the heel, the sides, the ankle, and the top of the foot. A folk-remedy variation is to place a wooden rolling pin on the floor and roll the soles of the feet across it, applying as much pressure as possible, for three minutes each night just before bed.

Nerve Pressure

Unless otherwise indicated, press each point for 10 seconds, release for 10 seconds, and repeat three times.

- Use the thumb and index finger to squeeze and press just above the bridge of the nose for 10 minutes.
- Press a point 1 inch behind each earlobe.
- Press a point in the center of the chest.
- Press 1½ inches toward the elbow from the largest crease on the inner wrist, directly in line with the middle finger.
- Use the thumbnail to press the wrist crease against the bone leading to the little finger.
- Press a point on the abdomen 1½ inches directly below the navel.
- On each foot, press just below the lower corners of the toenails of the second and fourth toes, on the side toward the little toe.
- Place the thumb below the ball of the foot in line with the third toe. Press in while inhaling slowly, release pressure gradually as breath is exhaled. Repeat 10 times on each foot.

Relaxation

Practicing any favorite relaxation technique (see pages 9-10) until the sensation of complete relaxation is firmly established makes it possible to merely point the conscious mind in that direction and have the muscles relax. Yogas believe that gazing at a lighted candle for 10 minutes before retiring will quiet the mind and the nervous system. Saying aloud, "I will fall asleep more quickly tonight and will awaken refreshed at the sound of the alarm," and then repeating it silently a few times is a form of autosuggestion that weakens negative expectations. When sleep does not immediately follow physical relaxation, there are numerous alternatives to counting sheep.

- Inhale deeply through the mouth, then exhale through the nose. Repeat five times, or until yawning.
- Take four deep breaths. With the lungs empty, refrain from breathing to the point of discomfort, then take four more deep breaths and repeat for four cycles. As explained in *Somniquest*[292], this utilizes the body's natural reserves of carbon dioxide to create drowsiness.
- There are several options for blocking the entrance of disturbing thoughts or unpleasant emotions:

  Think of yourself as a child, sitting in a swing on a pleasant day. Visualize yourself swinging back while you inhale and think the word "sleep." Then exhale and swing forward while mentally counting "two." Inhale and swing back on the count of three, forward with an exhalation on "four." Repeat until sleep comes.

  With the eyes closed, imagine entering an elevator on the hundredth floor. Watch the indicator above the elevator door and mentally recite the numbers as it slowly descends to the ground.

  Imagine a blackboard with the number 100 written on it inside a large circle. Mentally erase the number and write the next lower number, then write the words "deep sleep" beside the circle. Continue erasing, renumbering, and writing over the words as long as necessary.

- Sounds soothe many people to sleep and keep them sleeping. Electric fans, soft music, or ticking clocks were used before the advent of "sleep sound" recordings of rain, ocean waves, trickling brooks, or waterfalls were available.

Warm Baths

Warm or hot baths relax the muscles and produce a state of mental drowsiness. Soaking for 20 minutes in a hot tub, with or without a handful of epsom salts, is soothing. Following a hot bath or shower with 30 seconds of cold water often calms the nervous system enough to make relaxation possible. If a full bath is inconvenient, a hot footbath is believed to draw the blood from the brain, making it sluggish and inducing sleep. When all else fails, the ultimate resort is to fill the bathtub with warm water, add all the salt that will dissolve (besides being soothing, this prevents sinking and drowning) then go to sleep in the tub.[160]

Sources (See Bibliography)

4, 9, 10, 13, 24, 30, 34, 37, 43, 45, 52, 53, 62, 63, 65, 67, 68, 78, 81, 88, 89, 92, 142, 147, 151, 154, 156, 160, 165, 168, 174, 176, 178, 180, 181, 184, 190, 191, 208, 211, 226, 227, 228, 241, 243, 252, 254, 257, 261, 269, 270, 288, 289, 290, 292, 297, 298, 305, 315, 318, 319, 325, 330, 333, 335, 349, 353.

KIDNEY AND BLADDER PROBLEMS AND STONES (See Also Infections)

Maladies of the urinary system may stem from problems with either the kidneys or bladder and should be diagnosed by a physician. "Kidney trouble" describes a variety of disorders: inflammation of the kidneys (Bright's disease, nephritis, or pyelitis), dropsy (see Edema), or kidney stones (renal calculi). Because of anatomical differences, infections of the urinary tract are more frequent in females than males. "Honeymoon cystitis" may originate from the beginning of sexual experiences. Bladder inflammation can be provoked by pregnancy or allergies or, in older persons, by problems of elimination. Bladder or kidney irritation can lead to the formation of stones that usually migrate to the bladder from the kidneys. More men than women are afflicted with these stones and there appears to be a genetic tendency for both bladder inflammations and stone formation.

The kidneys may be adversely affected by alcohol, overuse of aspirin, cortisone or hypertensive drugs, chemicals used in dry cleaning, dehydration, enlargement of the male prostate gland (see Prostrate Problems), immobility, infection in other parts of the body, or by nutritional deficiencies. According to current medical belief, high blood pressure (which see) is a causative factor in practically all kidney disease.

The following suggestions are offered for chronic bladder conditions: drink cranberry juice and extra fluids but restrict tea and coffee, drink a full glass of water just before retiring, take showers in preference to tub baths, urinate frequently, void after intercourse, wear cotton underwear, exercise regularly to strengthen abdominal muscles.

Most kidney stones are formed around crystals of calcium combined with phosphorus and/or oxalic acid, but there is little relationship between the amount of calcium ingested and the quantity that appears in the urine. In rare cases, excess uric acid (see Gout) or the amino acid cystine is responsible for the stones. Chemical analysis of a passed stone is required to determine the preventive measures required to avoid recurrence. Simply supplementing the diet with magnesium and vitamin B-6 has dissolved many kidney stones and prevented recurrence in 80 to 90 percent of patients in clinically controlled studies (*American Health,* November/December, 1982). Large stones may require surgical removal, but, with immediate care and natural remedies, most bladder and kidney abnormalities can be rectified.

Diet and Supplements

Drinking two to three quarts of liquid each day dilutes the urine, helps prevent bladder and kidney maladies, speeds recovery, and sometimes flushes out stones and gravel. Including at least two glasses of cranberry juice is recommended by folk healers and physicians alike. According to *Archives of Physical Medicine and Rehabilitation* (December, 1975), hospital studies have shown that drinking four glasses of cranberry juice helped prevent kidney stones from forming and helped clear other problems of the urinary tract—including urgent or too-frequent urination. Other juices with diuretic properties (see Edema) reduce urine concentration and provide nutrients, but much of the fluid intake should be plain water. European doctors advise women subject to cystitis to drink two glasses of water after intercourse. Some American physicians recommend that kidney-stone formers set an alarm clock in order to drink several additional glasses of water during the night.

Authorities agree that acidifying the urine inhibits infection and the formation of calcium-oxalate stones. Cranberries, eggs, meats, natural cheeses and whole grains are acid-forming foods. During acute episodes, vegetables and citrus fruits should be avoided. (If uric-acid kidney stones have been diagnosed, an opposite program should be followed. The acid foods should be restricted and the alkalinizing vegetables and citrus fruits stressed.)

Brown rice, cantaloupe, celery, cucumber, garlic, grape juice, honey, horseradish, onions, parsley, parsnips, strawberries, watercress and watermelon are considered excellent for urinary disorders. Asparagus, bananas and papayas are believed to have a healing effect on the kidneys. Eating five or six small meals rather than two or three large ones is considered beneficial. Some nutritional experts recommend that nothing but raw fruits and vegetables be eaten for one day of each week to cleanse and rejuvenate the urinary system.

Dietary regimens for stone-formers are controversial. The traditional "low-protein, low-calcium, no oxalate-containing foods" diet is now considered unnecessary and possibly harmful by many doctors. When there is an intake of less than 40 grams of protein a day, so much body protein must be broken down that even more urea is formed than if a high-protein diet were eaten. (One boiled egg contains 6 grams of protein; one hamburger patty, 21.[189]). At least 70 grams of protein is usually recommended, and, except for cases threatened by uremic poisoning, even more is believed beneficial. Studies have shown that patients with kidney disease recovered much more rapidly when 150 to 200 grams of protein were eaten daily.[76,89]

While milk, other dairy products, and high-oxalic foods such as chocolate, rhubarb, and spinach may need to be avoided during a kidney-stone attack, many experts question the value of restricting them permanently. As explained in the *Harvard Medical School Health Letter* (March, 1983), a reduction of calcium in the diet may result in increased absorption of oxalate and the formation of kidney stones. Normally, 99 percent of all calcium passing through the kidneys is absorbed back into the blood.[18] Adequate magnesium plus vitamins D and E are necessary for this resorption. If they are undersupplied, or if over 5,000 units of synthetic vitamin D are taken per day, large amounts of both calcium and phosphorus pass into the urine.[89] Aspirin and other drugs also increase the urinary losses of calcium and phosphorus. Calcium deposits in the soft tissues become worse when the diet is low in calcium. Continued bed rest can cause calcium to be drawn from the bones into the urine even though no calcium at all is ingested.[4] Most of the urine's oxalate is synthesized by the body itself—only about 2 percent of the oxalates eaten reach the urine—and ample magnesium plus vitamin B-6 usually keeps the calcium oxalate soluble so it is less likely to precipitate into stones.

Sodium restriction also is being debated. Too much salt holds water in the tissues, causing dropsy, but too little dehydrates the system and predisposes to kidney stone formation. According to most authorities, at least 500 milligrams of sodium (the amount in one-fourth teaspoon of table salt) should be obtained daily. Some physicians prescribe generous amounts of potassium (up to 12 grams daily) to cause salt to be excreted and make restriction unnecessary.

The quantity of fluids required during treatment can wash vitamins and minerals out of the body. Dietary limitations can create nutritional deficiencies. So, for general health, a multi-vitamin-mineral tablet is generally recommended in addition to supplements for therapeutic purposes.

Vitamin A—25,000 to 75,000 units daily for three months, then 10,000 units per day as maintenance. Besides being needed for the prevention and cure of infections, vitamin A is essential as an aid in preventing clogging of the kidneys with dead cells from mucous membranes. A deficiency of vitamin A has been shown to induce both bladder and kidney stones.

Vitamin B-6 and Magnesium—10 to 100 milligrams B-6 plus 200 to 500 milligrams magnesium, taken in two divided doses daily. The most effective natural remedy for calcium-oxalate kidney stones, this combination developed by physicians and scientists has been used with success since 1960. Stone-formers appear to have an exaggerated need for B-6 to control the body's production of oxalic acid and to work with magnesium to prevent, dissolve, or avoid recurrence of kidney stones. Results may be speeded by including 1,000 to 4,000 milligrams of vitamin C daily to maintain an acid urine.

Vitamin C—1,000 to 4,000 milligrams daily, increased to 1,000 to 2,000 milligrams per hour (plus 500 milligrams of bioflavonoids) for two or three days during bladder infections or nephritis. Well known for its ability to combat infections, the "excess" vitamin C "wasted" in the urine not only detoxifies the poisons causing cystitis and other genito-urinary maladies, but makes the urine so acid that formation of stones is practically impossible and many existing stones are dissolved. Vitamin C also encourages urination so there is less chance for urine to remain in the bladder to cause infection or stones. Vitamin B-6 helps counteract the gas, diarrhea, and high levels of oxalate which occasionally develop when over 8,000 milligrams of vitamin C are taken daily. For the few who are beset by uric-acid stones and need to maintain an alkaline urine, vitamin C may be taken as sodium ascorbate or accompanied by a small amount of baking soda to neutralize its acid.

Calcium and Magnesium—

Dolomite—For cystitis or bladder infection, taking six dolomite tablets with plenty of water several times each day often brings relief in as little as 24 hours. Taking two dolomite tablets before retiring may solve the problem of interrupted sleep due to frequent trips to the bathroom. The use of at least four dolomite tablets daily by those with kidney-stone problems is recommended by experts who believe this calcium-magnesium combination offsets the high phosphorus intake from meats and whole grains, and prevents the formation of stones.

Magnesium—Some authorities prefer that no supplementary calcium be used by stone-formers and advise that only chelated magnesium be taken. As reported in *Journal of the American College of Nutrition* (Vol. 1, 1982), 200 milligrams of magnesium per day resulted in a 90-percent reduction of kidney stones for a test group of kidney-stone formers over a five-year period. Other long-term studies involving hundreds of patients who had repeatedly been afflicted with kidney stones showed stone formation to be reduced even more than the 90 percent by daily doses of magnesium plus B-6. (See Vitamin B-6 and Magnesium, above.)

Choline and/or Lecithin—1,000 milligrams choline taken in divided doses daily, and/or one to six tablespoons lecithin granules. (Lecithin capsules may be substituted, but one 1,200-milligram capsule contains only 40 milligrams of choline while one tablespoon of the granules provides 400 milligrams.) Diets high in calories, especially when much alcohol or refined sugar is included, increase the need for choline to prevent dropsy or kidney damage.

Vitamin E (see Caution, page 6)—300 to 1,000 IU daily. Vitamin E helps prevent the formation of kidney stones caused by toxic substances, and has brought relief from Bright's disease and dropsy as well as preventing bladder scarring from cystitis. Alpha tocopherol restores normal capillary permeability and has cleared cases of acute nephritis in a matter of days.[301]

Potassium—The inability to pass urine following extreme stress or surgery can often be corrected with supplements of potassium. In some cases, additional vitamin B-2 and pantothenic acid are required to relieve paralysis of the bladder muscles.

Tissue Salts recommended for specific problems with urination:

Frequent or copious—Take 12X Nat. Mur. and Nat. Phos. alternately, twice each day.

Interrupted, with inflammation—Take three daily doses each Ferr. Phos., Kali. Mur., and Nat. Sulph.

Scalding or burning—Take three alternating daily doses of 6X Ferr. Phos., Kali. Phos., and Nat. Mur.

For adult incontinence from muscular weakness—Take 12X Ferr. Phos. three times daily. If the incontinence is from nervousness, take 12X Kali. Phos. on the same schedule.

For incontinence in children—One dose each 3X Kali. Phos. and Nat. Phos. three times a day until the condition is normal.

For retention in adults—Dissolve three tablets of 3X Mag. Phos. in hot water and take frequently until corrected.

For retention from chilling or in children—Take 3X Ferr. Phos. frequently until normal.

Folk Remedies

Apple Cider Vinegar—Stir one or two teaspoons apple cider vinegar in a glass of water and drink with each meal. This was believed to not only acidify the urine to prevent the growth of infectious bacteria but to counteract the alkalinity of the blood produced by large amounts of protein.

Fruits—

Apples—Simmer the peels from washed apples in water, strain, and sip throughout the day to energize the kidneys.

Cherry Juice—Drinking one glass daily has reportedly regulated bladder problems requiring urination as often as once every hour.

Cranberries—In addition to the now medically sanctioned cranberry juice, ground raw cranberries mixed with honey and/or yogurt are considered beneficial.

Lemon—Drinking the juice of one or two large lemons each day has been credited with dissolving existing kidney stones and preventing the formation of new ones.

Peach Leaves—An infusion made from crushed peach tree leaves and boiling water was believed to cure all manner of bladder and kidney inflammations if taken several times each day.

Strawberries—Eating fresh strawberries was said to prevent the formation of kidney stones.

Herbs (see Edema for additional diuretics)—

Camomile—Considered both cleansing and soothing.

Catnip—The tea may be sipped for kidney stones or used as an enema in cases of retention.

Cornsilk—To soothe irritation from infections and stones.

Couchgrass—To stimulate bladder and kidney activity.

Dandelion Root—Used as a diuretic and kidney stimulant.

Juniper Berry—The berries may be chewed or made into a tea for cystitis or for eliminating gravel and stones.

Parsley—This familiar diuretic was believed to help dissolve kidney stones.

Sage—Has a mild sedative effect and was thought to purify the kidneys.

Slippery Elm—Soothing in cases of scalding urine.

Spearmint—Advised for suppression of urine and problems with urinary gravel.

Uva Ursi—Recommended for incontinence, painful urination, or stones in the bladder or kidneys.

Watermelon Seed Tea—Dried, ground watermelon seeds steeped in boiling water were used as a curative for bladder and kidney problems as well as being a standard diuretic.

Honey—Used as a sweetening agent and taken by the spoonful, honey is recommended during inflammations of the kidneys to hasten the release of urine and create a beneficial antiseptic reaction. Hippocrates advised honey mixed with milk for patients with kidney trouble.

Vegetables—

Asparagus—One-fourth cup cooked, pureed asparagus (diluted with hot water for a beverage, if desired) taken twice daily has been used to dissolve kidney stones since the 1800s.

Carrots—Drinking three cups a day of the water in which chopped carrots and their tops were simmered was first recommended by an Oriental physician in 1550 and was used by folk healers as a bladder and kidney rejuvenator.

Garlic—For cystitis or urinary infections, mince and swallow three cloves of garlic three times a day for five days.

Horseradish—Minced and eaten raw or cooked with an equal amount of mustard seed and strained to sip three times a day, horseradish is a classic treatment for abolishing small stones and gravel.

Kidney Bean Pods—Considered the most effective folk medicine for all kidney and bladder disorders, 2 ounces of kidney bean pods (without the beans) should be simmered in one gallon of water for four hours and strained, then one glass of the liquid taken every two hours during the day for four to eight weeks.

Parsnips—For gravel in the urinary tract, boil ½ pound chopped parsnips in one quart of water. Strain and drink one cup of the liquid each morning and evening for six weeks.

Hot Baths or Packs

Reclining in a sauna or tub of hot water for half an hour twice a day often relaxes muscles causing urine retention. It is also beneficial during early stages of kidney disease as some of the wastes in the blood can be released through the skin. The pain from kidney stones may be relieved by covering the area with a towel wrung out of plain hot water or a ginger-water solution made by simmering 1 ounce of fresh ginger in one quart of water for five minutes. Some folk practitioners used a poultice of wheat bran stirred into hot water. Others preferred heating chopped onions, dropping them in a cup of white wine, and saturating a small towel in the mixture. The onions were to be folded inside the towel before it was placed over the painful area.

Nerve Massage

For cystitis or bladder inflammation—Massage the center of each inner wrist. Then massage the inner edge of each foot near the heel.

For pain connected with the bladder—Wind rubber bands around the thumbs and first two fingers of both hands several times daily for from three to 20 minutes. (Remove the bands when the fingers begin to turn blue.) Another option is to bite the tongue and lip for several minutes.

For kidney infections and stones—For no longer than one minute at a time, massage the center of the palms, then rub back and forth from the center of the palms to the inner wrists. Or, massage the thumb, index, and middle finger of each hand or apply clothespins to the tips of these fingers. Or, massage under the arch of each foot, then back and forth to the beginning of the heel pad.

Nerve Pressure

For all bladder and kidney problems, press each point for 10 seconds, release for 10 seconds, and repeat three times.

- Press the end of each cheekbone just in front of the upper part of each ear.
- Press the center of the small depression about 1 inch below the top of the breastbone.
- Hook the fingers along the inside of the ribs approximately two-thirds of the distance down from the end of the breastbone toward the lowest rib, then press inward and upward.

Sources (See Bibliography)

3, 4, 12, 13, 18, 25, 28, 34, 37, 43, 52, 53, 63, 64, 68, 76, 84, 88, 89, 92, 113, 134, 142, 151, 152, 153, 154, 156, 165, 168, 171, 173, 174, 175, 176, 180, 190, 201, 208, 226, 228, 243, 251, 253, 254, 260, 261, 269, 270, 288, 289, 293, 297, 301, 305, 309, 315, 330, 333, 334, 335, 350, 353.

LOW BLOOD SUGAR (FUNCTIONAL OR SECONDARY HYPOGLYCEMIA)

A relative newcomer as a recognized malady, low blood sugar was first separated from diabetic reactions in 1924 and remains the subject of much controversy. One medical contingent contends that it exists only as the rare primary hypoglycemia caused by an insulin-secreting tumor, while another group believes that at least one-fourth of the American population is suffering from secondary or functional hypoglycemia (low blood sugar).[210]

Low blood sugar involves an increased output of, or increased sensitivity to, the insulin produced in the body. There are still some practicing physicians who were indoctrinated according to earlier theories and prescribe candy bars for the physical fatigue and mental confusion engendered by this condition as if it were the same as diabetic insulin shock. In spite of the similarity of symptoms and the fact that uncontrolled hypoglycemia can lead to diabetes, the two are exact opposites. In diabetes, the pancreas cannot produce sufficient, assimilable insulin to cope with a normal amount of carbohydrates and must be assisted by oral anti-diabetic agents or insulin injections. When an excess of insulin is supplied, "insulin shock" can result, and a piece of candy or a glass of orange juice will restore the balance and rescue the diabetic. In hypoglycemia, the pancreas over-reacts to carbohydrates and releases more insulin than is needed. Additional sugar in any form will give a few minutes of temporary relief, but, when new insulin is released, all the new sugar is swept out of the bloodstream and, along with it, some of the small amount of sugar that was present in the beginning—leaving the individual with even more pronounced symptoms. The effects are cumulative as the cycle continues; the ups are higher and the downs are lower. If left unremedied, this imbalance may lead to degenerative diseases or addictive drinking.

Case History

Cindy B. did not tell anyone about her first blackout. She assumed it was her own fault for not following her doctor's instructions about eating a candy bar whenever she felt wobbly—her "slightly low" blood sugar required reinforcing! Cindy was so determined to make it on her own with her first job away from home that she risked possible weight gain by eating extra candy whenever she felt tired. However, after her second and third blackouts occurred in supermarkets and necessitated embarrassing assistance plus calling a cab to get back to her apartment, Cindy did telephone her mother for advice. Her nutritionally aware mother immediately mailed her the basic outline for a hypoglycemia diet, and suggested she adhere to it until she was transferred to a larger city where she could have another blood-sugar test. Cindy still has not been transferred; but the high-protein, no-sugar diet has been so successful that she has not had any more blackouts, and has so increased her mental and physical prowess that she has been promoted to a position as area manager.

Since the brain requires an even level of blood sugar to maintain emotional health, the fluctuations resulting from low blood sugar can be misdiagnosed as anything from brain tumors and depression to "just nerves." The physical symptoms of fatigue, headache, nausea, night sweats, trembling, etc. may also be accounted for by other abnormalities. The most reliable method of diagnosis is the six-hour glucose-tolerance test. Another method is to have blood drawn at the moment symptoms are experienced following a meal. But, even with these tests, expert analysis is required. As Carlton Fredericks explains in *Low Blood Sugar and You*[129], blood sugar levels within the normal range may be responsible for hypoglycemic symptoms.

Exercise is an important part of the treatment for hypoglycemia because physical activity helps control blood-sugar fluctuations. Outdoor activity may be particularly valuable since lack of sufficient exposure to sunlight is another possible contributory factor in low blood sugar. During strenuous exercise such as jogging or tennis, a snack of protein plus carbohydrate every 20 minutes is suggested. (Peanuts are easy to carry in a pocket.) Chronic stress can induce hypoglycemia by making excessive demands on the adrenal glands. In addition to exercise, a few minutes of deliberate relaxation and positive thinking (see pages 9-10) often proves beneficial.

Despite its possibly serious consequences, low blood sugar is one ailment for which home-testing is safe. The basic treatment for functional hypoglycemia is diet plus vitamin supplementation, and a week or two of following the regimen should bring relief from the symptoms. If not, medical help should be obtained. Low blood sugar may originate from allergies, lack of stomach acid, or other deficiencies that require extensive blood, urine, and hair analysis tests for identification.

Diet

Whatever the contributing factors, diet is always involved. The amount of sugar consumed annually by Americans has risen from 5 pounds to a total of 150 pounds per person in 300 years—46 pounds of that increase during the past 12 years.[24] (This may account for much of the increased incidence of hypoglycemia as excessive demands for insulin can cause the pancreas to become oversensitive.) At least half that annual sugar comes from nonsweet sources: bottled, canned, and packaged gravies, ketchup, lunchmeats, mayonnaise, sauces, soups, vegetables, etc. There is no specific dietary need for sugar. The body's nutritional need for glucose can be met by many other carbohydrates. Refined flour increases the workload of the pancreas because its starch is changed to sugar by the body more quickly than that of whole grains and, therefore, requires a surge of insulin. Recent research at the University of Colorado and the University of Toronto indicates further differences in blood-sugar reactions to individual foods. As reported in the public media in July, 1983, some complex carbohydrates were found to raise blood sugar as rapidly as sweets. In these university tests, carrots, corn, corn flakes, honey, parsnips, white potatoes, and white rice had an even faster blood-sugar response than ordinary table sugar. High-carbohydrate foods with the slowest blood-sugar reactions were apples, dried legumes, fructose, milk, oatmeal, peanuts, spaghetti, and yogurt. Even sugar-free coffee, tea, and caffeine-containing soft drinks aggravate the situation. Artificial colorings, flavorings, and additives are not recommended as they can precipitate hypoglycemic symptoms for some individuals, as can tobacco in those who are susceptible. (Nicotine can stimulate the adrenal glands to cause a temporpary rise in blood sugar, then a corresponding drop, so even "light" cigarettes should be used with moderation.)

A hypoglycemia-control diet, however, is nothing to be dreaded. Its frequent mini-meals and snacks with their high-protein, accent-on-natural-foods approach is the same nutritional program recommended for everyone who wants optimum health. (The body depends on protein for an even flow of energy without depleting the blood-sugar level[280].) Sugar in all its forms must be avoided but protein and fat do not trigger insulin, small amounts of carbohydrate are required with each meal or snack, and fruits are allowed, so there need be no feeling of deprivation. Eating several small meals instead of two or three large ones each day helps maintain even blood-sugar levels. The precise schedule varies with individuals. There are a few who are comfortable with nothing more substantial than a glass of milk between three regular meals. Others may need seven or eight mini-meals during the day and then rouse to eat something in the middle of the night to prevent morning headache, nausea, and weariness. For most people, a pre-breakfast glass of juice or milk and three standard meals plus mid-morning, mid-afternoon, and before-bed snacks are satisfactory.

The original Seale Harris diet, made famous in the book *Body, Mind and Sugar*[2], called for one-half cup fruit juice upon arising, three high-protein meals at normal intervals, with one-half cup juice in the middle of the morning, one glass of milk three hours after lunch, one-half glass of juice an hour before dinner, one glass of milk two hours after dinner, and one-half cup milk or a small handful of nuts every two hours until bedtime. One slice of bread was allowed with each meal but bananas, dried fruits, pastas, potatoes, rice, any form of sugar, caffeine, and alcohol were absolutely forbidden.

Dr. Airola details a vegetarian diet for low blood sugar in his book *How to Get Well*[13] and Dr. Pritikin, Director of the Longevity Research Institute in California, also stresses cooked grains in his diet, but the majority of hypoglycemic diets rely on meat as the principal source of protein. Carnitine, a substance found in animal proteins and synthesized by the body from the amino acids lysine and methionine, is necessary for the body's utilization of stored fats for energy. As reported in the September, 1983 issue of *Prevention Magazine,* it was stated at a recent meeting of the American Diabetes Association that hypoglycemia was an early and treatable symptom of systemic carnitine deficiency. The amino acids, lysine and methionine, are generously supplied by animal proteins but poorly supplied by plants.

In *Low Blood Sugar and You*[129], Carlton Fredericks and Herman Goodman each give their version of a basic diet. Abram Hoffer[171] found that some of his patients developed allergies to dairy products while on a high-protein regimen, so now advises simply eliminating all refined foods from the normal diet. Frank Hurdle[175], on the other hand, believes a hypoglycemic diet should consist of four times more protein than fat and twice as much protein as carbohydrate. Robert Atkins[24] would limit the total carbohydrates to 40 grams daily. A dozen other variations are proffered in as many books, but most of the suggested diets are high in protein, moderate in fat, call for generous amounts of vegetables, forbid sugar, and limit carbohydrates to approximately 100 grams daily. Some persons with low blood sugar can tolerate more than the 100 grams of carbohydrate and even use a little fructose, honey, or molasses. (Fructose releases less insulin over a longer period of time than cane or beet sugar. Honey and brown sugar have the same type of insulin-releasing effect as the sucrose from cane or beet sugar. All should be avoided during testing and severely limited thereafter.) There are others who must reduce their daily carbohydrate intake to less than 100 grams in order to be symptom-free. The total carbohydrates ingested daily by average American adults is estimated at 300 grams. A rough formula for relating ounces, grams, and calories is:

    1 ounce = 28.35 grams
    1 gram of either carbohydrate or protein = 4 calories
    1 gram of fat = 9 calories
    4 ounces or ½ cup cooked vegetables = approximately 100 grams

For weight maintenance, an average adult requires 10 calories per pound of body weight per day, plus three calories per pound for light activity, five calories for moderate activity, and 10 calories for strenuous activity. Individual adjustments may be made after experimentation with the sample 100-carbohydrate-gram diet which follows.

For the first week's experiment, drink one glass of milk or unsweetened juice (fortified with brewer's yeast or protein powder, if desired) immediately upon arising. Then divide the "required daily foods" among three meals and three snacks so there are an ounce or two of meat or cheese plus some bread, milk, or fruit with each one. Both the quantity of food and an evenly spaced schedule of eating should be carefully adhered to while the body becomes accustomed to the smaller, more frequent meals. Earl Mindell's *Quick and Easy Guide to Better Health*[228] recommends one-fourth cup of the following protein drink every two hours: one to one and one-half cups milk, fruit or vegetable juice, or water (whirred in an electric blender with one tablespoon milk-and-egg protein powder), one teaspoon each acidophilus, brewer's yeast, vitamin C powder, lecithin granules, and vegetable oil. (If available, one drop of niacin may be included.)

The constant hunger and craving for sweets which accompany the onset of hypoglycemia can result in the accumulation of unwanted pounds. Those who wish to lose weight should use the smallest amount given for each item, forego the optional butter and mayonnaise, use skim milk, and have no more than one ounce of cheddar-type cheese or one-fourth cup cottage cheese daily. For weight maintenance, very active people may need to increase even the largest amounts shown but should keep the same proportions for dietary balance.

Daily foods, required

11 to 14 ounces meat, poultry, and/or seafood (cooked weight of edible portion, not breaded).

1 or 2 eggs (1 or 2 additional ounces of meat may be substituted for each egg).

1 to 3 tablespoons cold-pressed vegetable oil.

2 to 5 cups of any vegetable except beets, carrots, cooked dried beans or peas, corn, parsnips, potatoes, pumpkin, rutabagas, turnips, or winter squash.

3 slices whole-grain bread (once each day, one-half slice bread may be replaced with one-half cup of any vegetable listed above as an exception).

2 servings fruit (fresh or unsweetened canned or frozen).

2 glasses milk. (If milk cannot be tolerated, substitute a calcium supplement, 3 ounces meat or its equivalent, and 24 grams carbohydrate from the charts which follow. For instance: one glass tomato juice, one boiled egg, two wheat crackers, and a 300-milligram calcium tablet would equal the protein, carbohydrate, and calcium in one glass of milk.)

Daily foods, optional

Clear broths, homemade or canned.

Butter or margarine and sugar-free mayonnaise. (As far as other dietary considerations allow, sensible amounts of fats are recommended for those with hypoglycemia. Fats slow the digestive process and help equalize blood-sugar levels.)

2 ounces natural Swiss or cheddar-type cheese and/or ½ cup cottage cheese or plain yogurt. (Any of these may be used to replace 2 ounces of meat.)

2 tablespoons natural peanut butter. (May replace 1 ounce meat, if desired.)

Lemon juice and vinegar.

Spices and herbs—Basil, marjoram, oregano, and thyme are especially recommended.

Unflavored gelatin—A rich source of the amino acid, glycine, which is of special importance for some hypoglycemics. (Gelatin should always be used with other foods as it is an incomplete protein.)

1 serving pudding or gelatin dessert made with artificial sweetener.

1 glass sugar-free, caffeine-free soft drink. (Both desserts and soft drinks should be limited because the pancreas sometimes reacts to the sweet taste and sends out insulin even when no sugar is present.)

Decaffeinated coffee—The caffeine in regular coffee, tea, colas, or other soft drinks creates an adrenalin rush that makes blood sugar rise just as if a full meal or a sweet dessert had been eaten, then plummet to an even lower low. (Weak pekoe tea is relatively low in caffeine, so may be used occasionally.)

Case History

Roger M. had always been outgoing and even-tempered. His wife, Polly, began to worry about his taciturn moodiness; wondered if he had become a secret drinker when she noticed his shaky hands; and feared that the unexplained depletion of their savings account indicated Roger was having an affair. Polly was actually relieved when Roger admitted he had gambled away the money and, when his annual check-up revealed high blood pressure and a need for weight loss, thought their problems were solved. She bought decaffeinated coffee, and prepared low-calorie meals. Roger took his blood-pressure medication, and lost 10 pounds, but his mood swings and shakiness persisted. Then one evening before dinner, Roger blacked out. He attributed his dizzy spell to hunger—to keep his weight down he had been skipping lunch, and getting through the work day by drinking "regular" black coffee in the mornings and caffeine-containing sugar-free colas in the afternoons. Polly, however, refused to ignore the episode. A friend, recently diagnosed as a hypoglycemic, loaned her a book about low blood sugar. Polly convinced Roger, and his doctor, that a long glucose-tolerance test was in order. Roger's blood sugar was so low that the test had to be discontinued after five hours. His reaction to proper dietary treatment, including the avoidance of caffeine, was almost miraculous. Within weeks Roger's fingers steadied, his temporary penchant for gambling disappeared, his ebullient good nature returned, and their problems really were solved.

Herbal Teas—Alfalfa, camomile, comfrey, dandelion, juniper berry, licorice root, peppermint, rose hips, and spearmint are recommended, but any caffeine-free herb tea is allowed. Saffron is believed to help metabolize milk sugar and may be included with other teas.

If improvemnt is noticed after the first week, continue with the pre-breakfast drink and the basic diet for another three weeks, adding "optionals" as weight loss permits and adjusting the time schedule if necessary. Then, while still following the outline of required foods and frequent eating, it is usually possible to add variety to the diet and gradually include favorite dishes. Anything sweetened with sugar, corn syrup, honey, maple syrup, molasses, etc., or made with all-white flour is not for most hypoglycemics. But an enjoyably satisfying diet can be assembled from other foods— and a surprising number of delicious desserts contrived from eggs, milk, cottage cheese, gelatin, naturally sweet fruits, and an occasional drop or two of artificial sweetener. Tupelo honey contains a different type of sugar from other honeys and small amounts have been used without ill effects by many people with low blood sugar.

No elaborate bookkeeping system is necessary with this diet. Ninety grams of carbohydrates are accounted for by the Required Daily Foods: 3 slices bread, 3 cups "allowable" vegetables, 2 servings fruit, and 2 glasses of milk. (No insulin is needed for proteins and fats.) The following generalized charts of carbohydrate content (compiled from *Hypoglycemia Control Cookery* [275] and *Nutrition Almanac*[189]) make "spending" the other 10 bonus-grams of carbohydrate a simple matter.

At least one slice of the bread should remain with the Required Foods, but considerable wheeling and dealing can be accomplished with the 24 grams of carbohydrate from the other two slices and the 10 "bonus" grams. Besides trading a half-slice of bread for one-half cup of the vegetables listed with the Daily Foods, there can be a daily exchange of one slice of bread for one serving of pasta or rice, or a corn tortilla, or peanuts, popcorn, or crackers as part of a snack. Sauces and gravies can be made with one tablespoon whole-wheat flour (5 carbohydrate grams) for thickening; meat, poultry, or sea food can be breaded with cornmeal, wheat germ, or ground oatmeal—the possibilities are practically endless.

Alcoholic beverages must be used with caution and are sometimes forbidden. (Alcohol contains no carbohydrates but affects metabolism as if it did, in much the same way as caffeine and nicotine for susceptible people.) Many doctors feel the tranquilizing effect of a drink or two of gin, vodka, whiskey, or other nonsweet liquor before dinner or bed is beneficial. A glass of dry wine (5 carbohydrate grams for 4 ounces) with a meal, or a glass of "light" beer (2 to 4 grams of carbohydrate for 8 ounces) with a handful of peanuts or a few cheese cubes for a snack do not upset blood-sugar levels for most hypoglycemics, if the necessary Daily Foods are eaten at frequent intervals, the carbohydrates evenly distributed, and their total kept near 100 grams.

CARBOHYDRATE CONTENT OF COMMON FOODS

15 carbohydrate grams
½ cup cooked rice, macaroni, noodles or spaghetti—preferably brown rice or whole-wheat pasta. (Cooking the pasta for an extra minute or so before draining and rinsing may upset some "al dente" enthusiasts and wash out a few vitamins, but it reduces the carbohydrates by up to one-fourth and makes an even trade for a slice of bread.)

½ cup cooked dried beans or peas.

½ cup mashed potato or 1 small-medium baked potato.

½ medium banana.

¼ cup dry oatmeal.

1 cup plain, whole-milk yogurt.

1 cup popped corn.

⅓ cup peanuts or sunflower seeds.

7 carbohydrate grams

1 cup creamed cottage cheese.

½ cup cooked beets, carrots, onions, green peas, turnips, or winter squash.

½ medium-large avocado. (Avocados contain a type of carbohydrate that actually depresses insulin release and are, therefore, ideal for hypoglycemics.[128])

Many hypoglycemia diets do not even count the remaining vegetables as part of the carbohydrate quota. Lettuce and other raw greens have approximately 2 grams per cup, while the listed vegetables average less than 3 grams for each cooked, one-half-cup serving.

3 grams (or less) carbohydrate per ½ cup cooked (practically free food)

Asparagus	Eggplant	Mushrooms
Beans, green or wax	Greens:	Okra
Broccoli	Beet	Peppers
Cabbage	Chard	Radish
Cauliflower	Mustard	Sauerkraut
Celery	Spinach	Summer Squash
Cucumber	Turnip	Tomatoes

Dietary Supplements

Many vitamins and trace elements have been found to mediate glucose metabolism. Hypoglycemia usually requires vitamin and mineral supplementation in addition to a correct diet because a stress reaction is set off each time blood sugar falls below normal. This increases the need for nutrients and can create deficiencies which further affect the body's utilization of sugar. A comprehensive, high-potency multi-vitamin-mineral tablet daily is suggested. Those who cannot assimilate vitamin B-12 when taken orally may require an injection every week or two. The following additional supplements have proven beneficial in many cases and may be experimented with on an individual basis.

B Vitamins help metabolize carbohydrates, build up the adrenals, and are necessary for combating stress. Deficiencies of B-2 and pantothenic acid can prevent the liver from producing enzymes to inactivate insulin, thus causing the blood sugar level to fall. Taking up to 600 milligrams B-2 per day has decreased the craving for sugar. Equally large amounts of pantothenic acid have also proven helpful. Both Jonathan Wright[353] and H.L. Newbold[238] have found that 1,000 to 1,500 milligrams niacinamide, accompanied by an equal amount of vitamin C, taken with each of three daily meals has reduced depression and tension as well as other symptoms of low blood sugar.

Brewer's Yeast is a source of high-grade protein plus B vitamins and chromium. Taking one teaspoon to one tablespoon between meals has restored energy and mental efficiency, and impeded other hypoglycemic symptoms.

Vitamin C—1,000 to 5,000 milligrams in divided doses, daily. Vitamin C helps normalize sugar metabolism and protects against stress.

Calcium—Two or more bone meal or dolomite tablets per day. Scientific tests have shown that a high protein diet including two glasses of milk each day resulted in a bodily loss of 58 milligrams of calcium each day.[256] (The acid ash of the protein is responsible for this calcium loss which can cause osteoporosis if not overcome by extra calcium.)

Chromium—250, or more, micrograms daily. Inadequate chromium is believed to be a common cause of blood-sugar problems. Chromium is the active component of the glucose tolerance factor (GTF) which is essential for carbohydrate metabolism and maintenance of even blood sugar levels. Accompanying chromium supplements with brewer's yeast has been shown to increase their effectiveness.

Vitamin E (see Caution, page 6)—100 to 1,600 IU daily. In addition to its other capabilities, vitamin E improves sugar storage in the liver and prevents bodily oxidation of vitamin A and the vitamin E from vegetable oils.

Magnesium—200 to 500 milligrams daily. Magnesium is involved in the metabolism of carbohydrates and is required for the utilization of B vitamins. (Dolomite tablets contain both magnesium and calcium.)

Potassium—Low blood sugar creates stress conditions that can cause retention of sodium and water, and potassium loss. Using a salt substitute containing potassium may prevent blackouts due to hypoglycemia. In *Let's Get Well*[89], Adelle Davis suggested carrying potassium tablets to chew when a blackout threatened and appropriate food was not available. For hypoglycemic headaches and trembling, many authorities recommend 200 milligrams of potassium daily in divided doses with meals, but continual use should have medical supervision.

Zinc—10 to 30 milligrams per day, if not included in the daily multiple supplement. Zinc is used by the body in dealing with all carbohydrates, and is particularly effective in relieving the symptoms of hypoglycemia when accompanied by vitamin B-6 and manganese.[7,256]

Sources (See Bibliography)

2, 3, 4, 6, 7, 9, 13, 23, 24, 39, 41, 42, 48, 52, 54, 62, 80, 88, 89, 93, 105, 124, 126, 128, 129, 143, 154, 156, 171, 174, 175, 189, 194, 208, 210, 228, 229, 238, 250, 252, 254, 256, 257, 261, 269, 272, 275, 279, 280, 282, 284, 287, 305, 315, 325, 326, 350, 353, 354.

MENIERE'S DISEASE AND VERTIGO

Technically termed "endolymphatic hydrops," characterized by a whirling dizziness called vertigo and a ringing in the ears called tinnitus (see Hearing Loss and Tinnitus), Meniere's disease is occasioned by excess fluid in the inner ear or "labyrinth." It rarely affects people under 30 or over 60. Attacks may be accompanied by hearing impairment and nausea. Symptoms wax and wane, usually in accordance with illness, stress, or general physical well-being. Labyrinthitis (an inflammation of the inner ear which can create a sensation of vertigo for a few weeks) usually follows a viral infection or large doses of aspirin, quinine, or certain of the "miacin" antibiotics. Occasional dizziness may originate from high blood pressure or other maladies. Both vertigo and chronic Meniere's disease warrant medical diagnosis.

Prosper Meniere, who first described the symptoms in 1861, believed there was an association between migraine headaches and Meniere's disease. Modern otologists agree that the spasm of a blood vessel with its subsequent stretching and increased flow of blood, is the first stage of both. But, in the Meniere syndrome, there is an accumulation of fluid in the labyrinth that disturbs the delicate balance mechanism to produce vertigo and other symptoms. Alcohol, allergy, eye strain, mental or physical stress, or tobacco may serve to trigger these spasms. Anything (such as cigarette smoking) which causes constriction of the small blood vessels should be avoided. When mental stress is the suspected cause, practicing deliberate relaxation and positive thinking (see pages 9-10) for a few minutes each day may be helpful. Drugs (see above) that might aggravate inner ear disorders should not be used, and there should be no sudden movements when turning the head or rising from a seated or reclining position.

Allergic reactions or childhood virus infections may be responsible for defective fluid absorption in the inner ear. In these cases, limitation of both salt and fluid intake is advised and the B-6, pantothenic acid plus vitamin C combination used for hay fever (which see) may prove helpful. Other causes may be adrenal gland exhaustion (possibly from ACTH or cortisone medication) which causes too much salt to be excreted and excessive fluid to pass into the tissues of the ear. To counteract this condition, Adelle Davis[89] recommended a high-protein diet with plenty of salt, a daily B-complex tablet, and 3,000 milligrams vitamin C plus 600 milligrams pantothenic acid taken in divided doses during the day.

Recent research has developed further information regarding both the cause and cure of Meniere's disease. According to *Medical World News* (June 8, 1981), many specialists now believe that impaired circulation from too much insulin in the blood (low blood sugar) is the primary cause of Meniere's disease. Tests have shown an abnormal concentration of insulin to be closely related to high levels of cholesterol and fats in the blood—with obesity a contributing factor. (The loss of excess weight often allows insulin to enter the cells and establishes normal metabolic activity.) The good news is that blood-sugar levels and body weight can usually be controlled by adhering to the diet for hypoglycemia (see Low Blood Sugar).

A few weeks of personal experimentation with natural remedies may resolve the problem without extensive medical tests. If the condition persists, professional help should be obtained because either chronic Meniere's disease or labyrinthitis can become incapacitating and lead to progressive deafness.

Diet and Supplements

In keeping with the low-blood-sugar theory, *Dr. Heimlich's Home Guide to Emergency Medical Situations*[156] states that an occasional attack of dizziness can be overcome by drinking a glass of orange juice. Some cases of chronic dizziness have responded to one or two weeks of treatment with 2,000 to 20,000 milligrams of bioflavonoids taken in divided doses daily. (Strong catnip tea was the folk remedy for vertigo.) For Meniere's disease, most physicians recommend a low-sodium, low-carbohydrate diet high in manganese and potassium (from bananas, leafy green vegetables, etc.) without any alcohol, coffee, tea, or other caffeine-containing beverages.

Besides a nutritious diet, vitamin supplementation is often necessary to abolish the annoying symptoms of Meniere's disease and effect a cure. Doctors have found that most patients with Meniere's disease have B-vitamin deficiencies. Even after relief is achieved, the large amounts of these vitamins required to prevent recurrence suggest some defect in utilization or metabolism. One comprehensive, high-potency B-complex tablet one to three times daily is recommended in addition to any individual B-vitamins used.

B-6 and Pantothenic Acid—Divided daily doses of 100 milligrams B-6 have cleared the nausea which sometimes accompanies Meniere's disease, and, when 100 milligrams of pantothenic acid are taken at the same time, both dizziness and noises in the ears have been relieved.[89]

Niacin or Niacinamide—25 to 100 milligrams taken with meals one to three times each day. Niacin may produce a temporary sensation of flushing or itching, but has a vasodilator action recognized as effective in controlling Meniere attacks. For some persons, taking 50 to 100 milligrams niacinamide three times daily has reduced vertigo without producing any side effects.

C Complex and Vitamin E—Taking 1,000 milligrams vitamin C plus 500 milligrams of bioflavonoids and 400 IU vitamin E (see Caution, page 6) daily is often beneficial.

Nerve Pressure for Dizziness and Vertigo

Apply pressure for 10 seconds, release for 10 seconds, and repeat for a total of 30 seconds pressure once each day.

- With the thumb and index finger, firmly pinch the area between the eyebrows.
- With the thumbnail, firmly press between the first and second metatarsal bones, 2 inches toward the ankle from the point where the big toe and second toe meet on the right foot. Repeat with the left foot.

Sources (See Bibliography)

13, 19, 24, 36, 52, 67, 75, 76, 84, 88, 89, 129, 156, 168, 189, 229, 239, 261, 280, 288, 298, 315, 328, 349, 353.

MENSTRUAL DIFFICULTIES AND MENOPAUSE

The unpleasant symptoms of monthly irritability, water retention, abdominal pain, breast soreness, and backache are so prevalent that, when not related to obvious physical causes, they are usually regarded as being either normal or "all in the mind."

Yet many women advance comfortably from puberty through menopause. (Healthy females in uncivilized countries like Hunza and Central America reportedly have no such problems.) Menstrual irregularities may be instigated or aggravated by emotional strain or constipation (which see), but, according to biochemists and orthomolecular physicians, most menstrual and menopausal difficulties are caused by nutritional deficiencies that can be corrected within a few months—with natural remedies providing interim relief. Exercise helps strengthen abdominal muscles to prevent pain during menstrual periods and physical problems during menopause. When unusually frequent, heavy, painful, or scanty periods of menstrual flow persist, medical attention should be sought as physical abnormalities may be present.

The delicate hormonal system can be drastically altered by inadequate nutrition, and set right again with proper diet. A few physicians share Dr. Ruben's theory[273] that vitamin and mineral supplementation is unnecessary for menstrual difficulties but most have found a natural high-protein, low-carbohydrate diet plus a daily multi-vitamin-mineral tablet advantageous. Protein and B vitamins are needed by the liver to process the hormones released prior to menstruation. Too much dietary sugar may upset the natural balance to cause premenstrual tension, bloating, cramps, irregularity, or heavy and prolonged periods. Because of the hidden shortcomings of processed foods, most women between 15 and 50 need to fortify their diets with additional iron, extra vitamin C to help absorb the iron, and the B-complex vitamins to help build blood. It has been estimated that two-thirds of menstruating women have at least mild iron deficiencies.[261] Additional amounts of vitamins B-6 and C are required when oral contraceptives are used. The amount of calcium in a woman's blood decreases before and during menstruation. If calcium supplements are not taken on a regular basis, starting them the week before the anticipated period and continuing until menstruation has ceased may reduce nervous tension and painful cramps. Many menstrual difficulties may be related to a shortage of magnesium, which must be present in order for the body to utilize either B-6 or calcium.

Abstaining from salt and sugar for the week before a period may help avoid the nervousness and pain from difficult menstruation. Nutritionists suggest including "dark" juices such as cherry, grape, prune, and red beet, as well as ample amounts of cooked greens, broccoli, cabbage, mushrooms, whole grains, and two to three daily tablespoons of brewer's yeast in the diet.

Stimulating two nerve-pressure points until slight pain is felt, then repeating the pressure three times at 10-second intervals is believed helpful for all "female troubles." 1) Press a point on the abdomen 1½ inches directly below the navel. 2) Press the depression in the shinbone about 4 inches above the ankle on each leg.

Additional treatment varies with the specific difficulties although there may be an overlap of both symptoms and remedies.

Irregular or suppressed menstruation (amenorrhea)

It is not uncommon to skip one or two periods during times of stress. Amenorrhea can also be brought about by anemia, illness, overly vigorous physical training, or malnutrition from "reducing" diets. As explained in Dr. Goodenough's 1904 *Home Cures and Herbal Remedies*[142], "By stopping the loss of blood, Nature tries to reserve the forces of the patient." Restoring the general system is still the advocated method of re-establishing regular menstrual periods.

Decreased or irregular menstrual flow may be an indication of vitamin deficiency that frequently responds to daily supplements of 200 milligrams B-2, 50 to 150 milligrams B-6, 400 to 800 micrograms folic acid, and up to 600 IU vitamin E (see Caution, page 6). Drinking a tea made from dried marigold petals, eating several garlic cloves, or taking a daily teaspoon of kelp granules has relieved some cases of suppressed menstruation. Folk healers recommend drinking the boiled-down liquid from cooked beets, or teas made from basil, camomile, catnip, celery, fenugreek seeds, ginger, juniper berries, marjoram, parsley, rosemary, sage, tarragon, white mustard seed, or wintergreen.

Hot baths, especially when fortified with dried camomile, juniper needles, or ground mustard seeds, are an ancient formula. Alternating hot and cold baths each morning and evening are also suggested. Applying hot towels over the lower back for at least 10 minutes three or four times a day has induced menstruation. Unless pregnancy is suspected, using the broad handle of a tablespoon to press as far back on the tongue as possible without gagging has been known to start menstruation within a few minutes.[63] When other natural remedies have not been successful and no physical abnormality accounts for the menstrual irregularity, burning a 25-watt light bulb in the sleeping room from the fourteenth through the seventeenth nights following the first day of the last menstrual period may solve the problem by replacing the moonlight exposure of primitive women.

Premenstrual tension (PMT)

Nervousness, water-retention and breast sensitivity may be average but are not necessarily normal. Vitamin A (10,000 to 25,000 units daily) may help relieve general symptoms associated with premenstrual tension. Stabilizing blood sugar by following the Low Blood Sugar diet (which see) is often helpful. Vitamin B-6 is regarded as a natural miracle-worker for premenstrual problems. Countless clinical tests have shown that B-6 works better for premenstrual fluid retention, tension, and acne than commercial diuretics, tranquilizers, or facial scrubs and creams. Taking a B-complex tablet containing 50 milligrams of B-6 each morning and a 50-milligram tablet of B-6 each evening, then increasing the B-6 to 150 milligrams during the ten days preceding menstruation has proven very successful. Combining the B-6 regimen with a high-protein, low-carbohydrate diet plus extra supplements of calcium, magnesium, and zinc often eliminates involuntary muscle spasms of the legs, tenderness of the breasts, and other PMT difficulties.

If there has been a long-standing calcium deficiency, increasing the intake of vitamins C, D, and pantothenic acid plus calcium and magnesium may be useful. Even a mild deficiency of calcium in the blood can be responsible for uncontrollable temper outbursts.[71] According to the *American Journal of Clinical Nutrition* (November, 1981), the premenstrual syndrome can drain the body's stores of magnesium. Chewing several dolomite tablets often reduces tension headaches and breast tenderness, especially when 400 to 600 milligrams of this calcium-magnesium combination are taken daily for the week before an expected period.

Restricting fluids and salt for several days before the symptoms are anticipated may help prevent the bloating and emotional irritability related to fluid pressure on the brain. Nutritionally oriented physicians and folk practitioners recommend garlic to relieve premenstrual problems. Minced fresh garlic mixed with honey and swallowed by the teaspoonful, garlic capsules, or garlic tea made by stirring one teaspoon garlic powder in a cup of hot water and adding honey to taste are considered equally beneficial. Camomile, comfrey, and spearmint teas are also believed helpful.

A popular European remedy for PMT, Oil of Evening Primrose, is now available in American health food stores. As reported in *American Health* (January/February, 1983), evening primrose oil gave complete relief of premenstrual tension symptoms to 62 percent and partial relief to another 22 percent of the women involved in a recent study in London. The usual dosage is two capsules taken twice daily for three days before the expected onset of the symptoms. The nerve-pressure remedy of pressing the deep hollow just below the collarbone for 10 seconds, releasing, and repeating three times on both sides has nullified premenstrual discomfort in many instances.

Painful menstruation (dysmenorrhea)

Primary dysmenorrhea, which begins at puberty, may benefit from postural exercises and vanish with childbirth.

Case History

Brenda L. was ready to give up. Coping with menstrual pain in addition to her commitments as a full-time student and a part-time bookkeeper was just too much. She still had work to make up from the classes she missed last month; her employer was displeased with her poor attendance record; pain pills upset her stomach; and she was so miserable that all she wanted to do was curl up in bed with a heating pad. A co-worker suggested a simple exercise she had found effective for preventing menstrual discomfort. Realizing that she had been using her busy schedule as an excuse for not exercising, Brenda wrote down the directions for this one and tucked the slip of paper in her purse before she rushed off to class. When she got home, she fastened the note to her bedroom mirror and each night during the cycle between her menstrual periods Brenda faithfully followed the instructions:

1) Stand beside a wall, with feet parallel to the wall but about 6 inches away from it.
2) Place the forearm and hand (of the arm nearest the wall) flat against the wall at shoulder level.
3) Bring the hip in to touch the wall three times.
4) Turn around and repeat the process.

Brenda's next monthly period was less troublesome than usual; the period that followed was practically pain free.

Secondary dysmenorrhea begins later in life. Both should be medically diagnosed to rule out physical causes. Nervous tension or anxiety may cause painful menstruation by producing spasms of the uterus. A few minutes of daily relaxation (see pages 9-10) may bring some relief. Oral contraceptives reduce dysmenorrhea because they suppress ovulation, without which cramps do not occur. Sedentary women are more subject to menstrual cramps than those who are physically active, so daily walking or other outdoor exercise is recommended. Other standard remedies include a well-balanced diet with plenty of fiber to avoid constipation, and the application of heat to either the lower back or the abdomen. Before the advent of heating pads, hot salt, a mustard poultice, or towels wrung out of hot water and sprinkled with turpentine were used to provide lasting warmth. Alternating heat on the abdomen with an ice pack over the lower back each 10 minutes for an hour has relieved menstrual pain. Hot mustard footbaths were also believed to alleviate abdominal and lumbar discomfort.

Since blood calcium levels begin to decrease before menstruation and drop sharply the first day of the period, taking a balanced calcium supplement and increasing the intake of calcium-containing foods such as milk, cheese, canned salmon, or sardines, and eating leafy greens should be helpful. If cramps do occur, one or two dolomite or bone meal tablets every hour often bring relief. From 1,000 to 5,000 units of natural vitamin D are needed daily to assure absorption of the calcium.[89] Magnesium also is necessary for calcium utilization, plays a role in regulating female hormones, and is a mild diuretic. According to *Annals of Clinical and Laboratory Science* (July/August, 1981), painful menstruation can be avoided by taking 400 milligrams of magnesium every day, or by taking 600 milligrams daily for five days before and during the period. In *Extraordinary Healing Secrets from a Doctor's Private Files*[325], James Van Fleet suggests taking 15 dolomite tablets for painful or heavy menstruation, repeating the dosage in one hour, and then taking 2,000 milligrams of the calcium-magnesium combination every day for maintenance. Adding 100 milligrams of B-6 each day improves the effectiveness of the magnesium.

Increasing regular daily vitamin supplements to include a high-potency B-complex tablet and 50 to 600 milligrams B-6, 1,000 milligrams vitamin C, and 400 to 800 IU of vitamin E (see Caution, page 6) often helps regulate the secretion of estrogen and prevent menstrual pain. (The cutoff of blood and oxygen to the uterus during contraction is partially responsible for cramps—vitamin E increases the oxygen supply.) Hourly doses of the tissue salts, Calc. Fluor. and Mag. Phos. in the 6X potency, often relieve painful menstruation. Additional doses of Mag. Phos. dissolved in hot water may be taken to remedy spasmodic or convulsive pains.

Herbal teas used for relieving menstrual cramps are: camomile, catnip, comfrey, ginger, licorice root, mint, parsley, red raspberry, saffron, sage, thyme. More potent folk remedies for the "monthly miseries" are gin in which juniper berries have been steeped, and "Ozark Stew"—a mixture of corn whiskey, ginger, and a modicum of hot water.

To relieve menstrual pain with nerve massage: thoroughly massage both sides of both wrists, then the hollows beneath the inner and outer ankle bones. Rubbing a point in the middle of the back (about an inch to the right of the spine) is said to reduce pain in the abdomen after 30 seconds and abolish it after three or four minutes of massage.

Stimulating any, or all, of these nerve-pressure points has brought relief from menstrual pain in many instances. Unless otherwise indicated, pressure should be exerted for 10 seconds, released for 10 seconds, and repeated three times.

- With a tongue-depressor or popsicle stick, press three-quarters of the way back on the tongue. Hold firmly for two or three minutes, then move the pressure from one side to the other.
- Use fingers or clothespins to exert pressure on the thumbs and first and second fingers of both hands.
- On the right hand, press the fleshy area formed between the thumb and index finger when the two are pushed together. Repeat on the left hand.
- Press 1½ inches toward the elbow from the center of the largest crease on both inner wrists.
- Press 1 inch above and to both sides of the navel.
- With the thumb and index finger, squeeze the web between the big toe and the one next to it. Repeat on the other foot.

Excessive or prolonged menstrual flow (menorrhagia)

A medical examination to rule out physical causes is wise, but heavy or prolonged menstruation usually indicates vitamin and mineral deficiencies. Taking 10,000 units of vitamin A two or three times a day, plus 400 to 600 IU vitamin E (see Caution, page 6), and supplements of iron and zinc has corrected the condition in one to three months.[53,254] Heavy menstrual flow accompanied by continual fatigue may be caused by poor iron absorption due to lack of vitamin C. Hospital tests reported in *Family Practice News* on March 15, 1974, showed excellent results when 2,000 milligrams of vitamin C plus 1,000 milligrams of bioflavonoids were taken daily for two or three months. Taking 100 micrograms of vitamin K or one teaspoon kelp granules each day has also served to relieve excessive menstruation. The tissue salts for menorrhagia are 6X Calc. Phos., Ferr. Phos., and Kali. Sulph. taken alternately in three daily doses. When the latter part of the period is accompanied by nervous depletion, three daily doses of 12X Kali. Phos. have been helpful. Eating small, frequent meals helps prevent the low blood sugar (which see) that is common during menstruation, and iron-rich foods such as apricots, blackstrap molasses, eggs, milk, nuts, and whole grains are advised.

Folk remedies for excessive menstruation include bed rest during the menstrual period (in extreme cases, elevate the foot of the bed), applications of cold cloths over the abdomen, and drinking the juice of one lemon in a glass of cold water three times a day. Stirring two teaspoons apple cider vinegar (plus an equal amount of honey, if desired) in a glass of water and sipping with each meal is said to reduce a profuse flow to normalcy within three months. Natural teas of cinnamon, plantain, strawberry leaf, or uva ursi are believed to decrease menstrual flow. A Japanese cure for prolonged menstruation is to eat a handful of dried aduki beans (small red beans available in health food stores) each day.

Three nerve pressure points are used to relieve excessive menses. Each point should be pressed for 10 seconds, released for 10 seconds, and the cycle repeated for a total of three pressures on each point.

- Directly below and to the corner toward the thumb of the middle fingernail on both hands.

- The web of skin between the big toe and the second toe on each foot.
- Directly below the toenail on the big toe of each foot, on the side toward the little toe.

Menopause (climatric or change-of-life) and hot flashes

At the end of the reproductive period the ovaries gradually become inactive and estrogen production ceases. The adrenal glands, however, begin providing a hormone which takes over all the functions of estrogen, except for the menstrual cycle, and often the transition can be symptom-free. (Surgical removal of the ovaries before the natural menopause may not prevent a second menopause when the chronological time arrives.[312]) Emotional stress, poor diet, and lack of exercise may exaggerate the discomforts of menopause. Relaxation techniques (see pages 9-10) and a regular program of physical activity can resolve some of the problems. Menopause and hypoglycemia (see Low Blood Sugar) share a myriad of symptoms, many of which are amenable to the same dietary treatment.

A natural diet with adequate protein and little refined carbohydrate is advised. Many foods and herbs contain natural estrogen that can help compensate for the diminished supply. Bananas, bee pollen, raw nuts, seeds, sprouts, and whole grains are recommended along with herbal teas of alfalfa, elder, licorice root, red clover, sage, sarsaparilla, and sassafras. Grating 1 ounce of nutmeg in a pint of rum and taking one teaspoon three times each day was believed to reduce menstrual flow during the climatric. To relieve hot flashes, folk healers suggest using natural honey, chervil, chives, garlic, horseradish, nutmeg, shallots, and tarragon—either as seasonings or teas.

Menopause slows the metabolic rate so fewer calories are required to maintain normal weight. Inactivity of the reproductive system further reduces caloric requirements for a total reduction of 40 to 45 percent.[285] Eating less to avoid adding unwanted pounds makes vitamin and mineral supplementation practically mandatory for proper hormonal function and the prevention of hot flashes, insomnia, and the demineralization of bones. Besides a daily multiple-vitamin-mineral tablet, specific supplements may be of value.

Vitamins C and E and certain B vitamins (B-6, B-12, folic acid, PABA, pantothenic acid) have properties which intensify the effect of existing estrogen and stimulate its production. From 1,000 to 10,000 milligrams of vitamin C are suggested to assure proper adrenal function during menopause. When taken in divided doses with bioflavonoids, vitamin C has relieved hot flashes. Vitamin E, in large doses, is a natural substitute for estrogen. Reputable researchers have found 400 to 800 IU of mixed tocopherols daily (see Caution, page 6) the most effective treatment for menopausal hot flashes and nervousness.[261, 285] In some cases, results have been apparent in two days when 800 IU vitamin E was accompanied by 3,000 milligrams vitamin C and 1,000 milligrams calcium—all in divided doses daily. Once the hot flashes have subsided, the vitamin E intake can be reduced to 400 IU each day. If estrogen has been prescribed, even more vitamin E is required[238], but the two should be taken several hours apart. When both vitamin E and B vitamins are taken, it may be possible to reduce or gradually eliminate the estrogen supplement. Combining a 1,000-

milligram capsule of ginseng (which contains estriol, a variant of estrogen) with daily vitamin E therapy has been found to limit hot flashes to a period of two weeks.[294]

Vitamin E and the B complex are also necessary for an adequate supply of pituitary hormones. One daily B-complex tablet plus 50 to 100 milligrams B-6 has been found to allay depression, help control hot flashes, and improve menopausal arthritis of the fingers. PABA and pantothenic acid (100 milligrams of each daily) helps delay menopause and stimulates adrenal function.

The diminishing amounts of sex hormones decrease the body's absorption of calcium. Unless a combination of milk, cheese, and supplements provides 1,400 to 2,000 milligrams of calcium each day, nervousness, irritability, insomnia, headaches, leg cramps, depression, and the fragile, shrinking bones of osteoporosis can result. A two-year study published in *Annals of Internal Medicine* (December, 1977) showed that women who took 1,400 milligrams of calcium each day had no bone loss. (According to the June, 1976 issue of *Postgraduate Medicine,* postmenopausal women without calcium supplementation may lose from 1 to 6 inches in height.) When taken with vitamin E, calcium has been effective in relieving hot flashes. To assure calcium absorption, each 500-milligram calcium supplement requires 250 milligrams magnesium, 500 to 1,000 milligrams phosphorus, and up to 2,000 IU natural vitamin D. Even after the cessation of menstruation, a pseudo-menstrual cycle can usually be observed and the calcium intake should be increased at such times to prevent calcium-deficiency symptoms.

Most menopausal women have been found to be low in zinc and manganese. If not included with the daily supplement, at least 10 milligrams of each may be beneficial. One to two grams of the amino acid, tryptophan, and 500 milligrams niacinamide are often successful in relieving depression. The tissue salt, Ferr. Phos., may provide immediate relief from hot flashes. The dosage is three tablets of the 6X-potency dissolved under the tongue every 10 minutes until normal. If nervousness accompanies the hot flashes, add three tablets of 6X Kali. Phos. each day until improved. Alternating hot and cold sensations, pains in the arms or legs, or headaches may be cleared by taking 6X Kali. Sulph.

Nerve massage has been successfully used to stimulate the production of hormones and relieve menopausal symptoms.

- **To relieve hot flashes**—Massage the inside of both wrists from side to side.
- **To restore pituitary hormone circulation**—Massage the thumbs of both hands and/or the under-center of each big toe.
- **To help restore ovarian function**—Massage the outside of each foot just under the ankle bone.

Sources (See Bibliography)

3, 4, 8, 13, 19, 22, 24, 34, 37, 43, 52, 53, 54, 62, 63, 64, 68, 71, 81, 82, 88, 89, 91, 98, 101, 105, 113, 121, 128, 139, 142, 152, 154, 156, 168, 173, 174, 175, 180, 184, 189, 190, 199, 226, 229, 242, 250, 253, 254, 255, 256, 260, 261, 270, 273, 282, 284, 285, 288, 293, 294, 297, 299, 312, 315, 325, 353.

MOTION SICKNESS (See Also Nausea and Vomiting)

Triggered by an inner-ear balance mechanism that reacts to stimulation from the movement of an airplane, boat, or car, motion sickness occurs most frequently among those who are also subject to high blood pressure or migraine headaches, and/or have a B-vitamin deficiency. Merely taking a 100-milligram B-complex tablet the night before and the morning of the trip has avoided queasiness for many travelers. Other susceptible people have found that taking a B-complex tablet plus extra B-6 and eating brewer's yeast daily for at least two weeks before an anticipated trip prevented all discomfort. Possibly because of an antihistamine effect, taking 500 milligrams vitamin C, 100 milligrams pantothenic acid, and 50 milligrams B-6 before a trip, 30 minutes after starting and again in four hours, thwarts motion sickness for some individuals.

As reported in *Lancet* (March 20, 1982), taking two or three capsules per hour of powdered ginger (available in health food stores) has been found to be almost twice as effective as dramamine in preventing the nausea of motion sickness. The tissue salts, Kali. Phos. and Nat. Phos., act as a preventive when two 12X tablets of each are taken before starting and every two hours during travel. For acute motion sickness, the same dosage may be taken at 30-minute intervals.

Evacuating the bowels and eating lightly before leaving decreases the likelihood of an attack. An empty stomach succumbs more easily but heavy foods with rich sauces or large amounts of sugar or salt should be avoided. Beef or chicken broth, one tablespoon of brewer's yeast stirred in a glass of tomato juice, or an egg white whisked with the juice of a lemon may be beneficial when taken just before embarking.

Reading while in motion is not advocated, but keeping mentally occupied with anything else distracts the mind and often averts motion sickness. Leaning back with the head supported minimizes the effect of movement on the inner ear. Sitting in the front seat of a car and watching the road, or in the center of a boat or ship and fixing the eyes on the horizon, aids stabilization. When traveling by air, the motion is less pronounced in the center of the plane over the wings.

Folk Remedies

Castor Oil—Taking a tablespoon of castor oil the night before going aboard was believed to prevent seasickness.

Cayenne Pepper—To alleviate the nausea, stir as much ground red pepper as can be borne into a cup of hot broth and sip slowly.

Celery—Slowly and thoroughly chewing and swallowing small pieces of raw celery often quells the queasiness of motion sickness.

Cinnamon—Sipping cinnamon tea or eating cinnamon sticks steeped in red wine often checks the nausea and vomiting.

Cloves—Chewing one or two whole cloves may relieve nauseous sensations.

Egg White—For prolonged seasickness, take the white of one egg beaten in cold water.

Gingerale—Sipping gingerale over crushed ice was a favorite shipboard remedy for seasickness.

Grapefruit Peel—Thoroughly chewing one-half teaspoon shredded, dried grapefruit peel sometimes quells motion-sickness queasiness.

Green Tea—Drinking as much strong green tea as the stomach would tolerate was another favored remedy.

Heat—Lying quietly in the berth with a hot water bottle on the abdomen and another at the feet was an old restorative for seasickness.

Herbal Teas—Anise, basil, camomile, caraway seed, clove, ginger, goldenseal, marjoram, peppermint, sage, or savory tea often calms a stomach upset by motion sickness.

Lemon or Lime—Sucking a lemon at the first sign of nausea is the oldest remedy for seasickness. Sipping fresh lemon or lime juice during an attack of any form of motion sickness is also recommended.

Mint or Sage—Chew a sprig of fresh mint or a few sage leaves to counteract the nausea.

Pressure—For any type of motion sickness, tighten a wide belt (or a strip of cloth or a towel) around the waist for 30 minutes.

Water—Taking sips of warm water between deep breaths is said to help allay queasiness.

Case History

Virginia T. was excited about going to see her new grandson, and had been looking forward to taking her first trip on a plane. As she fastened her seat belt, Virginia enjoyed the sensation of butterflies fluttering in her stomach—it had been a long time since she had experienced this feeling of happy anticipation. By the time the plane was in the air, however, her pleasure began to turn into panic. The internal flutterings were no longer those of exuberant expectancy; Virginia was more than queasy, she was nauseous. The stewardess observed her discomfort, and, when told the reason for it, promptly handed Virginia a paper cup filled with cool water. She suggested that Virginia take tiny sips of the water, lean back, and try to relax. The nausea gradually lessened, but Virginia continued to sip the water every few minutes throughout the remainder of the flight. The stewardess's explanation for the success of this simple remedy was that sipping the water affected the barometric pressure in the ear. She advised Virginia to request a cup of water as soon as she boarded the plane for the return flight, and to start sipping it before takeoff. Virginia followed these instructions and had a pleasant flight home—with no nausea to mar her memories of the wonderful visit with her daughter and the new baby.

Nerve Massage

- Massage the hollow at the base of the skull and along the edge of the mastoid bone behind each ear. Then, rub, squeeze, and tap the back of the neck.
- Massage the last two fingers on both hands for 10 minutes. If no relief is felt, massage the thumbs and first two fingers on each hand, including the webs at the base of the fingers.

- Using the fingernails of the opposite hand, scratch the thumb and index finger of the left hand and the first three fingers on the right hand, as well as the webs between. When possible, scratching the corresponding toes is also believed helpful.
- Massage both kneecaps for three minutes.

Nerve Pressure

Press each point for 10 seconds, release for 10 seconds, and repeat three times.

- Use the index fingers to press 1 inch behind each earlobe. Then press just below the earlobes where the jawbones end.
- Press and massage each inner arm 2 inches toward the elbow from the base of the thumb.
- Press a point 1 inch below the bottom of the breastbone, and another point 2 inches above the navel.
- Press the upper surface of the shinbone, 3 inches up from the anklebone, then use the thumbs to press parallel points on the inside of each leg.

Sources (See Bibliography)

3, 13, 18, 20, 34, 52, 62, 63, 67, 68, 89, 142, 168, 173, 211, 215, 226, 227, 229, 236, 254, 261, 288, 312, 315, 318, 319.

MOUTH AND GUM PROBLEMS—PYORRHEA (See Also Cold Sores and Toothache)

A sore mouth can be caused by a variety of factors: allergies, decayed teeth, poor oral hygiene, malocclusion, teeth grinding, improperly fitted dentures, or inadequate nutrition. Proper care of "baby teeth" is necessary to prevent future malocclusion, and daily cleansing plus regular dental checkups are recommended, but, since mouth tissues give early warning of nutritional deficiencies, many problems can be prevented or corrected with dietary supplements. Herbal teas of red raspberry or sage can be used as natural mouthwashes for all mouth problems.

Burning sensations in the mouth may be corrected by taking a B-complex tablet plus 50 to 100 milligrams B-6 daily. Additional B-2 may be helpful in some cases.

Coated tongue may indicate that putrefactive bacteria are inhabiting the intestines. This usually clears when a B-complex supplement plus acidophilus yogurt (or acidophilus capsules) are taken with each meal.

Cracks at the corners of the mouth or sore lips may be caused by lack of B vitamins. Taking a 50-milligram B-complex tablet three times a day may suffice. If individual B vitamins are preferred: one B-complex tablet plus 400 micrograms folic acid, 100 milligrams pantothenic acid, and 50 milligrams each B-2 and B-6 are suggested. Adding one tablespoon cold-pressed vegetable oil to the daily diet or taking several capsules of vitamin F may be beneficial.

Dry mouth—Up to 25,000 units of vitamin A each day is sometimes helpful for increasing the amount of saliva. As reported in the *Journal of the American Medical Association* (July 29, 1974), many diabetics and hypoglycemics suffer from dry mouths as a result of blood-sugar imbalance. The condition is relieved when the blood-sugar problem is controlled (see Diabetes and Low Blood Sugar). A dry mouth may also be the result of taking drugs which stop the flow of saliva, or it may be due to a depressed mental state that can be alleviated by taking extra B-complex tablets or practicing deliberate relaxation and positive thinking (see pages 9-10). Immediate relief may be obtained by gargling with honey and water to increase the secretion of saliva.

Inflammation of the mouth (stomatitis, trench mouth, or Vincent's disease)—Poor sanitation in the trenches during World War I gave the name "trench mouth" to ulceronecrotic gingivostomatitis or Vincent's angina. Mouth irritation may be caused by allergy, decaying teeth, excessive medication, or appear as a complication of gastric or intestinal diseases, so should have medical attention if persistent. Stomatitis usually disappears when 10,000 to 25,000 units vitamin A, a B-complex tablet, 150 milligrams niacinamide, and 1,000 milligrams vitamin C are taken each day. Including orange or tomato juice and brewer's yeast in the diet is advised. Rinsing the mouth every half hour with a solution of one or two teaspoons baking soda or one-half teaspoon salt in a glass of water, strawberry-leaf tea (with or without a pinch of alum), or a mixture of one tablespoon hydrogen peroxide with two tablespoons of water may be beneficial. Trench mouth (Vincent's disease) is a severe form of stomatitis and is contagious, so eating utensils should be sterilized and intimate physical contact avoided.

Loss of sense of taste—If not due to nerve damage, this may be normalized by taking 50 milligrams of zinc daily for a few weeks, then reducing the dosage to 15 milligrams for maintenance.

Case History

Elizabeth B., an accident victim confined to a wheelchair, was devastated by the death of her husband. The couple had remained exuberantly happy and self-sufficient by taking care of each other through years of poor health. Even after they were housebound they maintained an extensive correspondence with residents of nursing homes throughout the country, cheering those they considered less fortunate than themselves—now Elizabeth had given up. In a letter to a friend she apologized for not sending a Christmas card, explaining that she was now bedfast and being cared for by a woman who came in daily. Still attempting to accentuate the positive, Elizabeth mentioned that her pastor had arranged for her to have meals delivered daily, but admitted that she was eating very little, was too lethargic to bother with taking any vitamins, and was losing weight because nothing tasted good. Elizabeth's friend was a retired nutritionist who believed this "state of decline" could be remedied by the addition of a dietary supplement. She promptly mailed a month's supply of 50-milligram zinc tablets to Elizabeth, and insisted that Elizabeth take one each day with one of the multiple-vitamin-mineral tablets she already had. By the end of the month Elizabeth had regained her sense of taste and her appetite, gained both weight and strength, and was again able to maneuver her wheelchair. She reduced her daily dosage of zinc to 15 milligrams a day, cancelled her meals-on-wheels and, before Eastertime, had written over 200 cheerful notes to accompany her cards to "the less fortunate."

Sore mouth from dental work can often be relieved by applying aloe vera gel (available from health food stores) or vitamin A (squeezed from a pierced capsule) directly to the sore spots several times each day.

Sore mouth due to wearing dentures—Once the dentures are correctly fitted, a 50-milligram B-complex tablet, 1,000 milligrams vitamin C, and 1,000 milligrams of calcium with magnesium (dolomite) plus 400 IU natural vitamin D taken daily usually relieves the problem. Adding 25,000 units of vitamin A and 50 milligrams of zinc for a few days helps speed the healing of any raw areas. Studies reported in *Journal of the Amrican Dental Association* (January, 1976) and the *Journal of Prosthetic Dentistry* (January, 1979) showed that an over-balance of phosphorus in the diet caused shrinkage of the jawbone and difficulty with dentures even when the calcium intake appeared to be adequate. Researchers have found a one-to-one ratio of phosphorus and calcium with half as much magnesium more effective in controlling bone loss than the former ideal ratio of two to two and one-half times as much phosphorus as calcium. One glass of whole milk contains 291 milligrams calcium, 228 milligrams phosphorus, and 33 milligrams magnesium. In meat, the phosphorus-calcium ratio is 20 to 1, refined cereal products are about 6 to 1, and potatoes 5 to 1.[339] Soft drinks also contain large amounts of phosphorus. Dolomite or magnesium supplements help offset this phosphorus imbalance.

Sore tongue (glossitis or glossodynia) usually indicates a lack of B vitamins. A purplish tongue is a sign of B-2 deficiency; a painfully red one, a lack of niacin; a smooth, shiny tongue an undersupply of folic acid or B-12; and a sore, swollen tongue may result from lack of B-1, B-2, B-6, or pantothenic acid. If taking a 50-milligram B-complex tablet three times a day with meals does not remedy the problem, a medical examination is in order as a sore tongue can arise from allergic reactions or iron-deficiency anemia. A burning tongue may also result from a strong dentifrice, excessive use of alcohol or tobacco, or overly hot or spicy foods. In older women, a burning tongue may be due to a lack of hydrochloric acid in the stomach and remedied by taking a betaine hydrochloride tablet with each meal.

Teeth grinding (bruxism)—According to the *Journal of the American Dental Association* (January, 1971), teeth clenching or grinding can cause damage to the gums, jaws, muscles, and teeth. Numerous tests have shown that a 50-milligram B-complex tablet each morning and evening, plus 100 milligrams pantothenic acid and two bone meal and dolomite tablets before bed ameliorate the problem.

White patches on the lining of the mouth (leukoplakia or thrush) is common in persons taking large doses of antibiotics for long periods of time but may result from gastrointestinal problems. This condition often responds dramatically to a 50-milligram B-complex tablet and acidophilus yogurt (or acidophilus capsules) taken with each meal. Folk remedies for these white patches included covering them with mashed raw garlic, rubbing them with alum, or rinsing the mouth with a mixture of one-fourth cup each apple cider vinegar and water plus one teaspoon salt and pinch of black or red pepper.

Gum Problems—Periodontal Disease—Pyorrhea

"Periodontal" refers to the gums, bone, and tissues surrounding the teeth. Problems generally appear after the age of 35 and account for more teeth lost after middle age than do dental caries. Periodontal disease commonly becomes noticeable with inflammation and bleeding of the gums (gingivitis), followed by recession of the gums and the bony structure supporting the teeth. Aggravated by tartar and plaque at the gum line, infected pockets form between gums and teeth (pyorrhea), and, if left untreated, the teeth become so wobbly they either fall out or must be removed.

There is controversy over the direct cause of pyorrhea. One view is that poor dental hygiene and lack of vitamin C cause inflamed, spongy gums that allow bacteria to infiltrate the teeth sockets and create bone loss. Another theory is that insufficient dietary calcium forces the body to borrow calcium from the bones to supply the nerves, that the jawbone is the first affected, and that poorly supported teeth instigate the irritated, receding gums. According to research reported in *Your Health* (September, 1982), sugar may be responsible for periodontal disease. Sugar (not the carbohydrates from starches) has been found to interfere with the constant bone formation necessary to prevent the bone loss around the roots of the teeth which leads to gum inflammation and loose teeth.

Regardless of origin, both the prevention and treatment of periodontal problems call for periodic tooth-cleaning sessions in a dental office plus daily brushing and flossing to prevent tartar build up. Many dentists recommend the Bass Technique, developed by Dr. Charles C. Bass at Tulane University Medical School in 1948, for dislodging plaque and restoring health to puffy gums. Twice each day the gums and teeth are brushed with soft, round-tipped nylon bristles arranged in a straight line. With the brush across the teeth and the bristles at gum line, wiggling the brush back and forth loosens the plaque. Then the biting surfaces of the teeth are cleansed by brushing lengthwise. Brushing too hard or with bristles that are too stiff may actually force the gums away from the teeth and create tooth sensitivity—especially if a highly abrasive toothpaste is used.

Many clinical studies have shown that large doses of vitamin C, preferably with bioflavonoids, cure "pink toothbrush" while firming and tightening teeth and gums. The August 14, 1981 issue of the *Journal of the American Medical Association* reported that taking 2,000 to 3,000 milligrams of vitamin C daily provided protection against the bacteria causing periodontal disease.

Vitamin A, with vitamin E for stabilization, and extra zinc combat gum infection. Calcium supplements balanced with magnesium and phosphorus, plus vitamin D to assure absorption, have not only arrested bone erosion and tightened teeth, but have been shown by x-rays to have caused the hollow sockets around the teeth to fill in with new bone.[52] The daily supplemental amounts suggested are:

Vitamin A—50,000 units for three weeks, then 10,000 to 25,000 units.

B Complex—One comprehensive, high-potency tablet.

Vitamin C—1,000 to 10,000 milligrams plus at least 500 milligrams of the bioflavonoid complex (citrus bioflavonoids, hesperidin, and rutin).

Calcium and Vitamin D—2,000 milligrams of calcium in bone meal and dolomite tablets (or calcium carbonate or gluconate plus magnesium and phosphorus supplements) plus 400 to 1,000 IU vitamin D. Taking some form of acid with the calcium—apple cider vinegar in water, vitamin C, or a hydrochloric acid tablet—is believed to increase calcium absorption.

Vitamin E (see Caution, page 6)—100 to 400 IU. (The capsules may be punctured and rubbed on the gums before swallowing for even more rapid improvement.)

Zinc—15 to 150 milligrams to speed healing.

Emphasizing crunchy foods such as raw fruits and vegetables while cutting down on sweet, mushy ones often helps tone up soft, inflammation-prone gums. For further stimulus by friction, the old-fashioned method was to rub the gums with a rough cloth or massage them with salt. Using baking soda and salt as a dentifrice was also recommended. For the sodium-conscious, epsom salts could be substituted for the salt. Other folk remedies for bleeding gums or pyorrhea include:

- Apple Cider Vinegar—Each night and morning, stir one teaspoon apple cider vinegar in one cup water. Use a little as a mouthwash, then drink the remainder.
- Eat generous amounts of cooked Brussels sprouts, raw cauliflower, and watercress.
- Rinse the mouth several times a day with camomile tea or use either of these two natural mouthwashes every hour. 1) Steep one-fourth teaspoon each dried anise, mint, and rosemary in three-fourths cup boiling water for 10 minutes and strain. 2) Boil two tablespoons dried, ground pomegranate rinds in three cups water until reduced to two cups.
- Cook figs in milk, rub the figs on the sore gums, and drink the liquid.
- Use lemon juice as a dentifrice and/or cut lemon into strips and apply the inside of the rind to the gums and teeth.

Sources (See Bibliography)

3, 4, 6, 7, 8, 13, 22, 24, 52, 53, 75, 76, 78, 84, 89, 92, 99, 110, 128, 142, 168, 174, 184, 189, 215, 223, 226, 227, 228, 229, 242, 254, 256, 261, 270, 281, 288, 293, 305, 312, 315, 316, 325, 335, 349.

MUSCLE CRAMPS, SPASMS, TICS, AND TREMORS—INTERMITTENT CLAUDICATION

The former theory that tics and twitches were expressions of neurosis has generally been forsaken. Muscles are controlled by electrical impulses from the nervous system which depends on B vitamins for proper functioning. Increased amounts of these vitamins are needed during periods of emotional stress. A few minutes of daily mental and physical relaxation (see pages 9-10) may also be helpful. Nerve impulses are conducted by minerals. Any deficiency or imbalance of calcium, magnesium, phosphorus, potassium, etc. can cause muscle spasms, tics, or tremors. Alcohol, allergies, antacids, diuretics, tranquilizers, or other medication can upset the mineral balance but most of these muscular problems are believed to be the result of vitamin and mineral deficiencies.

Exercising in heat and humidity can cause cramps from a depletion of sodium that can be replenished by eating salty foods. Painful muscular contractions and stiffness arising from unaccustomed exercise can usually be prevented by taking 500 milligrams of vitamin C before, each hour or so during, and immediately after the strenuous activity. If a "charley horse" does attack, it may be eased by pushing the foot against resistance, gently massaging the affected muscle, and applying heat or ice.

Restless legs syndrome (nighttime leg cramps or jerking) is a common complaint, but, according to the *Harvard Medical School Health Letter* (December, 1982), is seldom associated with serious blood vessel disease. Supplements of calcium and/or vitamin E usually resolve this problem within a few weeks but additional vitamins and minerals may be necessary. Low Blood Sugar (which see) can be a contributory factor—almost half the individuals with hypoglycemia are troubled by nocturnal leg cramps.[171] The leg cramps suffered by women during pregnancy, menstruation, or menopause can frequently be relieved by taking 1,000 milligrams calcium, 500 milligrams magnesium, 400 IU vitamin D, and 50 to 150 milligrams vitamin B-6. Tremors and facial tics have reportedly been corrected by the same supplementation plus several tablespoons of brewer's yeast or comprehensive B-complex tablets.

Tic Douloureaux (facial twitching and pain) may be occasioned by a dental problem that requires surgery, but some cases have cleared when all forms of caffeine were eliminated from the diet. (This would include caffeine-containing medications and soft drinks as well as coffee, tea, chocolate, and cocoa.) In other cases, a daily multi-vitamin-mineral tablet plus extra C, E, and 1,000 micrograms of B-12 have done away with the problem.

Poor circulation can contribute to muscle cramping. Intermittent claudication (leg cramps and pain that occur during walking but not while resting) is caused by narrowed blood vessels providing insufficient oxygen-rich blood to the legs. Large amounts of vitamin E often correct this condition in a matter of months, particularly when vitamin C and lecithin are added (see Hardening of the Arteries). Some cases of Intermittent claudication have improved after one month of taking 1,600 IU of vitamin E daily[325] (see Caution, page 6). Some have found relief only after three months of daily therapy with 8,000 milligrams vitamin C, 800 IU vitamin E, 100 milligrams B-15, and 50 milligrams zinc. Others have found 3,000 milligrams vitamin C, 2,000 IU vitamin E, 2,000 micrograms chromium, 200 micrograms selenium, and 150 mlligrams zinc to be more effective.[353]

If left untreated, reduced circulation to the legs can result in Buerger's disease—an inflammation of the blood vessels with clot formation. Even more vitamin E is then indicated, along with a week's bed rest, to dissolve the blood clots without their breaking loose to cause a stroke or other blockage that might result in gangrene. Massive amounts of vitamin E should be used only under a doctor's supervision, and any muscular irregularity that does not respond to natural treatment should receive medical attention as it might be indicative of a serious disorder.

Diet and Supplements

Even in the 1850s it was recognized that spasmodic muscles were caused by irritation of the nerves controlling them and a more nutritious diet was recommended. Adequate nourishment is important for proper muscle functioning, and extra amounts of protein are needed for tissue rebuilding after a severe charley horse or cramp. Fresh vegetables and whole grains provide magnesium, phosphorus, and potassium as well as other nutrients. Beet, carrot, and cucumber juices are believed especially beneficial for muscular health. Apple and most other fruit juices improve the absorption of calcium as do the fatty acids (vitamin F) in buttermilk and unsaturated oils. Dr. Jarvis, author of the famous book on folk medicine[181], recommends two teaspoons honey (or two teaspoons each honey and apple cider vinegar) stirred in a glass of water and sipped with each meal to correct either twitches or leg cramps. Although honey does contain a little potassium, sugar requires potassium for conversion to glycogen within the body. A tic or twitch may be instigated by potassium depletion resulting from over-ingestion of sugar.

A well-balanced diet usually prevents muscular abnormalities, but, when the cramps and tremors do appear, digestive enzymes or betaine hydrochloride tablets at mealtime may aid the assimilation of nutrients, extra antioxidants (see page 3) are often helpful, and therapeutic amounts of specific supplements may be required.

> **B Complex**—One comprehensive tablet daily plus additional B vitamins as appropriate: 100 milligrams B-1 daily for facial neuralgia, numbness, or "pins and needles" in the hands or feet. Up to 50 milligrams niacin three times a day to inhibit the chemical activity possibly responsible for tremors. Up to 150 milligrams B-6 each day to prevent nocturnal leg cramps, numbness, tingling, and cramping of fingers and toes. 100 to 300 milligrams pantothenic acid two to four times a day for relief of muscle spasms due to strain and tension.
>
> **Vitamin C and Bioflavonoids**—At least 500 milligrams vitamin C (preferably with bioflavonoids) three times a day. Vitamin C is responsible for the health of the body's connective tissues. It often prevents stiffness when taken before and during arduous activity, relieves leg cramps, and reduces tremors and shaking. Taking 4,000 milligrams of vitamin C each day has alleviated some cases of Parkinson's Disease, and 1,000 milligrams of bioflavonoids three times a day has eased painful joints[7].

Case History

John and Lorna G. decided to forego their usual vacation trip, stay home, and build a backyard patio. They solicited advice from experienced friends, and among the tips on types of paving blocks and roofing material was the suggestion that they take extra vitamin C to avoid muscle stiffness. John and Lorna followed all the instructions as they tamped sand, carried bricks, balanced on sawhorses to paint rafters, and boosted roof panels into place. Every time they paused for a break, they each took a 1000-milligram tablet of vitamin C with bioflavonoids, and they took more vitamin C before they went to bed at night. They had scheduled the completion of their project for several days prior to returning to their desk jobs because neither of them were accustomed to such strenuous activity and they would need some time to recuperate from the anticipated muscle soreness. Amazingly, there was no stiffness. The natural preventive-remedy was so effective that John and Lorna spent their final vacation days transplanting shrubs to landscape their new patio.

Calcium—800 to 1,200 milligrams daily. Calcium is as vital for the soft tissues as it is for maintenance of bones and teeth. A lack of absorbable calcium is frequently responsible for the intermittent muscle cramps or spasms called "tetany." Vitamins A and D plus the proper proportions of magnesium and phosphorus must be present in order for the calcium to be fully utilized. Milk contains all these nutrients and "balanced" calcium supplements are available. Taking calcium-magnesium-phosphorus tablets with each meal and with a glass of milk before bed often eradicates the problems of leg cramps during sleep or exercise, muscular spasms of the feet and toes, and spastic contractions of the fingers.

Vitamin E—300 to 1,000 IU d-alpha tocopherol daily for nocturnal leg cramps and twitching, jerking muscles. 1,200 to 2,400 IU for intermittent claudication. Those with uncontrolled hypertension or diabetes requiring insulin should begin with no more than 100 IU daily and gradually increase the amount while their condition is monitored by a physician (see Caution, page 6). Vitamin E improves glycogen storage in the muscles to prevent middle-of-the-night muscular abnormalities when blood sugar is at its lowest ebb, enables the body tissues to make better use of the oxygen they receive, increases the blood supply, and is helpful whenever circulation is impaired. Taking vitamin E each morning and calcium plus magnesium before retiring has solved the problem of restless nighttime legs for many, and alleviated muscular ache-all-over discomfort for others.

Magnesium—500 to 800 milligrams daily. Magnesium is necessary for absorption of both calcium (see above) and vitamin B-6, and is a major factor in transmitting nerve impulses and relaxing muscles. Magnesium deficiencies are quite common. When severe or prolonged, they can cause leg and foot cramps, muscle jerkiness, or tremors that can be relieved with a day or two of magnesium supplementation.

Phosphorus is essential for the assimilation of calcium, but too much phosphorus can take calcium out of the body. When using calcium supplements, the proper proportions of phosphorus-magnesium-calcium can be maintained by taking a combination rather than relying solely on any one form—bone meal, dolomite, calcium gluconate, lactate, etc.

Tissue Salts

For muscle cramps or spasms with numbness—Take three or four tablets of 6X Calc. Phos. three times a day.

For pain and muscle cramps following exercise—Take 6X Calc. Fluor., Calc. Phos., and Mag. Phos. every 20 minutes for the first two hours, then a dose of each remedy once every two hours.

For nocturnal leg cramps or muscle spasms—Take three tablets of 6X Silicea plus supplements of calcium, magnesium, and vitamin B-6 before retiring.

Exercise

Walking as far as can be tolerated, resting while the pain fades, then walking again is part of the treatment for intermittent claudication. The cramps caused by wearing high-heeled shoes may be prevented by devoting a few minutes twice each day to stretching out the legs, extending the heels as far as possible, and bending the tops of the feet toward the body. A "stitch in the side" is often alleviated by forcefully blowing the air out of the lungs, bending over, raising the knee on the painful side, and pushing against the "stitch" with the hand.

Regular exercise improves muscle tone and lessens the tendency for muscular stiffness or cramping. Some physical activity is essential for the absorption of calcium. Hospital tests with bed-fast patients have shown that regardless of the amount of vitamins, calcium, and other minerals given, none of the calcium was retained unless the body was in an upright position for at least a few minutes each day.[8] Sitting motionless for long periods retards circulation—occasional movement or gentle rocking can counteract this. Sleeping with the feet elevated on a pillow may help return blood from the legs to the heart and avoid nocturnal leg cramps.

Folk Remedies

Drinking three cups of comfrey tea each day or eating two teaspoons of honey with every meal were considered preventives for muscular problems. Aside from advising a careful diet, thorough elimination, fresh air, and moderate exercise, most other rustic remedies were limited to easing their painful aftermath. The favored treatment for muscular tics and twitches was one teaspoon apple cider vinegar stirred in one-half cup grape juice, diluted to taste with water and taken twice each day between meals. According to Carolyn Niethammer's book, *American Indian Food and Lore* (Macmillan, 1974), cooked wild rose hips were eaten by the Pueblo Indians for relief from muscular pains.

Covering the afflicted muscle with hot, moist towels or a compress of salt heated in a dry skillet and placed in a cotton sack was recommended by many folk practitioners. Sore leg muscles were relieved by wrapping first with thin cloths squeezed out of cold water, then with a thick layer of dry material. Rubbing the aching parts with slices of raw potato or raw onion was believed to ease the pain. Plain turpentine was sometimes used, but the standard "muscle liniment" was prepared by warming one-half cup each turpentine and apple cider vinegar with one tablespoon ground red pepper. After cooling, the mixture was shaken with one-half cup rubbing alcohol and allowed to stand for three days before straining and bottling.

Nerve Massage

For cramping muscles—Massage the outer edge of the bottom of the right foot from 1 inch below the little toe to the center of the arch.

Nerve Pressure

For facial twitches or neuralgia—Wind rubber bands around the joints of the thumb and index finger of the left hand for up to 10 minutes, removing the moment the fingers start to turn blue. Repeat every half hour while acute, then gradually reduce the treatments to once each day.

Hand tremors have reportedly been relieved by putting clothespins on the tips of the fingers for 15 minutes (or until the fingers begin to change color) once or twice each day for one week.

Sources (See Bibliography)

3, 4, 7, 8, 9, 13, 24, 34, 52, 63, 64, 68, 70, 78, 81, 88, 89, 113, 114, 139, 142, 152, 156, 168, 171, 174, 181, 185, 189, 198, 226, 227, 229, 241, 249, 252, 254, 256, 257, 260, 282, 288, 293, 299, 301, 302, 305, 306, 315, 325, 328, 353, 354.

NAUSEA AND VOMITING (See Also Indigestion, Motion Sickness, and Pregnancy)

One of the most common signs of digestive disturbance, vomiting that follows eating tainted or overly rich food, is a naturally protective measure. If an emotional upset is responsible, deliberate relaxation (see pages 9-10) accompanied by positive statements such as "My stomach is relaxing and I will feel fine in a few minutes," may quell the queasiness. Some cases of nausea may be related to Constipation (which see). When an infection is the cause, diarrhea often occurs. Severe or persistent nausea should receive professional attention as it might be a symptom of low blood sugar or serious gastrointestinal disorders. Occasional periods of nausea or vomiting accompanying indigestion usually respond to rest and natural remedies.

Diet and Supplements

Fluids lost through vomiting can be replaced by sucking on ice chips if it is impossible to keep other liquids down. As soon as anything can be retained, Dr. Sehnert[297] recommends the following mixture, chilled and sipped during the day: one package unsweetened soft-drink mix, two tablespoons sugar, one tablespoon salt, and two teaspoons baking soda in four cups boiled water. If solid foods are minimized following a nauseous episode, broths, custards, and gelatins can be used to provide nutrients. Midnight or early-morning nausea may be due to Low Blood Sugar (which see) and corrected by eating a protein snack before retiring. Nausea following surgery may be prevented by having a large amount of sugar in the body to help metabolize stored fat. In *You Can Get Well*[89], Adelle Davis suggests eating 1 pound of fat-free candy (gum drops, jelly beans, marshmallows) the day before surgery. Post-operative nausea can sometimes be alleviated by taking one teaspoonful of honey or sweetened orange juice every 15 to 30 minutes.

B Vitamins and Magnesium—Frequent nausea and vomiting may be indicative of a deficiency of vitamins B-1, B-6, and/or magnesium. A daily B-complex supplement plus dolomite or magnesium tablets often corrects the problem.

Vitamin C—For immediate relief from an occasional bout of nausea and vomiting, one-half teaspoon vitamin C powder (2,000 milligrams) dissolved in one-fourth cup fruit juice or water and taken by the teaspoon each half hour is often effective.

Tissue Salts—Take two tablets each 6X Kali. Phos. and Nat. Phos. every 20 minutes for an hour, then repeat each hour until relieved. If the nausea is bilious, two tablets of 6X Nat. Sulph. may be included with the dosage.

Folk Remedies

Apple Cider Vinegar—Stirring one teaspoon apple cider vinegar in a glass of water and drinking it before ingesting any questionable food was believed to prevent the unpleasantness of mild food poisoning. The same mixture (plus one teaspoon salt, if desired) was used as an after-the-fact remedy for nausea and vomiting. One teaspoonful was to be taken each five minutes until the situation appeared under control, then reduced to one swallow every 15 minutes.

Apples—During an extended period of nausea, shredded raw apple mixed with raw honey (with or without goat's milk) has been retained by those who could tolerate no other food.

Cayenne Pepper—Eating a bowl of hot soup with as much ground red pepper as can be borne is said to make nausea disappear.

Celery—To calm an unsettled stomach, slowly eat small pieces of raw celery.

Cinnamon—A favored folk remedy, ground cinnamon was made into a tea or used as a poultice over the stomach. Cinnamon sticks steeped in red wine were believed to allay nausea and vomiting.

Chicken Gizzard—Cook one chopped chicken gizzard with two chopped lemons. Drink the liquid and, if possible, eat the gizzard.

Cloves—Drinking clove tea or chewing one or two whole cloves often relieves queasiness. Simmering two teaspoons ground cloves in one cup milk and taking one tablespoon each 15 to 30 minutes was another standard remedy.

Egg Yolk and Rum—Downing one raw egg yolk blended with two tablespoons rum was believed to stop persistent vomiting.

Garlic—An old remedy revived, one teaspoon minced fresh garlic or two garlic perles taken after meals proved effective in relieving chronic nausea for 75 percent of the patients tested in a hospital study.[3]

Gingerale, Champagne, or Carbonated Water—Sipping any of these liquids over crushed ice may check queasiness while replacing fluids lost through vomiting.

Grapefruit Peel—Slowly chewing one-half teaspoon dry, grated grapefruit peel often settles an upset stomach.

Grass—A pioneer remedy was to pound grass blades to a pulp, cover with boiling water, and sweeten with brown sugar. The mixture was strained and taken by the spoonful each 10 minutes to stop vomiting.

Herbal Teas—Basil, camomile, ginger, licorice root, mace, nutmeg, or peppermint. A potent mixture of allspice, cinnamon, cloves, and ginger in boiling water was used to stop vomiting. Warm peppermint tea with a little brandy was believed to calm the stomach after an episode of vomiting.

Hot Water—Sipping one tablespoon scalding water every few minutes is the easiest of all natural remedies for quieting an agitated stomach.

Ice Pack—Applying cold cloths or an ice pack to the back of the neck sometimes settles the stomach.

Mint—Placing a poultice of the crushed leaves over the stomach or chewing a few fresh sprigs was another favorite remedy for nauseous conditions.

Mustard—In severe cases, a paste of dry mustard and egg white or water was applied to the stomach, then removed before blistering occurred.

Onion—To control incessant vomiting, the instructions were to peel a large onion, cut it in half, and place one section in each armpit.

Nerve Massage and Pressure

- Massage the thumb and first and second fingers of each hand.
- With the fingernails or a comb, gently scratch the thumb and index finger of the left hand and the first three fingers of the right hand, as well as the webs between those fingers. Scratching the corresponding toes is also believed helpful.
- With the index finger, press 1 inch to the left of the center of the chest for 10 seconds. Release for 10 seconds, and repeat three times.
- Press the inside of each arm 2 inches toward the elbow from the center of each wrist. Exert pressure for 10 seconds, release for 10 seconds, and repeat three times. According to *Medical Update* (Vol. 6, 1982), this technique is successful for postoperative nausea as well as that created by chemotherapy treatments for cancer.
- Using the knuckle of the index finger, firmly press and roll the area between the ball of the foot and the beginning of the arch on both feet.

Sources (See Bibliography)

3, 7, 13, 18, 19, 34, 43, 52, 63, 64, 68, 88, 89, 92, 129, 142, 152, 156, 165, 168, 173, 174, 181, 206, 211, 226, 227, 254, 284, 293, 297, 305, 312, 318, 319, 325, 328, 333.

NOSEBLEED

Whether called epistaxis by a doctor or a bloody nose by a scuffling youngster, nosebleeds are common mishaps. They usually result from an injury to the nose, too much or too hard blowing of the nose, or scratching the interior of a nostril with a finger or other object. The tiny arteries and veins imbedded in the center partition of the nose are so fragile that spontaneous nosebleeds may occur following excessive sneezing or coughing due to a cold or hay fever, or exposure to extremely dry air. Most nasal hemorrhages respond to home treatment but if the bleeding persists more than 20 minutes, or a fracture is suspected, the assistance of a physician should be sought. Recurrent nosebleeds also warrant medical diagnosis as they might be an indication of concussion, high blood pressure, or faulty blood coagulation.

Antibiotics, ACTH, or cortisone therapy may deplete the friendly intestinal bacteria responsible for synthesizing vitamin K and controlling blood clotting. Eating generous amounts of acidophilus yogurt, broccoli, cabbage, spinach, and other green vegetables often prevents recurrent nosebleeds, but supplements of vitamin K or acidophilus capsules may be necessary. Taking one or two teaspoons of apple cider vinegar in a glass of water three times a day is a folk remedy for frequent nosebleeds. Increasing the daily intake of vitamin C and the bioflavonoids to 500 to 5,000 milligrams vitamin C and 500 to 1,000 milligrams bioflavonoids strengthens the walls of the capillaries and blood vessels so there is less chance of spontaneous nosebleeds. The bleeding tendency of dry membranes in the nose may be corrected by coating the inside of the nostrils several times a day with mineral oil (or vitamin E squeezed from a capsule) on a cotton swab.

Ancient folklore advised applying sliced onions or the leaves of beets, cabbage, lettuce, or turnips to the back of the neck to quell nasal hemorrhages. Those suffering from frequent nosebleeds were instructed to wear a bright silk ribbon around the throat or an iron key between the shoulder blades. However, most folk remedies for arresting a nosebleed bear a remarkable similarity to modern first-aid treatments. Once the bleeding has ceased, it is wise to refrain from stooping over or blowing the nose for an hour or so.

> **Pressure**—Almost all nosebleeds respond to simple compression of the soft part of the nose with the thumb and first finger. The pressure should be maintained for five to 15 minutes while sitting quietly in a chair. (Sitting up decreases blood flow to the head and causes draining blood to run out the front of the nose rather than down the back of the throat.) Pressure should be released slowly to avoid disturbing the newly formed clot. If the bleeding has not stopped, pressure should be reapplied for another five minutes. Applying pressure with one hand while raising the arm on the same side as the bleeding nostril, or using a clothespin to apply pressure while holding both hands over the head or clasped behind the neck is successful for some. Others prefer pressing on a roll of paper or gauze placed above the teeth under the upper lip.
>
> **Chilling**—Research has shown that cooling the skin of any part of the body causes a reflex contraction of blood vessels in the nose and helps stop the

bleeding.[241] Placing the feet in a bucket of cold water while pressing the nose closed may reduce bleeding time. (Soaking the feet in hot water while drinking a cup of cayenne-pepper tea was the folk method for drawing blood away from the head.) Applying cold packs to the nose, forehead, back of the neck, or under the lower jaw while maintaining pressure on the nose is usually the speediest method of abating the blood flow. Holding a sliver of ice inside the nose and a large piece against the side of the nose and forehead is another option.

Case History

After he slipped and banged his face against the boulder, 15-year-old Brad L. realized that he had been showing off. His parents had insisted he participate in this family picnic—it really hadn't been too bad, he had sort of enjoyed playing tag and hide-and-seek with his younger cousins who were pretty neat kids—but he just couldn't resist demonstrating his manly prowess by attempting to climb to the top of the rocky ridge behind their picnic spot. Now he was the center of attention all right. The blood spurting from his nose drew cries of consternation from everyone except his mother. She scooped the last of their picnic-chest ice into a plastic bag, wrapped it in a towel, placed it on the back of Brad's neck, and told him to lean back against the boulder. Then she extracted the only remaining frosty object in the ice chest and pressed it against his bleeding proboscis. No one laughed at him, and the bleeding soon ceased, but, thought Brad as he held the package of semi-frozen peas over his nose, so much for manly prowess.

Nasal Plugs are sometimes preferable to pressure and may be used in combination with the ice packs. During the 1800s, filling the nostril with bacon grease (or inserting a piece of fat bacon cut to fit the nostril) and holding a lump of ice in the mouth was recommended. Plugging the nostril with facial tissue, gauze or a clean handkerchief may be more convenient. Saturating the dry packing substance with lemon juice, mineral oil, Vaseline, vinegar, or vitamin E oil increases effectiveness and helps prevent fibers being caught up in the clot.

Tissue Salts—For a common nosebleed, take three tablets each 6X Ferr. Phos. and Kali. Phos. at 10-minute intervals until the bleeding stops. If the blood is black and clotted, substitute three tablets of 6X Kali. Mur.

Sources (See Bibliography)

7, 19, 28, 53, 68, 81, 89, 98, 111, 121, 142, 156, 174, 180, 226, 227, 254, 270, 289, 293, 297, 305, 312, 315, 316, 318, 345, 353.

POISON IVY AND POISON OAK (Contact Dermatitis)

Reactions to these irritants are considered allergy-related since some people are completely immune, some develop the blistering rash only after a second exposure, and others are so susceptible that they react to the smoke from burning plants a long distance away. The irritating substance (urushiol) is in the leaves, flowers, fruit, stems, bark, and roots of buttercup, primrose, and sumac as well as poison ivy and poison oak. It can be passed from one person to another when the oily sap is on the skin, or it can be contacted by petting a cat or dog that has recently rubbed against the plants. Clothing or tools can become contaminated and spread the irritant from one user to another.

The itchy blisters may require from six hours to six days to make an appearance. Whenever exposure is suspected, it is wise to thoroughly cleanse the area with soap and water and wash all the outer clothing. Lathering four or five times with bar laundry soap, then rinsing with rubbing alcohol and again with water is the surest method of removing all the irritant from the skin.

Case History

Rosemary K. insisted that she looked like an upended turnip during this last month of her pregnancy; but she felt great, accepted her mother-in-law's invitation to the family's end-of-summer picnic, and donned her maternity shorts. However, the festivities came to a screeching halt when Rosemary's husband noticed that the wildflowers she was gathering were in the midst of a bed of poison ivy. Rushed home, Rosemary obediently stripped, scrubbed down with brown soap, and showered in the basement laundry room. The next day her legs were fine but her red-rashed, itchy behind necessitated a visit to the local physician. The doctor wanted to know everything she had done during the preceding few days. While recounting the events following her encounter with poison ivy at the picnic, Rosemary remembered that she had piled her clothing on a chair before showering, then sat down on the garments while she re-dressed. No serious damage resulted—Rosemary survived her itchy discomfort and delivered a healthy baby—but she did learn that home remedies as well as prescriptive ones should be followed to the letter for total success.

Taking 1,000 to 2,000 milligrams vitamin C plus 100 to 300 milligrams pantothenic acid and 50 to 100 milligrams B-6 immediately following exposure and each four or five hours thereafter may be beneficial because of their antihistamine and detoxifying effects. Combined with the cleansing, they may prevent a rash from appearing.

Traditionally, the rash gets worse for five days, then better for five days, but the process may be speeded by utilizing natural remedies. Once the rash becomes apparent, taking two or three dolomite tablets, applying vitamin E squeezed from a capsule, and swallowing the remainder sometimes alleviates the pain and itching. Applying a paste of powdered vitamin C mixed with water has been known to effect a cure within 24 hours when at least 10,000 milligrams of oral vitamin C was taken in divided doses during the day.[350] Three tablets each of the tissue salts, Kali. Sulph. and Nat. Mur. in the 6X potency, dissolved under the tongue every few hours, has also proven helpful. Taking one or two tablespoons brewer's yeast mixed with warm water and honey every two hours for the first day, then each three or four hours for the next few days often speeds the drying-up process.

Folk Remedies

Over 2,000 years ago oriental physicians used crushed crab as a remedy for poison ivy. Other folk remedies for the discomfort of poison ivy or poison oak include a wide assortment of washes, rubs, compresses, and pastes.

Aloe vera gel, alum water, ammonia, apple cider vinegar, a solution of baking soda or salt and water, whole-milk or buttermilk (mixed with vinegar and salt or one-half teaspoon baking soda per cup, if desired), a strong epsom-salts solution, herbal teas of golden seal or white oak bark, kerosene, lemon juice, witch hazel, or the water from cooked oats may be sponged over the rash at frequent intervals.

A piece of chalk can be pulverized, mixed with a pint of water, and applied with a clean cloth. The blisters can be smeared with olive oil and, in severe cases, one teaspoon to one tablespoon of the oil taken internally every three hours. The inside of banana peels, orange slices, raw rhubarb, or the juice from green tomatoes rubbed over the area each hour are said to inhibit itching and speed healing.

Rubbing a mixture of epsom salts and baking soda, plain salt, linseed oil, or white shoe polish on the poisoned area, or dabbing on a solution of one-fourth bar brown laundry soap liquefied in two cups hot water, three or four times a day, was believed to hasten recovery.

Pastes made from cornstarch or baking soda and water, applied directly to the rash, were standard remedies. Poultices of mashed fresh catnip leaves, boiled oatmeal, crushed raw garlic, ground green-bean pods, or bruised blades of grass were also used to relieve itching and promote healing.

Sources (See Bibliography)

3, 7, 13, 19, 28, 52, 53, 62, 68, 76, 81, 89, 98, 152, 153, 156, 168, 184, 190, 226, 228, 288, 305, 312, 315, 325, 328, 345, 350.

PREGNANCY

Having a competent obstetrician and following his advice is the prime prerequisite for a successful pregnancy. This is one instance where "old wives' tales" should yield to scientific progress. Recent studies correlating prenatal nutrition with infant development and intelligence, as well as the prevention of maladies common during pregnancy, offer exciting possibilities for self-help to augment professional care.

Adults can subsist on a "fair" diet, but optimum development of an embryo depends on a complete range of nutrients. The stringent dietary regimens of the past decades are being scuttled in favor of generous amounts of wholesome foods, vitamin-mineral supplements, and a weight-gain of 24 to 32 pounds. Many studies have shown that babies weighing in at over 7 pounds have a lower rate of infant mortality, fewer physical handicaps or behavioral problems, and higher IQs than smaller infants. Traditional oriental physicians believe that a hereditary "weak constitution" can be modified by the mother's diet during the fetus' first months in the womb. Among some primitive tribes, up to six months of special feeding for the bride is required before marriage—on the assumption that pregnancy will soon follow. Modern medical nutritionists recommend that both the prospective parents upgrade their diets for several months before a planned pregnancy.

The blueprints for all the baby's organs are laid down early in pregnancy, which may explain why thalidomide was disastrous when taken during the first few months but was harmless when taken later. Sexual deviations may result from inadequate vitamin A and niacinamide. The formation of permanent teeth begins five months before the infant is born. Not only are the number of brain cells determined prenatally but tests have shown that character traits can be controlled and IQs raised by the inclusion of essential elements in the mother's diet.[306] Heredity alone accounts for only 20 percent of the 200,000 infants born every year with some form of mental or physical deformity. Many of these possible "congenital errors" can be prevented since even genes and chromosomes require nutrients for their development.[89, 261]

No human mother has ever deliberately been nutritionally deprived in the interest of scientific research, but, in laboratory tests with animals, every birth defect known to humans has been produced at will by withholding specific nutrients during certain periods of gestation.[348] Harvard University conducted an extensive study which showed that 95 percent of women with good prenatal diets had babies born without complications and in good-to-excellent condition, while women with poor prenatal diets had results that were almost exactly the opposite.[48] Dozens of other studies have borne out these findings. From clinics across America and Europe come substantiated reports that the discomforts of pregnancy (nausea, leg cramps, excessive water retention, etc.) can be avoided, and that practically all maternal deaths and human reproductive failures (premature deaths, still-births, malformed or mentally retarded babies) can be prevented by nutritional means.

Even in "well-fed" America, the tragic results of pregnancy-malnutrition are now acknowledged by organized medicine. The low-calorie, low-protein, low-salt diets once prescribed to limit weight gain and produce small babies are now considered at least partially responsible for the tremendous number of slightly damaged youngsters. Neither mentally retarded nor abnormal in the textbook sense, these children are prone to physical illness and psychological disturbances which cause problems at home and at school. They are labeled hyperactive or learning-disabled, and relegated to already overcrowded classes for their education.[261, 306]

Diet

Human beings are more susceptible to their environment during the nine months between conception and birth than at any other time of life. What a mother eats can have lasting effects on her child. Experimental research has shown that an unborn baby must compete with its mother's body for nutrients. While the pregnant woman may incur assorted discomforts, it is more likely to be the baby who will suffer permanent damage if the mother's nutrition is inadequate.

Current recommendations are for a diet of natural, unprocessed foods with a minimum of sugar. (Pregnancy is frequently the overwhelming stress which touches off hypoglycemia in those who are both susceptible and improperly fed.[125]) Chemical additives or colorings should be avoided. Even those "generally recognized as safe"

(GRAS) may damage rapidly growing human cells in subtle or minor ways.[306] Recent evidence indicates that while all nutrients are essential for optimum development, prenatal protein deprivation not only reduces production of the normal number of brain cells but may affect the amount and distinctive structure of chromosomes and genes which determine character and personality.[261, 306]

The weight gained from protein and high-nutrient foods represents an increase in tissue rather than the accumulated fat and fluid resulting from low-nutrient, high-calorie foods. (Only about 5 pounds is the mother's, the rest of the weight gained is the child plus the fluids and tissues that hold it in place and are discharged at birth.[254])

Pregnancy increases the body's need for both potassium and sodium. Including moderate amounts of iodized salt along with potassium-rich foods is generally recommended. Since salt and potassium work together to regulate fluids within the body, the anti-salt regimens of the past are now thought to have been responsible for much of the toxemia of pregnancy as well as the leg cramps frequently experienced by pregnant women on low-sodium diets.[88, 125, 261]

While the old rule of "eating for two" need not be followed, there are additional nutrient needs. The following calorically generous, daily-diet pattern, plus vitamin and mineral supplements, is suggested by many authorities.

1 to 2 quarts milk (or equivalent in calcium supplements, protein, and liquid)
1 or 2 eggs
6 to 8 ounces lean meat, poultry, or fish
2 cups cooked vegetables
1 cup raw vegetables
1 baked potato (or 1 serving brown rice or whole-wheat pasta)
4 slices whole-grain bread
1 serving sugar-free, whole-grain cereal
2 servings fruit (Research has indicated that sharp fruit juices withdraw oils from the skin and contribute to stretch marks, so whole fruits rather than just their juices are suggested.)
1 custard, fruit dessert, gelatin, or pudding
Butter or margarine, vegetable oil, preservative-free salad dressings, yogurt, cottage cheese, or other natural cheeses are optionals to be included as desired and weight permits.

As outlined, this diet provides 70 to 100 grams protein and at least 2,000 milligrams calcium, so it is not necessary to weigh foods or tally their nutritional values. Vegetarians should pay particular attention to combining foods for complete protein. Both calcium and protein are so vital during pregnancy that these statistics compiled from *Nutrition Almanac*[189] may be useful when making substitutions or combination dishes.

	Calcium [milligrams]	Protein [grams]
1 cup milk (whole, skim, or reconstituted dry)	291	8.5
1 cup plain, low-fat yogurt	415	12
1 cup creamed cottage cheese	126	26

	Calcium [milligrams]	Protein [grams]
1 ounce cream cheese	17	2
1 ounce cheddar cheese (1/4 cup shredded)	211	7
2 tablespoons grated Parmesan cheese	138	4
1 large egg	31	7
1/4 pound lean ground beef, raw (protein value is not affected by cooking)	13	23
1/2 cup canned chicken	21	22
1/2 cup tuna, canned in water	16	28
1/4 pound flounder or sole	13	19
1 slice rye or whole-wheat bread	trace	2
1/2 cup cooked oatmeal	11	2
1 large baked potato	14	4
1/2 cup cooked, drained kidney beans	35	7
1/2 cup cooked, drained soy beans	65	10
1/2 cup baked custard	148	7
2 tablespoons full-fat soy flour	18	3.2
1/4 cup raw wheat germ	18	6.6

The *Complete Handbook of Nutrition*[243] advises two glasses of fresh juices daily—preferably 6 to 8 ounces of carrot juice combined with any mixture of apple, beet, coconut, cucumber, orange, and spinach juices. Herbalists recommend one to three daily cups of camomile, comfrey, peppermint, or red raspberry leaf tea. Comfrey tea (which contains allantoin, a substance related to the process of growth) is believed especially helpful during pregnancy and while the infant is being nursed. Taking one teaspoon apple cider vinegar in a glass of water with each meal is a folk-medicine prescription for easy labor and healthy babies. While the possibility of caffeine-induced fetal damage is being studied, coffee, tea, chocolate, and cola beverages should be limited.

Possibly harmful substances to be avoided or severely limited—Any non-nutritive chemical (alcohol, drug, food additive, nicotine) may affect the fetus and interfere with its delicately balanced growth factors. Taking drugs, particularly diuretics, can increase the risk of nutritional inadequacy. Cigarette smoking, stimulant drugs, tranquilizers, and amphetamine-containing appetite suppressants also have the potential for damaging rapidly growing human cells. Those who are accustomed to smoking and drinking are usually permitted an occasional glass of beer or wine and up to 10 cigarettes per day. According to *How to Be Your Own Doctor (Sometimes)*[297], the risk to the baby seems to disappear if the mother stops smoking about the fourth month.

During the final months of pregnancy, stomach capacity may shrink as the baby grows larger. Dividing the daily foods into six or seven small meals may prove more comfortable than the traditional three.

Dietary Supplements

Pregnancy should be a period of happy fulfillment, unencumbered by scientific pill-taking at precise intervals. However, accumulated evidence indicates that the combination of soil depletion and nutrient losses during harvesting, storage, and food preparation necessitates supplementing even the most wholesome diet. Since all the nutrients important to health are not yet known, adding supplemental foods such as brewer's yeast, kelp, lecithin granules, soy flour, and wheat germ to appropriate foods is recommended by many nutritionists. A daily multi-vitamin-mineral tablet may be sufficient but additional supplements may be beneficial. The goal is to provide the endocrine system with all the elements needed for maternal health and optimum fetal development.

> **Vitamin A**—10,000 units daily. In *Nutrition Against Disease*[348], Roger Williams reports that experiments with animals fed a diet deficient in vitamin A during early pregnancy showed birth defects in every animal in the litters, but when the same animals were fed the same diet plus adequate vitamin A, there were no abnormalities in any of the litters. Vitamin A plus the B-complex vitamins (especially niacinamide) offer protection for the sexual integrity of the unborn child. The sex of the fetus is determined at the time of conception but the hormones required for male or female body development are not synthesized without the proper nutrients. Genetic sex deviations have become so common that, since 1972, women athletes competing in the Olympic Games are required to have a chromosome test and are disqualified if their cells contain the masculine "Y" chromosome.[250, 261]

> **B Complex**—One comprehensive tablet with breakfast and dinner each day. All the B vitamins are needed to reduce the possibility of fetal abnormality. A study at Columbia University[128] showed that pregnancies generously nourished with B-1 produced babies with higher IQs than those minimally supplied. B-2 aids the absorption of iron and is involved in the reproduction process as a preventive of congenital malformations. B-12 is vital for the prevention of anemia and for proper growth of the fetus. Since meats are the principal source of B-12, vegetarians may require supplements during pregnancy.

> - **B-6**—50 to 600 milligrams daily. A natural diuretic as well as being supportive of the nervous system, B-6 has been used to prevent or correct many of pregnancy's common maladies: anemia, foot and leg cramps, headaches, hemorrhoids, nausea, nervousness, retention of water, and even toxemia. Nursing mothers should limit B-6 supplements to no more than 10 milligrams daily—200 milligrams taken three times a day has been as effective as estrogen in shutting off normal lactation.[353]

> - **Folic Acid**—1,600 micrograms daily. The mild deficiencies of folic acid common during pregnancy may be responsible for anemia in the mother or fetal malformations which may not be apparent until the baby reaches adulthood. The grayish-brown skin pigmentation called "pregnancy cap" often disappears when 5 milligrams (5,000 micrograms) of folic acid are taken after each meal for a few weeks.

> - **Niacinamide** (not niacin, which may cause flushing)—25 to 500 milligrams daily. This B vitamin works with vitamin A to help prevent birth defects and assure sexual integrity.

- **Pantothenic Acid**—20 to 100 milligrams daily. Roger Williams[348], who first identified this vitamin, believes 50 milligrams a day would substantially reduce the possibility and severity of reproductive failures.
- **Vitamin C**—500 to 15,000 milligrams in divided doses daily. As reported in *Journal of the International Academy of Preventive Medicine* (Spring, 1974), over 300 consecutive obstetrical cases showed increased vitamin C demands up to 15,000 milligrams per day. In numerous clinical studies, pregnant women taking optimal amounts of vitamin C experienced no anemia, few stretch marks or varicose veins, brief and less painful labor, and no infections. Vitamin C increases iron absorption and is essential for the utilization of folic acid. Taking bioflavonoids (500 to 1,000 milligrams daily) in concert with the vitamin C strengthens the small blood vessels, and, when other vitamins and minerals are adequate, has been beneficial in cases where there was a history of previous spontaneous abortions or miscarriages. There is no danger to either mother or baby from high doses, but, if the infant is not nursed, a little powdered vitamin C should be mixed with the formula to allow a gradual readjustment.
- **Calcium, Phosphorus and Magnesium**—1,300 to 2,000 milligrams of calcium are required for healthy tissues and nerves as well as preservation of the mother's bones and teeth while the baby develops. Calcium cannot be utilized without phosphorus and magnesium. The National Research Council recommends that during pregnancy the amounts of calcium and phosphorus should be equal, with half that amount of magnesium.[8] One quart whole, fortified milk contains 912 milligrams phosphorus, 1,164 milligrams calcium, and 132 milligrams magnesium.[189] Meat and whole grains are high in phosphorus but low in magnesium. Most nutritionally oriented obstetricians recommend 500 milligrams of supplemental magnesium to maintain the correct balance. Dolomite provides both calcium and magnesium and is available in either tablets or powder.

Vitamin D—Calcium cannot be absorbed without vitamin D. One to three is the usually prescribed ratio (one glass of pasteurized, commercially fortified, vitamin-D milk contains 100 IU vitamin D and 291 milligrams calcium). However, research at the Henry Ford Hospital in Detroit showed the amount of calcium absorbed from one quart of milk to be greatly increased when 4,000 IU of vitamin D were taken with it.[88, 256] Natural vitamin D from fish liver oils is identical to the substance the human body manufactures from sunlight so is unlikely to have the toxic effects that can result from large doses of synthetic vitamin D. As long as calcium consumption is adequate, there is now believed to be little danger of adult vitamin-D hypervitaminosis from an increased ratio of natural vitamin D.

Vitamin E (see Caution, page 6)—100 to 400 IU daily. Insufficient vitamin E can cause muscular weakness resulting in leg cramps, varicose veins, miscarriage, premature birth, or difficult delivery. Muscular weakness can also affect the babies of E-deficient mothers, causing them to be slow in sitting up and walking. Supplemental iron can destroy vitamin E unless the two supplements are taken at least eight hours apart. Applying vitamin E oil, or the oil squeezed from capsules, to the abdomen and any existing stretch marks, often prevents new ones from emerging and sometimes makes the old ones disappear. When applied to the nipples and nursing pads, vitamin E oil has relieved pain during breast feeding.

Iodine—If iodized salt is being used, supplementation is usually unnecessary. When salt is limited, kelp granules or tablets offer a natural source of iodine. Requirements increase during pregnancy and a deficiency of this mineral can lead to deafness or other birth defects in the infant.[89]

Iron—At least 18 milligrams daily. Most obstetricians regard the risk of iron deficiency, particularly during the last six months of pregnancy, sufficient to merit supplementation. (There is no conflict when iron and vitamin E are supplied by natural foods, but the supplements interfere with each other's absorption and should be taken at least eight hours apart.)

Manganese—5 to 10 milligrams daily. A high calcium and phosphorus intake increases the need for manganese. Besides aiding the absorption of other nutrients, manganese is important for fetal inner-ear development and the body-righting reflexes as well as the production of sex hormones and maternal milk. In *Let's Eat Right to Keep Fit*[88], Adelle Davis cited references showing that certain congenital defects could be prevented by increasing manganese intake during pregnancy.

Tissue Salts are natural supplements that may be taken alone or in combination without fear of side effects. The usual dosage is two to four tablets of 3X or 6X potency dissolved under the tongue three or four times daily for several days, or until the condition is remedied.

- **Calc. Fluor.**—Gives elasticity to tissues, preventing problems with hemorrhoids, varicose veins, muscular weakness, and poor circulation.
- **Calc. Phos.**—Aids in assimilation of nutrients from foods and helps in renewing the teeth and bony structures of the body.
- **Ferr. Phos.**—A form of iron that does not replace iron supplements but does help oxygen reach the cells and tissues of the body to prevent sagging muscles.
- **Kali. Phos. and Mag. Phos.**—Nerve and muscle nutrients to be taken together for the relief of darting pains and cramps during pregnancy.
- **Nat. Mur.**—Aids in controlling the distribution of water in the tissues and in preventing or correcting varicose veins.
- **Nat. Sulph.**—Helps regulate intercellular fluids and prevent bilious conditions.

Zinc—20 to 30 milligrams daily during pregnancy, 30 to 50 milligrams during lactation. Zinc cannot work without other nutrients, including vitamins B-6 and C, but is needed for all growing tissues. An ample supply helps prevent nausea, stretch marks, and prolonged labor for the mother, as well as mental or physical abnormalities in the infant.[256]

Exercise

Appropriate exercise during pregnancy is generally favored by obstetricians. What is appropriate depends on the amount of physical activity before pregnancy. Even for the perennially sedentary, some exercise of abdominal muscles at this time is advisable, but the amount and intensity is an individual matter. Women pearl divers off the coast of Japan continue to work in frigid waters up to the time of delivery with no ill effects, but no unusually strenuous activity should be undertaken without medical approval.

Remedies for Pregnancy-Related Maladies

Edema (water retention)—Slight swelling of the extremities during pregnancy is considered normal and not to be confused with toxemia. Taking 50 to 100 milligrams B-6 each morning and evening provides a natural diuretic action. Increasing the amount of protein and using average amounts of salt frequently reduces puffiness of the ankles or other tissues.

Hemorrhoids—The hemorrhoids common during pregnancy are usually alleviated by increasing the amounts of vitamins B-6, C, and E (see also, Tissue Salts, above).

Leg Cramps (see Calcium-Phosphorus-Magnesium and Vitamin E, above)—Large amounts of meats, cereals, or calcium supplements without magnesium may result in an overbalance of phosphorus and leg cramps that vanish when magnesium is supplied.

Nausea (morning sickness)—Additional B-6 and zinc frequently correct this problem. The amount of B-6 required may vary from 50 milligrams daily to 200 milligrams taken three times each day. Its effectiveness is intensified when brewer's yeast is used daily. Zinc supplementation may need to be increased to 150 milligrams daily. No toxicity has ever been reported for either mother or baby from this dosage. Occasionally, 25 to 100 milligrams of vitamin B-1 in addition to vitamin C and a small amount of vitamin K has been required to bring relief.

Case History

Diana and Tom H. were thrilled over the prospect of becoming parents but the first few days of nausea made Diana dread the remaining months of pregnancy. Her family had a history of difficult pregnancies with all-day morning sickness and Diana feared she would not be able to accompany Tom on his two job-related trips as they had planned. Diana's Aunt Ruth came to her rescue. Ruth, interested in wholistic health, had been doing a lot of reading in connection with the nutrition course she was taking. She told Diana about a report relating the effectiveness of vitamins in combating the nausea of pregnancy. Diana's obstetrician, who had already prescribed a daily multiple vitamin plus a calcium supplement, doubted that additional vitamins would abate her nausea. However, since the B vitamins, zinc, and vitamin C would do no harm, he approved of her experimentation. The nausea disappeared after two days. Diana reduced the dosage to 50 milligrams of B-6, 30 milligrams of zinc, and 500 milligrams of vitamin C twice each day as a precaution against the return of day-long morning sickness. Diana and her Aunt Ruth believe the B-6 may also have been responsible for the fact that she had no problems with water retention during her pregnancy, not even swollen ankles after the days she spent sightseeing with Tom on his business trips.

Increased milk consumption may be responsible for stomach upsets because the milk sugar, lactose, is not always easily assimilated. Cheeses, cultured milk products (yogurt, kefir, etc.), or calcium supplements may be used to replace milk in the diet. Nibbling high-protein snacks throughout the day and before getting out of bed in the morning may allay nausea. Folklore has it that sipping a mixture of two-thirds sparkling water to one-third concord grape juice will not only provide temporary relief from "morning sickness" but guarantee long hair for the infant. Drinking a little lemon or lime juice, or a tea made by steeping two tablespoons regular rolled oats in a pint of boiling water for 30 minutes, may bring relief. (Other remedies are suggested with Nausea and Motion Sickness.)

According to *Medical Update* (Vol. 6, No. 1, 1982), pressing the inner forearms 2 inches toward the elbow from the center of each wrist dispels nauseous feelings. (The pressure should be maintained for 10 seconds, released for 10 seconds, and repeated three times.)

Pre-Eclampsia (toxemia of pregnancy)—Responsible for one-third of the maternal deaths and for some 30,000 still-births each year, pre-eclampsia occurs in late pregnancy and warrants medical diagnosis. It is characterized by excessive fluid retention, fever, and soaring blood pressure. Many medical nutritionists believe that adequate protein and salt in the diet will prevent this toxemia. (There is evidence that the rising blood pressure may be a result of the body's attempt to compensate for a falling blood volume caused by failure to retain needed salt and water.[261]) When pre-eclampsia does occur, *Dr. Wright's Book of Nutritional Therapy*[353] recommends raising the daily protein intake to between 100 and 150 grams, taking 200 milligrams B-6 four times a day, 500 milligrams magnesium three times a day, 3,000 milligrams vitamin C, and an additional B-complex tablet daily. When the condition improves, the B-6 should be taken only three times a day and the magnesium twice daily. If there is any diarrhea, the amount of magnesium should be reduced. Extra vitamin E has also proven helpful for the nonconvulsive type of pre-eclampsia.

Sources (See Bibliography)

3, 4, 5, 7, 8, 9, 17, 19, 44, 48, 50, 52, 53, 54, 59, 60, 68, 78, 88, 89, 90, 91, 99, 105, 125, 128, 129, 160, 162, 165, 180, 183, 185, 189, 193, 194, 209, 216, 221, 226, 228, 229, 231, 238, 240, 243, 250, 254, 256, 260, 261, 265, 270, 278, 288, 297, 305, 306, 343, 348, 350, 353.

PROSTATE PROBLEMS

Located just below the bladder and surrounding the urethra, the prostate gland is a common source of trouble in the male genital system. Prostatitis (prostate congestion, inflammation, or infection) is a malady of young and middle-aged men. Prolonged sitting, overuse of alcohol or coffee, too much or not enough sexual activity (particularly sexual excitation without a natural conclusion), bacterial infection from another part of the body, or venereal disease are possible causes. Enlargement or hardening of the prostate (hypertrophy) occurs most often in older men. This condition was rare 100 years ago, but now an estimated 60 to 75 percent of American men over 55 have some enlargement of the prostate—and, by age 80, the proportion rises to 95 percent.[261, 330] The generally accepted explanation for the increase is the dietary change from natural to processed foods with resulting deficiencies of vitamins and minerals. Antihistamines may be a factor since they restrict the elimination of urine and should be used with caution by men who have an enlarged prostate gland.

All prostatic problems warrant prompt diagnosis by a urologist. If neglected, the bladder obstruction and retained urine can lead to infections, bladder stones, kidney disease (see individual listings), or other serious ailments. While surgical removal of this gland affects only the ability to reproduce, not potency, many medical researchers believe hormones involved with general health and bodily functions are manufactured in the prostate and that it should be retained whenever possible. The human male is considered to be as young as his prostate gland—which can often be restored to normalcy by natural remedies.

Diet and Supplements

Worldwide studies have shown that men who are still virile in their eighties and nineties, without prostate problems, are those who subsist on diets rich in natural foods and conspicuously lacking in refined sugar and white flour. Ample fluid intake (up to two and one-half quarts per day) helps dilute urine and encourage its passage. Excessive amounts of alcohol or caffeine-containing beverages, condiments, and spices are often irritating. The traditional value of eating zinc-rich oysters is now under scrutiny due to the possibility of contamination from polluted waters. Cold-pressed vegetable oils, however, plus raw seeds and nuts, are still recommended. Vitamins and minerals recognized as helpful to prostate sufferers include the amino acids, glutamic acid, and glycine (present in beef, milk, and soybeans), and:

Vitamin A—10,000 to 25,000 units per day. Vitamin A is essential for the health of cells lining the prostate. A deficiency can cause these cells to proliferate and quickly die. The dead cells plus natural warmth and moisture create an ideal medium for bacterial growth and may be responsible for problems with the prostate gland.

B Complex—One comprehensive tablet plus 50 milligrams B-6 daily. B vitamins are necessary for a healthy prostate; when combined with zinc supplements, they have been known to restore potency.

Bee Pollen—One to two teaspoons granules or 3 to 9 tablets daily. Bee pollen is believed to contain hormones beneficial to the prostate and is a storehouse of nutrients, particularly those removed during the refining of foods. Legend refers to bee pollen and honey as the elixer of perpetual youth for men. Despite a substantial number of European clinical studies establishing its effectivenss for prostate problems, some controversy over its value remains. Bee pollen does not destroy bacteria but does strengthen the prostate's ability to combat infection. Tests have shown excellent results with continued use of bee pollen, especially when accompanied by at least 30 milligrams of supplemental zinc each day.

Vitamin C—100 to 5,000 milligrams in divided doses daily. As reported in the *Journal of the American Geriatrics Society* (Vol. 20, 1964) and substantiated by later studies, the pain of prostatitis may be a result of vitamin C deficiency. Taking 500 milligrams three times each day has brought relief in many cases, but an increased dosage may be helpful.

Vitamin E (see Caution, page 6)—400 to 1,000 IU daily. Vitamin E protects both vitamin A and unsaturated oils from destruction by oxygen within the body. Taking 800 IU per day has cured some cases of prostatitis[4]; others responded in a month when 400 IU of vitamin E plus 60 milligrams of zinc were taken every day.[52]

Vitamin F and Lecithin—3 to 6 capsules of pumpkin, safflower, sesame, soy or sunflower seed oil, and/or one to two tablespoons lecithin granules (or the equivalent in capsules) each day. The essential fatty acids (vitamin F) which cannot be produced by the body are highly concentrated in these substances. Tests have shown these supplements alone to reduce enlarged prostates, but more rapid results have been obtained when bee pollen and zinc were added to the daily regimen.

Magnesium—300 to 500 milligrams daily, either as an individual supplement or combined with calcium in dolomite tablets. A lack of magnesium is suspect in some cases of prostatic enlargement.[282]

Zinc—30 to 220 milligrams daily for three months, then a maintenance dosage of 15 to 50 milligrams per day. Numerous studies have shown that zinc deficiency causes changes in the size, structure, and function of the prostate gland. Zinc supplementation has reduced enlarged prostates and improved or abolished symptoms of chronic prostatitis—returning many to complete normalcy in from two weeks to four months. Fifty milligrams taken three times a day is the generally recommended dosage, but, since zinc is required for the detoxification of alcohol by the liver, those who imbibe should increase the amount. Zinc may be taken with any of the other suggested supplements to benefit all types of prostate problems. When combined with bee pollen and pumpkin-seed oil, it has proven a most effective natural remedy for simple prostate enlargement.[353]

Exercise

A sedentary lifestyle can encourage prostatic congestion. Walking for an hour or performing a few minutes of calisthenics each day is recommended, especially for those whose occupation requires a great deal of sitting.

- An exercise said to have the effect of prostate massage is to lie on the back on the floor, flex both knees, place the soles of the feet together, then slowly extend both legs as far as possible. The maneuver should be repeated 10 times each morning and night.
- A yogic position designed to transport blood to the prostate area and relieve congestion is to sit on the heels with the back straight, then slide the legs and feet out so the weight of the body brings the buttocks directly to the floor.
- In *A Country Doctor's Common Sense Health Manual*[174], Dr. Hurdle offers a more direct approach. Cover the index finger with a rubber finger from a pharmacy, spread with Vaseline, and insert about 1-1/2 inches into the rectum. Then gently milk down the enlarged prostate gland.

Folk Remedies

Although prostate problems are more prevalent than they once were, eating a handful of pumpkin seeds every day has long been advised as a stimulant for the male genital system. Generous use of garlic is another old standby. Teas made from corn silk, golden seal, juniper berries, parsley, slippery elm, or uva ursi were also recommended for maintaining virility and avoiding trouble with the prostate.

Nerve Massage

- Place the right thumb on the left wrist just below the thumb. Massage with a firm, rolling motion, working across the wrist toward the little finger. Repeat with the other hand.
- Position the palms one on top of the other over the navel. Keeping the hands stationary, massage with a deep circular motion for three to five minutes. Then push down with firm, but not painful, pressure for another three to five minutes.
- Use the thumb to massage the inner heel while the knuckle of the index finger presses from the opposite side—about 1/2 inch from the cord going up the back of the leg. Use a pressing, rolling motion and alternate feet every two minutes for a quarter of an hour each day.

Nerve Pressure

Unless otherwise indicated, once each day press each point for 10 seconds, release for 10 seconds, and repeat three times on both sides of the body.

- Using the thumbs, press each side of the chest 2 inches in from the center of the underarms in line with the nipples.
- Press a point the width of one hand directly above the navel, then another point 1-1/2 inches below the navel.
- Press a point the width of one hand down from the bottom of the kneecap and 1-1/4 inches toward the outside of the leg. Then press a point on the shinbone one hand's-width up from the top of the anklebone.
- Press the hollow behind and slightly below the inner anklebone.

- Using the tip of the thumb, press deeply at the edge of the bony prominence on the sole of the foot at the base of the big toe.
- If there is pain in the prostate, check for a tender spot on the wrist near the base of the thumb and exert steady pressure for 15 minutes.

Sitz Baths

Immersing the lower portion of the trunk in 6 inches of warm water (with a few camomile tea bags, if desired) for 15 to 20 minutes twice each day has a soothing effect and often reduces prostate swelling. An alternative method of applying heat is to fill an enema bag with warm water, insert the nozzle about 2 inches into the rectum, and allow the water to run slowly in and back out again—just far enough to deliver warmth to the enlarged prostate bulging into the rectal wall.

Sources (See Bibliography)

3, 4, 6, 7, 9, 12, 13, 14, 19, 34, 43, 48, 52, 53, 62, 63, 64, 67, 76, 78, 84, 88, 89, 142, 154, 156, 173, 174, 184, 189, 194, 205, 228, 234, 253, 256, 261, 270, 282, 286, 288, 312, 315, 325, 330, 334, 353.

PSORIASIS

While neither life-threatening nor fatal, the red, silvery-scaled patches of psoriasis are a discomforting and disfiguring malady afflicting at least 5 million Americans. Medical literature lists psoriasis (lepra alphos, seborrhea) as a chronic skin disorder of unknown origin with no cure, although temporary control and remissions are possible. Experimental treatments with professionally administered vitamin A-Acid have recorded successful results, but most drugs prescribed to control psoriasis produce unpleasant side effects.

Psoriasis usually affects the scalp, hands, elbows, knees, or base of the spine but may appear anywhere on the body. Some cases appear to be triggered by germs or viruses, instigated by nervous upsets, or aggravated by drugs (steroids, lithium, etc.) administered for other conditions. Heredity may be a factor. Approximately one-fourth of all psoriasis sufferers have a family history of the malady, and, according to the *Harvard Medical School Health Letter* of July, 1983, a parent with psoriasis has a 50-50 chance of passing it on to each child. One possible cause may be a genetic tendency for an acceleration of skin formation. Biochemists and orthomolecular physicians believe psoriasis to be the result of faulty metabolism, particularly of fats, and therefore correctable through natural means. Another possible cause is too-frequent bathing with the use of soap, but, during an acute phase of psoriasis, it is sometimes advisable to bathe daily and remove all scales by gently scrubbing the spots with a soft brush.

Diet and Supplements

Even though there are differences of opinion regarding the advisability of limiting red meats and condiments, a natural, high-protein diet is usually recommended. Eating turkey in place of meat, seafood, chicken, or eggs has corrected some cases of psoriasis in as little as one week.[9] (Most high-protein foods except turkey contain an amino acid, tryptophan, believed to worsen psoriasis.) Refined or processed foods, white sugar, and hydrogenated fats should be eliminated but two tablespoons cold-pressed, unsaturated oil should be used each day. Whole grains, raw fruits, vegetables, and seeds such as pumpkin, sesame, and sunflower are believed helpful. Some nutritionists advise against the use of citrus juices but fresh apple, beet, carrot, cranberry, cucumber, and grape juices are considered especially beneficial. For those who have neither diabetes nor low blood sugar, "juice fasts" of from one to three days may assist in clearing the condition. Interspersing four cups of herb tea and two glasses of water with two glasses raw vegetable juice and one glass of fruit juice during the day is the accepted formula.

Including one-fourth cup lecithin granules (or the equivalent in lecithin liquid or capsules) in the diet each day for two months, then reducing the dosage by one-half has effected relief in a number of instances.[166] Many cases of psoriasis are accompanied by high serum cholesterol levels and improve when cholesterol is lowered (see Hardening of the Arteries). If cholesterol is excessively high, up to one-half cup lecithin granules may be required for the first few days. (The phosphorus content of lecithin may necessitate extra supplements of calcium and magnesium to avoid the muscular cramps that can result from an imbalance of these nutrients.)

Many investigations have shown vitamin therapy to be helpful for psoriasis. In 1964, *Medical World News* reported that Russian physicians were getting excellent results with vitamins C, B-12, and folic acid given twice a day for alternate 20-day periods. In more recent studies, some cases of psoriasis have been alleviated by taking large amounts of inositol (a member of the B complex present in lecithin). Others responded to 1,000 micrograms of B-12 each day for a month.[4] (Injections may be required if oral B-12 is not well-assimilated.)

The vitamin-mineral combination generally suggested for psoriasis is:

Vitamin A—30,000 to 100,000 units daily for one month, then 25,000 units daily for three months.
B Complex—One comprehensive tablet once or twice daily, plus 100 to 200 milligrams B-6.
Vitamin C—500 to 5,000 milligrams in divided doses daily.
Calcium-Magnesium Tablets (dolomite) or 500 milligrams of each, daily.
Vitamin E (see Caution, page 6)—300 to 1,600 IU each day.
Zinc—50 milligrams every day.

Larger amounts of vitamin A have been taken daily for six months without any sign of toxicity but it is considered advisable to limit extended use to less than 50,000 units per day unless under medical supervision. If vitamin E is inadequately supplied, vitamin A is destroyed by oxygen in the body. What may appear to be a deficiency of vitamin A may actually be caused by a lack of vitamin E. Taking 1,500 IU of vitamin E daily, plus smoothing vitamin E oil from capsules over the afflicted areas has brought improvement in three weeks and complete clearing in less than two months.[325] Combining 50 milligrams of zinc with 400 IUs of oral vitamin E plus topical applications has corrected some forms of psoriasis even more rapidly. Applying vitamin E oil to the scaly patches often speeds healing and helps avoid scarring. A soothing, healing ointment recommended by Paavo Airola[13] can be prepared by blending one tablespoon each almond, avocado, olive, and sesame oil with 50,000 units vitamin A and 1,000 IU vitamin E from pierced capsules. (Synthetic vitamin A may be substituted for the natural form to avoid any fishy odor.)

Additional minerals may be obtained by taking two to three tablespoons bottled sea water (from health food stores) or sprinkling kelp granules on foods, or taking up to five kelp tablets daily. Three tablets of the tissue salt Kali. Sulph. in the 6X potency, dissolved under the tongue three times daily, has alleviated psoriasis in some instances. Daily supplements of 10 to 90 milligrams of zinc are recommended by many authorities. (A lack of zinc can create a skin abnormality similar to psoriasis.)

Folk Remedies

Apple Cider Vinegar—Take a weekly bath in a tub of tepid water to which one-
   half cup of the vinegar has been added.
Avocado Oil—Rub the afflicted areas with avocado oil several times each day.
Herbs

- Drink several cups of comfrey root, dandelion, saffron, or sassafras tea daily.
- Let two tablespoons sarsaparilla stand overnight in one quart of water, then boil for 20 minutes. Drink part of the resulting tea while hot and sip the remainder during the day. Improvement has been observed within one week but the tea should be used daily to prevent a relapse.[215]
- Boil three tablespoons comfrey root tea with one cup water in a covered container. Cool and strain, then apply to the affected spots once each day with a cotton ball.

Potato Skins—Scrub and peel five potatoes, discarding sprouts and green
   portions. Boil the skins in two cups of water in a covered container for 20
   minutes. Let stand until cool, then strain. Drink one cup of the liquid each
   morning and afternoon.

Sea Water Bathing

Ocean swimming is a time-honored remedy for psoriasis. As reported in *Prevention Magazine* (December, 1977), experimental studies at an Israeli Dead Sea Spa (Ein Bokek) showed either improvement or complete recovery for over 500 psoriasis patients when daily sea bathing was combined with exposure to sunlight. (The water in the Dead Sea is 10 times saltier than ocean water.) When ocean swimming is not possible, homemade sea-water baths can be made by dissolving 1 to 4 pounds of sea salt (available in health food stores) in a tub half-filled with cool water. Applying bottled sea water to the scaly patches several times each day with a cotton ball has also proven helpful.

Sunlight

Gradually increasing exposure to sunlight is beneficial to most psoriasis sufferers. (The ultraviolet component causes psoriatic skin to slow down its rapid proliferation.) Slight reddening of the skin is beneficial but a painful sunburn should be avoided because burn injury can stimulate psoriatic skin growth. Sunlight is most effective when the skin is coated with Vaseline or mineral oil following an ocean or salt-water bath. Deep breathing or other mild exercise with the affected parts exposed is recommended. Sun lamps or untraviolet treatments may be substituted for natural sunlight but should be carefully monitored. When at least 15 minutes of daily exposure to the sun is not possible, supplements of natural vitamin D are suggested.

Sources (See Bibliography)

4, 6, 9, 13, 19, 52, 53, 62, 68, 81, 82, 83, 84, 88, 89, 119, 152, 166, 171, 189, 214, 229, 254, 256, 257, 260, 261, 288, 305, 311, 312, 315, 325, 331.

SENILITY AND PREMATURE AGING

In the not too distant past, anyone over the age of 60 was considered old, "aged" was matched with "infirm" in word-association tests, and senility was regarded as an inescapable adjunct to aging. Life expectancy has risen from 22 years for Romans at the time of Christ to 70-plus for modern Americans, with 26 years of that increase achieved during the past century. Much of the credit for the rise goes to advances in sanitation and medical control of infectious diseases and infant deaths, but more and more individuals are living beyond the age of 85. Gerontologists now believe life expectancy can be extended by another 50 years. The quality of those added years is of even more importance than the quantity. Recent scientific research has demonstrated that, while there is no magic elixir or fountain of youth, the aging process can be controlled and most senility prevented or reversed by natural means.

People do not become frail or demented through inevitable change coupled with chronological age. Creativity and judgement increase with time—old dogs *can* learn new tricks. Although the efficiency of cell reproduction and nutrient absorption does peak shortly after adolescence and then start to decline, adequate nutrition plus mental and physical activity can impede degeneration. Neuro-anatomists have discovered that human brain tissue does not deteriorate until after the age of 80—providing it has been properly nourished and consistently used. The body's cells, except for those in the brain, divide to replace themselves. Most authorities agree that aging should be treated as just another malady. What we are accustomed to think of as normal old age is actually an abnormal, premature phenomenon, and inescapable senility merely a myth.

Longevity surveys involving thousands of volunteers over 90 showed heredity to be less of a factor than previously believed and established guidelines for healthy, productive, enjoyable old age. The three essentials are:

- Adequate nutrition through diet and supplements—without excessive weight gain.
- Maintaining a positive outlook and mental momentum through work or creative hobbies.

• Keeping physically active and obtaining sufficient rest and relaxation.

While it is never too late to start improving existing conditions, premature aging and senility are easier to prevent than cure. The title of Lawrence Welk's autobiography, *You're Never Too Young,*[341] exemplifies this—*now* is the time to begin preparing for a lusty old age.

Diet and Supplements

The human body is amazingly resilient. After years of struggling to function with marginal deficiencies, it will rejuvenate itself by replenishing porous bones, scouring the sludge out of clogged arteries, and reactivating mental circuits when it is supplied with the necessary raw materials. Optimum nutrition encourages the other two essentials of staying young. The tea-and-toast regimen of Victorian novels can lead directly to shawl and rocking chair.

Many older people are trapped in what appears to be a vicious dietary circle because evolutionary alterations have not caught up with increased life expectancy. Metabolism, the sum of all the body's chemical reactions, slows with age. Caloric requirements decrease up to 8 percent for each decade of life past 20. The cessation of the female reproductive system reduces the need for calories by another 10 to 15 percent. In order to avoid excess weight gain after the age of 55, it may be necessary to limit food consumption to not much more than half of what was normal at the age of 20, even when there is an equal amount of physical activity. Yet the need for nutrients increases due to poorer absorption. Intelligent food selection plus supplements offers an exit from the merry-go-round, with a brass-ring bonus of better health.

Unless specific restrictions have been medically imposed, current dietary guidelines published by the government are applicable to those of all ages. The suggested reduction of sugar, salt, and fat, while accentuating whole grains and other natural foods, is particularly important for senior citizens. As the ability to digest and absorb diminishes, it may be wise to increase the proportion of protein to assure enough amino acids to control aging.

If dental difficulties prohibit chewing fibrous foods it may be necessary to add a spoonful or so of wheat or oat bran to the daily diet. Eating (or juicing and drinking) some raw fruits and vegetables each day sparks the digestive-assimilative processes. Raw papaya and pineapple are believed to stimulate the immune system and dissolve any damaged protein tissue, but should not be used by those with ulcers as they could retard healing. Apples, bananas, grapefruit, and leafy green vegetables are considered especially beneficial. Yogurt aids digestion and is thought to contribute to longevity. It was called "the milk of eternal life" in sixteenth-century France and is a staple food in Soviet Georgia where most of the residents live well past the century mark. Other fermented lactic-acid foods credited with revitalizing the digestive system and helping rectify degenerative diseases are: kefir, sauerkraut, sour pickles, sour milk, and sourdough breads.[12]

Drinking several glasses of water each day is recommended. As reported by Carlton Fredericks in *Prevention Magazine* (April, 1982), water deficiency can cause senile behavior. (When water intake is inadequate, blood becomes thicker and reduces circulation to the brain.) The minerals in hard water provide protection against coronary disease and strokes. Home water softeners should not be attached to the tap used for drinking water. Bottled spring water (not distilled water unless the minerals in each gallon are replaced by adding two tablespoons bottled sea water from a health food store[78]) is suggested for those living in soft-water areas.

The caffeine in coffee, tea, or soft drinks can cause rapid or irregular heartbeat. Decaffeinated coffee is under scrutiny for possibly harmful side effects, so, even though adding lemon to tea (or taking a little vitamin C with each cup) protects the body against tannic acid, these beverages should be used in moderation. Herbal teas are pleasant substitutes as well as folk-medicine remedies for controlling the debilities of aging. Anise, asafetida, garlic (four cloves or one-half teaspoon powder per cup of boiling water), ginseng, juniper berry, peppermint, rose hips, rosemary, and sage are thought to be particularly helpful.

Another time-tested folk remedy for many of the discomforts of old age is sipping a mixture of two teaspoons each apple cider vinegar and raw honey in a glass of water three times a day, with or between meals. According to folk practitioners, this beverage not only aids digestion and reduces dizziness and joint soreness, but has been known to restore mental and physical vigor. An additional glass before bedtime may prevent nightly leg cramps and allow natural sleep undisturbed by frequent trips to the bathroom.[181, 293]

Alcohol poses a special risk for the elderly as slowed metabolic processes increase both its immediate effect and the amount of time it remains in the body. Moderate use of alcohol, however, has been shown to contribute to longevity. Numerous studies have shown that those who have one to four alcoholic drinks daily live longer and are less likely to suffer heart disease than either heavy drinkers or the totally abstemious. Wine contains modest quantities of essential nutrients, increases the absorption of minerals from foods eaten with it, and has long been considered a tonic for older people. (Four ounces dry table wine contains the alcoholic equivalent of one mixed drink or one 12-ounce can of beer—which also contains some nutrients.)

One theory of aging is that free radicals bond with vital protein tissue to prevent the normal rejuvenation process, causing inflexible joints, wrinkles, hardened arteries, and general deterioration. As explained in *Health and Longevity Report* (November, 1982), a free radical is a portion of a molecule that has broken loose and is free to unite with and nullify useful protein molecules. During youth, the body produces enough enzymes to quickly separate these bondings. Enzyme production declines with age, leaving the body vulnerable to damage by free radicals. Besides those released through the body's metabolic processes, other free radicals can be assimilated from external agents. In his book, *Secrets of Life Extension* (Bantam, 1983), John A. Mann lists a number of such agents, including cigarette smoke, polluted air, and rancid foods. Antioxidants are scavengers. They combine with free radicals, rendering them harmless and unable to attack the body. Vitamins C and E and the mineral, selenium, are the best known antiradicals. Other free-radical antagonists are: amino acids (arginine, cysteine, ornithine, phenylalanine, tyrosine), bioflavonoids, B-2, B-3, B-6, inositol, niacin, PABA, pantothenic acid, and zinc. Foods recommended for their antioxidant properties are: bananas and other fruits, celery, eggs, potatoes, and certain seasonings (see page 3). Synthetic antioxidants like the food preservatives BHA and BHT are suggested as supplements by a few health writers but most authorities advise against their use.

Appetite usually diminishes in proportion to the need for calories, so smaller portions present no problem. Eating four or five mini-meals instead of two or three large ones increases nutrient absorption. While it is possible to combat the ravages of aging by strict adherence to a carefully programmed diet, a combination of enjoyable foods plus supplements is preferred by most people. Taking Betaine HCL (hydrochloric acid) and a multiple digestive enzyme (papain for protein; cellulose for fruits and vegetables; pancreatin for fat, protein, and starch) with each meal often improves digestion and assimilation.

Individual nutritional needs vary but even the most orthodox physicians and dieticians agree that those over 65 require supplemental vitamins and minerals. Orthomolecular doctors, biochemists, and nutritionists have found that aging can be postponed, degenerative diseases impeded or rectified, and senility controlled or reversed by therapeutic dosages of specific vitamins and minerals. Laboratory tests with animals demonstrated life extensions of from 45 to 65 percent with no negative side effects when the following supplements (in equivalents for humans) were given daily in addition to a normal diet:[194]

Vitamin A—20,000 to 30,000 units

B Complex—One comprehensive tablet plus one or two tablespoons brewer's yeast

Vitamin C—3,000 to 5,000 milligrams

Dolomite Tablets—to supply 600 milligrams calcium plus 380 milligrams magnesium

Vitamin E—100 to 200 IU

Individual, optional, anti-aging supplements suggested by many experts:

Multi-Vitamin-Mineral Formula—One tablet with breakfast plus another with dinner if additional supplements are not being used.

B Complex—One comprehensive tablet and/or two tablespoons brewer's yeast daily. Many studies, including a recent one at a Philadelphia hospital[154], showed that there was marked improvement in memory and ability to think clearly after all the B vitamins were administered to elderly patients. Up to 1,000 milligrams of niacin have been given daily to increase the oxygen-carrying ability of red blood cells and forestall senility in its early stages. Twenty-five to 1,000 micrograms of B-12 have been of help in preventing the chronic fatigue and mental confusion that may evolve with age. Vitamin B-15 is seldom included in combination supplements but 50 milligrams daily is believed helpful in preventing premature aging.

Bee Pollen—1,000 to 3,000 milligrams in chewable tablets (or one teaspoon granules) daily. Mentioned in the Bible, Koran, Talmud, and other ancient writings as a source of perpetual youth and health, bee pollen has been found to contain nearly all the nutrients known to bring about internal revitalization.[330]

Vitamin C—500 to 4,000 milligrams, preferably in divided doses with bioflavonoids. Besides all its other virtues, vitamin C helps retard deterioration of disks, joints, and other tissues and delays old age because of its antioxidant properties. When taken with vitamin E and zinc, vitamin C has a rejuvenating effect on cell tissues and has been credited with reversing some cases of senile dementia.

Calcium—600 to 1,000 milligrams daily; 1,500 milligrams for women past menopause. As vital in advancing age as in childhood, calcium prevents osteoporosity and bone fragility, regulates heartbeat, and aids the body's utilization of iron. It also relieves many symptoms associated with aging: backache, bone pain, insomnia, loose teeth, and tremors of the fingers. As a general rule, less than one-fourth of ingested calcium is absorbed[8] and, to function properly, must be accompanied by vitamins A, C, D, and B-6 plus magnesium, phosphorus, and protein. A single supplement containing the correct proportions of everything except the protein may be taken with meals, or individual tablets of calcium, bone meal, and dolomite may be used to augment the calcium derived from dairy products and other foods.

Chromium—100 to 300 micrograms daily, with meals, to help combat mental changes accompanying aging, regulate sugar levels in the blood, assist in lowering high blood pressure, and aid in reducing cholesterol and hardening of the arteries.

Vitamin D—800 to 1,000 IU daily. The ability to manufacture vitamin D within the body declines with age and, without vitamin-D supplementation, much of the ingested calcium cannot be utilized.

Vitamin E—(see Caution, page 6)—100 to 1,000 IU daily. Considered by many to be the most potent single factor in warding off old age, vitamin E offers a practically endless list of benefits—including protecting red blood cells from destruction and tissues from aging. (Scientists have found that lifespans can be extended when cells continue to multiply by division. Laboratory experiments with human cells have shown vitamin E to increase the number of times cells divide by at least 50 percent.[194])

Glutamine—An amino acid considered to be an anti-aging, anti-wrinkling factor, glutamine is found in foods such as asparagus, beets, cabbage, carrots, celery, garlic, green beans, mushrooms, papaya, parsley, and salmon. As a daily supplement, 500 to 1,000 milligrams of L-Glutamine is suggested.

Kelp—One tablet with each meal or one-fourth teaspoon ground kelp sprinkled on foods. (Larger amounts should be used only with medical approval as the iodine in kelp could affect the thyroid gland.) Long believed to prolong health and vitality, fresh kelp is eaten as a food in many parts of the world. For American convenience, the seaweed is dried and compressed into tablets or powdered for table use. Its slightly salty taste makes it a healthful substitute for salt, and its high mineral and vitamin content offers a valuable supplement for the elderly.

Lecithin—One teaspoon to one-fourth cup (the equivalent of three to forty 1,200 milligram capsules) daily. Soybean lecithin has been shown to prevent, slow, or revoke the ravages of age. It maintains or improves memory by preventing nerve-sheath destruction in the brain and, since almost one-third of the brain's substance is composed of lecithin, can reverse the progress of senility.[331] According to a 1978 report in *Lancet,* a British medical magazine, even the early stages of Alzheimer's disease have responded to a daily dose of three tablespoons of lecithin granules.

The emulsifying action of lecithin is of special importance for oldsters as slowed digestive processes allow fats to remain in the blood for up to 20 hours longer than in younger people, thereby allowing that much more time to create liver and artery degeneration.[164] There is no evidence of risk in taking lecithin[219] but it is high in phosphorus, so extra calcium and magnesium may be required to avoid chemical imbalances and muscular cramps.

Selenium—50 to 200 micrograms daily. Selenium is an antioxidant that works synergistically with vitamin E to retard cellular aging. Formerly believed an unnecessary supplement, current research indicates that selenium is a keystone in slowing the aging process and that soil depletion has made it almost impossible to acquire the 250 to 350 micrograms needed each day without some supplementation.

Superoxide Dismutase (SOD)—1,000 to 2,000 units daily. An anti-aging enzyme only recently available as a supplement, SOD appears to be as valuable as vitamins C, E, and the mineral selenium in preventing damage to vital tissues by free radicals.

Tissue Salts—Taking three to four tablets of the applicable 6X tissue salt three or four times daily has reportedly brought rapid improvement.

Calc. Phos.—To improve circulation, reduce aches and pains in the bones, and restore health to tissues.

Kali. Sulph.—To renew mental vigor and improve memory, hearing, and circulation.

Silicea—To increase nutrient assimilation and revitalize the nervous system.

Zinc—15 to 50 milligrams daily. Zinc invigorates the substances controlling cellular reproduction, is essential for normal functioning of the prostate gland, has a regulatory effect on insulin in the blood, and often restores a failing sense of taste or smell. Several studies have associated zinc deficiency with mental problems of the aged. It is particularly effective when combined with supplements of vitamins C and E. The May, 1981 issue of the *American Journal of Medicine* reported tests in Belgium showing that 220 milligrams of zinc taken twice each day effectively improved the immune function of patients over 70, but such massive amounts should be taken only under medical supervision.

Case History

Born with a chest deformity, orphaned and adopted at the age of three, Mabel J. was a "sickly child" with poor eyesight. She contracted all the childhood maladies, developed rickets because she did not drink milk, and, at the age of nine was informed by a country doctor that she would be blind within 10 years, could never have a baby, and should not expect to live for too many more years. Despite her physical problems, Mabel was a bright, gregarious girl. She read voraciously, reveled in the beauties of nature, and resolved to make the most of each day. Still sighted in her twenties, she taught in a one-room schoolhouse until she married a man who cared more for her than for the prospect of progeny, and went overseas with him to teach in a church school. Four months after returning to the States for stomach surgery, Mabel amazed her physicians by delivering a healthy baby. Determined that her child would not suffer the deprivations she had encountered, Mabel attended classes in nutrition, and practiced sightless survival by coping with household chores while blindfolded. She utilized her knowledge of diet and supplements for a lot more "coping" through the years. She had allergies before they were popular, pernicious anemia before the advent of B-12, hypoglycemia before it was a recognized malady, a broken back with thought-to-be-permanent paralysis, and a supposedly-fatal massive coronary. Mabel ate wisely, took vitamins and minerals, and compensated for her ailments instead of allowing them to cause premature aging or interfere with her happy and productive life. Before her sight finally failed (over 80 years after the original prognosis), Mabel memorized telephone numbers. When another heart attack and additional back-fractures curtailed her volunteer activities, she became telephone secretary for her church and club groups, and for her daughter who worked at home. Mabel kept up-to-date by listening to "talking" books and news magazines, and used a tape recorder to write poetry and maintain an extensive correspondence. By combining nutrients for her body with a caring, positive, mental outlook, Mabel surmounted her physical difficulties and thwarted senility. The years of her life were not "too long." She was still cheering, comforting, and counseling others when a fall terminated her life at the age of 94.

Drugs

According to reports published in 1977 (*Postgraduate Medical Journal* for April and *Nutrition Reports International* for December), those over 65 constitute only 10 percent of the population, yet consume 25 percent of all drugs prescribed, and suffer more than 50 percent of all drug side effects. The action of drugs, even over-the-counter pain-killers and laxatives, can combine with the slowed metabolic process of age to produce symptoms of senility—anxiety, confusion, depression, irritability, loss of memory, and slurred speech. Aspirin blocks vitamin C from entering the blood; diuretics can cause mineral depletion. Constipation, insomnia, and many other maladies (see individual listings) can often be controlled by natural methods. When drugs are necessary, they should be used exactly as prescribed but taking additional calcium plus vitamins B, C, and D may help prevent any secondary problems created by antacids, barbiturates, tranquilizers, or sleeping aids.

Exercise

Physical activity is essential for good physical and mental health at every age. As reported in the September, 1983 *Journal of the American Medical Association,* from the medical point of view an active person of 70 is like an inactive person of 30. A sedentary lifestyle reduces the capacity to absorb oxygen and allows joints and muscles to stiffen from lack of use. Walking, swimming, mild calisthenics—any form of regular exercise—often eliminates minor aches and pains as well as chronic tension and weariness.

Nerve Massage

To stimulate circulation and rejuvenate the entire system, gently massage the bottom of each foot for two to five minutes once or twice each day. Rub each toe, the individual pads, arch, and heel, extending up both sides of the heel to just below the ankle bone. Using a different hand to massage each foot will serve to massage the thumbs and fingers, but the palms of the hands may be massaged with the opposite thumb if circulation is poor and the extremities chilly.

Sources (See Bibliography)

3, 4, 10, 12, 25, 34, 44, 47, 54, 55, 57, 61, 63, 64, 68, 71, 76, 78, 84, 87, 88, 92, 95, 99, 110, 125, 126, 128, 130, 132, 148, 154, 155, 163, 164, 165, 166, 170, 175, 181, 188, 189, 194, 195, 203, 204, 206, 208, 211, 215, 222, 224, 228, 229, 238, 242, 243, 249, 250, 252, 253, 257, 261, 269, 282, 284, 286, 287, 293, 296, 317, 319, 325, 330, 333, 334, 336, 341, 348, 353, 354.

SHINGLES

A viral infection (herpes zoster or zona) that inflames nerve endings, shingles erupts in blisters following nerve paths. The rash-like sores usually appear on the trunk of the body but may occur on the head, arms, or legs. If shingles emerge on the face, a medical specialist should be consulted immediately as sight or hearing could be endangered. Young people generally recover from shingles in a week or so, but those over 60 often suffer lingering pain (called postherpetic neuralgia) which may continue for months and recur for years.

Research scientists believe the same virus is responsible for both shingles and chicken pox. Anyone who has partial immunity to, or has ever had, chicken pox may retain this dormant virus. A weakening of the body's natural resistance through physical illness or mental stress can initiate an attack. Some physicians regard shingles as a communicable disease and warn against direct personal contact.[81] In severe cases, quiet and bed rest are advised. Exposing the blisters to the drying warmth of a heat lamp (or incandescent bulb in an unshaded holder) may alleviate pain and speed healing when carefully watched to avoid burning the skin. Chiropractic or osteopathic manipulation has proven beneficial in some instances but strengthening the body's defenses through nutritional therapy seems to be the most effective treatment.

Diet and Supplements

A natural diet stressing raw or lightly cooked vegetables, whole-grain cereals, and organ meats is recommended. (Desiccated liver is available as powder or tablets for those who do not enjoy eating liver.) The nutritional deficit created by shingles is so high that a daily multi-vitamin-mineral tablet, plus at least some of the following optional supplements, is often advised.

Vitamin A—10,000 to 25,000 units one to three times daily to promote healing of the skin lesions.

B Complex—One comprehensive, high-potency tablet each morning and evening. All B vitamins are important for proper functioning of the nervous system and prevention of recurrent shingles. The addition of one or two tablespoons of brewer's yeast daily plus these individual B vitamins are considered particularly helpful in combating the malady.

B-1, B-6, and Pantothenic Acid—5 to 100 milligrams of each taken with milk each two or three hours until the symptoms begin to subside, then once or twice each day. (A lack of B-1, in particular, may instigate shingles or their painful aftermath.[88])

B-12—500 to 1,000 micrograms daily until blisters are healed. (Injections produce speedier results—often providing relief from the excruciating pain in as little as two hours[260]—and may be necessary if B-12 is not well-assimilated when taken orally.) Vitamin B-12 therapy has been found even more effective when combined with 50 milligrams of oral B-1 each day plus topical applications of aloe vera gel and vitamin E oil.

Case History

Mary Ellen R. was so upset over the red rash covering half her face that she knew she could not possibly attend the holiday luncheon to which she had just received an invitation. She telephoned her regrets, explaining that the doctor had given her some ointment to control the itching of her shingles, but that the red blisters were continuing to spread and she looked too terrible to be seen. The disappointed hostess suggested that she ask her doctor about taking extra B vitamins—B-12 and B-1 had worked wonders for her daughter's shingles—and offered to bring her some of the 1,000-milligram B-12 and 50-milligram B-1 tablets she had left over. Mary Ellen accepted and, with the approval of her physician, took one of each of the tablets each day. By the date of the luncheon the red rash was receding rather than spreading, was faint enough to be cosmetically camouflaged, and she could enjoy socializing with her friends without any self-consciousness.

Vitamin C and Bioflavonoids—1,000 milligrams vitamin C plus 100 to 300 milligrams bioflavonoids every hour or two until the symptoms begin to subside. (The bioflavonoid, rutin, is believed particularly effective against shingles.) When taken at the onset, massive amounts of vitamin C have not only relieved pain, but, by saturating the tissues and entering the virus-infected cells, prevented their further activity in increasing irritated areas or creating postherpetic pain.[350] To avoid any recurrence, the dosages should be continued for several days after the symptoms disappear, then gradually reduced.

Calcium and Vitamin D—One or two calcium tablets with each meal and before bedtime. 1,000 IU natural vitamin D, one to three times daily, for five days only. Vitamin D assists absorption of the calcium which is needed to surround and protect sensitive nerve endings and reduce irritation of the nervous system.

Vitamin E (see Caution, page 6)—400 to 1,600 IU daily. According to *Archives of Dermatology* (December, 1973), pain and itching from most cases of shingles can be alleviated by a combination of oral and topical vitamin E. The suggested dosage is four 400-IU capsules taken four times each day plus vitamin E oil rubbed on the blisters. The treatment should be continued for several weeks after the symptoms have disappeared, then the local applications discontinued and the amount of oral vitamin E gradually reduced. (Besides speeding healing, vitamin E is believed to prevent nerve damage which can result in postherpetic neuralgia.)

Lecithin—One to two tablespoons granules (10 to 20 1,200-milligram capsules) daily to aid both skin and nerves.

Lysine—500 to 1,000 milligrams each morning and evening. A favored treatment for herpes simplex (cold sores), this amino acid has often been effective in quelling the itching and inflammation of herpes zoster.

Magnesium—100 to 500 milligrams daily if dolomite is not used as the calcium supplement. Magnesium not only aids calcium absorption but prevents alterations in nerve conduction.[261]

Tissue Salts—Several options are offered for using either 3X or 6X tissue salts to combat shingles.

Calc. Phos. and Ferr. Phos.—Two tablets of each, twice each day plus one tablet each Kali. Phos. and Nat. Mur. taken three times each day. If the temperature usually registers as sub-normal, add three daily tablets of Nat. Sulph.

Kali. Mur.—Two tablets, three times daily, to speed healing.

Kali. Phos., Mag. Phos., and Silicea—One tablet of each, three times each day. This treatment is most effective when acid foods and beverages are eliminated from the diet.

Zinc—10 to 30 milligrams daily to promote healing of the skin lesions.

Folk Remedies

The archaic fear that shingles encircling the body would be fatal has been dispelled, but some of the old remedies may provide symptomatic relief from itching and pain.

Aloe Vera—Applying the split leaves of the aloe vera plant (or the bottled gel) has long been used to relieve the pain of shingles. Drinking one cup of aloe tea (one tablespoon aloe vera gel per cup of boiling water) each day was believed to bring a speedy recovery.

Apple Cider Vinegar—Drench the blisters with undiluted apple cider vinegar several times each day.

Baking Soda—Every few hours, sponge the irritated area with a solution of one teaspoon baking soda to one cup water. Cover with gauze or clean cloth to exclude the air.

Golden Seal Tea—Drink one cup of golden seal tea before each meal, then rub cooled tea over the blisters several times each day and before bed. Reportedly, this treatment has caused shingles to improve almost immediately and completely disappear within two weeks.[3]

Honey—At least three times each day, spread raw honey over the painful rash.

Hot or Cold Packs—To ease the burning, wring towels out of either hot or cold water and apply to the afflicted area.

Sources (See Bibliography)

3, 4, 7, 13, 19, 52, 53, 68, 81, 88, 89, 142, 156, 168, 189, 204, 229, 251, 254, 256, 260, 261, 288, 300, 305, 309, 312, 315, 350.

SUNBURN AND HEAT EXHAUSTION

Although its acquisition may be more pleasant than painful, sunburn is a real burn that affects skin and underlying tissues with the same degrees as an injury from flames or scalding liquids. If sunburn is extensive or severe, bed rest and the attention of a physician may be necessary. Sunburn can be acquired without the presence of direct sunlight or a sun lamp. Ultraviolet rays are not obstructed by clouds and can reflect into filtered shade. Many chemicals increase skin sensitivity. Among these agents are antibacterial soaps, antibiotics, antidiabetic drugs, antihistamines, barbiturates and tranquilizers, diuretics, food additives, and dyes. A deficiency of, or increased need for, vitamin B-6 may allow severe burning following only a short time in the sun.

Aside from limiting exposure until the skin becomes thickened and tanned, PABA has been found the most effective means of preventing sunburn. As reported in the *New England Journal of Medicine* (June, 1969), applying a sunscreening lotion containing 5 percent PABA in ethyl alcohol provided better protection than any of 24 commercial products tested. Many lotions and creams containing PABA are now on the market. Taking 1,000 milligrams oral PABA each day enhances their efficiency.

Additional protection may be obtained from 25,000 units vitamin A plus several bone meal tablets daily. Of the 3,000 people involved in a British study, all but 15 had complete protection or suffered only very mild symptoms when this combination was used.[261] Taking extra vitamin A before spending a day at the beach also helps prevent the night blindness that often follows overexposure of the eyes to extremely bright light. People who sunburn easily may have a defect in their ability to prevent and repair ultraviolet light damage to the skin. Taking 25,000 units of carotene (which is transformed into vitamin A within the body) plus extra C, D, PABA, and pantothenic acid daily may correct this.[252]

The muscular weakness, blurred vision, and nausea of mild heat exhaustion often accompanies sunburn but may occur from indoor heat. Profuse perspiration causes the body to lose fluids as well as water-soluble vitamins and minerals to such an extent that there may be muscular cramps of the arms, legs or abdomen. The *Journal of the American Medical Association* (June 25, 1982) stated that antidepressants, diuretics, and tranquilizers can increase the possibility of heat stroke by interfering with the body's normal cooling mechanisms.

Taking an extra multiple-vitamin-mineral tablet for several days before and after exposure is advised. According to research studies cited in the *South African Journal of*

Science (August, 1977), at least 250 milligrams of vitamin C each day improves blood circulation close to the skin and decreases the possibility of heat exhaustion. During days of intensive heat, eating salty food with each meal, taking one-fourth teaspoon salt with each glass of water, or sipping a mixture of one and one-half teaspoons salt plus three-fourths teaspoon baking soda in one quart water is recommended to prevent heat prostration. Some fluid (fruit or vegetable juices are especially beneficial) should be taken every 30 to 45 minutes while working or exercising in high temperatures.

If the symptoms of heat exhaustion do appear, getting out of the heat and replacing fluids and sodium are of prime importance. Reclining in a cooler area with the feet elevated 8 to 10 inches is helpful. Taking one-half teaspoon salt, or three 12X tablets of the tissue salt Nat. Mur., every 15 minutes with one-half glass cool coffee, juice, or water usually corrects the problem. (Plain water or alcoholic beverages are not advised during heat exhaustion as they may aggravate the situation.)

In true heat stroke or sunstroke, the cool, clammy skin of heat exhaustion is replaced by hot, dry skin and a rising internal temperature as the heat-regulating mechanism of the body ceases to function. Medical assistance should be obtained as quickly as possible. In the interim, body temperature should be lowered with ice packs, cold food from a picnic hamper, or cloths dipped in water and whirled in the air until cool.

Severe sunburn should be treated as any other burn (see Burns and Scalds). The redness and discomfort of ordinary sunburn usually responds to immediate cooling and a covering of lotion or oil to exclude the air. When soaking in a tub of cool water is not feasible, applying a towel dipped in ice water or a cold compress wrung out of a solution of one quart water to two tablespoons rubbing alcohol is equally effective. The tender skin should be allowed to dry without rubbing. Smoothing on vitamin E cream (or the oil squeezed from capsules) relieves discomfort and helps prevent blistering. Blending the oil from punctured capsules of 50,000 units of vitamin A and 1,000 IU vitamin E with four tablespoons of vegetable oil makes a soothing, healing ointment.

In addition to the suggested 1,000 milligrams of PABA, the following daily supplements have been found to speed sunburn healing.

> One multi-vitamin-mineral tablet plus vitamin A to equal 25,000 units
> One comprehensive, high-potency B-complex tablet
> Vitamin C—500 to 5,000 milligrams in divided doses, preferably with bioflavonoids
> Calcium—One or two bone meal or dolomite tablets with each meal and before bed.
> Vitamin E—400 IU (see Caution, page 6)
> Zinc—15 to 50 milligrams

Folk Remedies

During the centuries before packaged vitamins and pre-mixed lotions were available, folk healers relied on other natural remedies for sunburn.

Apple cider vinegar, or raw egg yolk beaten with water, rubbed on the skin before exposure was believed to produce a healthy tan without burning.

When sunburn did occur, immediate cooling in a tub of water to which 1 pound of cornstarch or two cups of apple cider vinegar had been added was advised. When this was not practical, dousing the reddened area with apple cider vinegar or a solution of three tablespoons of baking soda in a quart of water, or applying compresses of either liquid were recommended options. For severe sunburn, compresses of cold milk, weak salt water, or a paste of baking soda or baking powder and water were used.

Coating inflamed skin with aloe vera gel is one of the oldest, and most effective, treatments for all types of burns. Covering the area with a towel soaked in a mixture of one cup skim milk, three cups water, and two cups cracked ice was another favorite remedy. (Fresh, cold towels should be applied every 15 minutes until relief is achieved.) Other options were to apply plain olive oil, a half-and-half mixture of olive oil and apple cider vinegar, Vaseline, heavy cream, or a beaten egg yolk which was to be rinsed off after 30 minutes.

To treat heat prostration accompanying sunburn during the 1800s, cool cloths were applied to the victim's head, mustard or turpentine to the calves of the legs and soles of the feet, and sips of whiskey diluted with water were administered.

Sources (See Bibliography)

4, 7, 13, 19, 52, 53, 68, 81, 88, 89, 98, 142, 152, 154, 156, 168, 174, 229, 260, 261, 288, 297, 299, 300, 301, 305, 312, 315, 328, 333, 335, 350.

TOBACCO AND ALCOHOL USE (Diet and Supplements for)

In this era of unprecedented environmental pollution and artificial foods, the added toxins of alcohol and tobacco are too much for the body to handle without creating deficiencies and diseases unknown to smokers and drinkers during previous centuries of clean air and natural diets. Numerous studies have shown that drinking a small amount of alcohol daily reduces the likelihood of circulatory or heart problems, but no health benefits are attributed to using tobacco. However, by analyzing the harmful consequences of overindulgence, medical scientists have convincingly demonstrated many nutritional methods of protecting the body from dangers inherent in their moderate use.

Nicotine is a mild stimulant, alcohol a mild depressant. Both are toxins and, when used together, alcohol potentiates the carcinogens (cancer-causing substances) in cigarette smoke. The nicotine from cigar, cigarette, or pipe smoking, plug tobacco, or snuff is absorbed equally by the system. As reported in the August, 1982 *Journal of the American Medical Association,* pipe-smokers who inhale are at greater risk than cigarette smokers.

Although the percentage varies with volume, one jigger of whiskey, 4 ounces of wine, or one 12-ounce bottle of beer contain the same amount of alcohol. The "light" beers, wines, and cigarettes now on the market require both careful selection and moderation in consumption to be of value in lessening possible damage. (Alcohol reduction ranges from approximately one-fourth to one-half; the nicotine and tar content of cigarettes has an even broader variance.) According to an article by Jerome H. Jaffe in the March/April, 1982 issue of *American Health Magazine,* in 1960 one regular cigarette contained more tar and nicotine than over two cartons of the new "ultra low" cigarettes. As explained in *The Harvard Medical School Health Letter* (July, 1983), blocking the air vents in the sides of low-tar cigarette filter-tips can transform "lights" to "mediums." Smoking only the first half or two-thirds of each cigarette, regardless of the number smoked, reduces the overall amounts of tar and nicotine reaching the lungs—as does not inhaling.

For those who are attempting to "cut down," regular exercise and minor dietary changes can reduce the craving for alcohol and tobacco. Ninety-five percent of addictive drinkers have abnormal sugar metabolism which causes blood-sugar levels to frequently fall below normal.[326] Nicotine further aggravates the problem with brief blood-sugar-highs followed by even lower lows (see Low Blood Sugar). Eliminating refined sugar (considered by some authorities to be even more damaging to the liver than alcohol) and adhering to a high-protein diet stressing B-vitamin-containing whole grains is recommended. Drinking a glass of orange or tomato juice blended with the juice of a fresh lemon and one teaspoon to one tablespoon brewer's yeast often eases the urge for an alcoholic beverage.

An alkalinizing diet emphasizing apples, bananas, Brussels sprouts, carrots, celery, cucumbers, lima beans, potatoes, raisins, spinach, and tomatoes helps maintain nicotine levels in the bloodstream to reduce tobacco requirements. The *Los Angeles County Medical Association Healthlines* (March, 1980) advocated munching raw sunflower seeds to decrease the desire for cigarettes, provide added nutrients, and keep the hands occupied. Sucking on whole cloves was the folk-practitioner's method of quelling tobacco cravings.

Even the wisest of diets seldom provides enough vitamins and minerals to compensate for tobacco and alcohol use. Extra vitamins A, B, C, E, and the antioxidants (see page 3) are needed to combat the potentially harmful results of smoking and drinking. In their book, *Life Extension*[252], Durk Pearson and Sandy Shaw advise those who drink to take choline, lecithin, and at least 100 milligrams pantothenic acid daily, plus large amounts of B-6 and C to counteract the effect of alcohol on the brain.

> **Vitamin A and Carotene**—10,000 to 25,000 units vitamin A, plus 10,000 to 25,000 units carotene. Vitamin A is well-known for preventing eye disturbances resulting from smoking. Investigations cited in the *International Journal of Cancer* (April, 1975) and the *Journal of the National Cancer Institute* (June, 1979) showed that a high intake of vitamin A appeared to protect against lung cancer at all levels of cigarette smoking regardless of age. Another study reported by the National Cancer Institute demonstrated that carotene (available in supplement form or from carrots and other vegetables for conversion to vitamin A within the body) reduced the risk of lung cancer for smokers by 40 percent. The problem of male sterility among heavy drinkers may relate to the need for increased amounts of vitamin A. (Alcohol inhibits the process whereby vitamin A is changed to the form necessary for creating sperm.[6])
>
> **B Complex**—One comprehensive, high-potency tablet daily, plus extra tablets before and after drinking (see Hangover). B vitamins are destroyed by alcohol to such an extent that there is a movement afoot to make their addition to alcoholic beverages mandatory.[172] The entire B complex reinforces nerves

against damage from smoking and drinking. Individual supplements offer specific benefits.

Moderate drinkers are believed to need at least 50 milligrams of B-1 daily. For heavy drinkers, 100 to 3,000 milligrams is recommended along with supplements of B-2, B-6, B-12, and folic acid.

Taking 50 to 100 milligrams of B-1 and pantothenic acid, plus extra vitamin C and the amino acid cysteine, often impedes or improves premature skin wrinkling caused by smoking.

PABA provides protection against damage to the lungs by cigarette smoke. Sufficient B-12 has been found to prevent Amblyopia (tobacco blindness also linked to excessive use of alcohol).[78]

Only recently available in the United States, B-15 is believed to have a detoxifying effect, reduces the likelihood of cancer, and increases internal oxygen for smokers. The usual dosage is 50 milligrams per day, but clinical tests here and in Russia have shown 100 milligrams daily to be completely nontoxic.[280]

Vitamin C—500 to 20,000 milligrams in divided doses daily, preferably with bioflavonoids. Vitamin C strengthens body tissues to fend off pre-cancerous conditions. It offers protection against acetaldehyde—a toxic substance in cigarette smoke which is intensified by the consumption of alcohol and may be involved in heart or lung disease. Adequate vitamin C, plus bioflavonoids, is believed to prevent the bladder cancer, early hardening of the arteries, and facial wrinkles that often beset confirmed smokers. Large amounts of vitamin C, particularly when accompanied by zinc supplements, lower the quantity of alcohol remaining in the bloodstream an hour after taking an alcoholic drink.[7] Cigarette smoking consumes enormous amounts of vitamin C from the body's stores. Twenty-five milligrams of vitamin C per cigarette smoked is the accepted ratio but Irwin Stone[309] believes smokers should take 3,000 to 5,000 milligrams with each pack of cigarettes. Sipping a glass of fruit juice or water in which one teaspoon powdered vitamin C has been dissolved often counteracts "smokers cough." For those who are attempting to cut down or stop smoking, taking vitamin C as sodium ascorbate (or with one-eighth teaspoon baking soda) eliminates its acidifying effect.

Calcium and Magnesium—4 to 6 dolomite tablets daily. For heavy drinkers, at least 700 milligrams of magnesium each day is recommended. Alcohol increases the excretion of magnesium, which is required for the assimilation of calcium to prevent jittery nerves from either alcohol or nicotine use. An article in *Archives of Internal Medicine* (Vol. 136, 1976) stated that certain types of osteoporosis (fragile, shrinking bones) were 76 percent more likely when middle-aged persons were heavy smokers.

Vitamin E (see Caution, page 6)—100 to 1,000 IU daily. The antioxidant properties of vitamin E protect vitamin A from destruction within the body, guard against cardiovascular or pulmonary difficulties due to lung damage from tobacco smoke, and help prevent blood clots resulting from temporary constriction of the small blood vessels by nicotine. In *Common Questions on Vitamin E and Their Answers*[299], Evan Shute states that at least 400 IUs of vitamin E are needed daily by smokers to replace the amount destroyed.

Lecithin—One or two tablespoons granules (or the equivalent in 1,200-milligram capsules at the rate of 10 per tablespoon) each day to protect smokers from eye or nerve damage and avoid loss of memory or brain damage from alcohol use. Lecithin also helps emulsify saturated fats created in the bloodstream by surplus calories from alcohol.

Selenium—100 to 200 micrograms daily. The antioxidant qualities of selenium help combat the harm from either tobacco or alcohol and increase the effectiveness of vitamin E.

Zinc—15 to 50 milligrams daily. Even though the slogan "zinc before you drink" has been questioned, zinc is an antioxidant that benefits both smokers and drinkers—yet alcohol prohibits its storage by the body.

Sources (See Bibliography)

4, 6, 8, 9, 23, 48, 53, 54, 72, 78, 84, 89, 105, 128, 166, 168, 171, 172, 174, 184, 194, 207, 208, 228, 229, 238, 248, 249, 251, 252, 254, 261, 269, 280, 288, 289, 297, 299, 301, 309, 326, 331, 334, 347, 354.

TOOTHACHE—DENTAL CARIES

Dental cavities require professional help. No amount of self-applied therapy can effect a permanent cure. Abscesses (infections at the roots of the teeth) also warrant immediate medical attention. Much can be done at home, however, to prevent dental caries, and, since toothache seldom strikes during office hours, alleviate pain until a specialist can be reached.

Although a cavity is the usual cause, toothache can result from an impacted food particle or nervous tension. Using dental floss to clean between the affected tooth and its neighbors relieves the pain from food pressure. Psychosomatic toothache occasionally occurs, and mental pressure has been proven a contributing factor in tooth decay. (Stress decreases the volume of tooth-protective saliva, causing it to thicken and become more acid.[88]) Practicing relaxation techniques (see pages 9-10) plus taking vitamins B and C help counteract the damaging consequences.

Ideally, teeth should be brushed after each meal or snack, but, when this is not feasible, rinsing the mouth with water is the next best thing. British schoolchildren taught to "bubble, swill, and swallow" three mouthfuls of water after eating reduced their incidence of dental caries by as much as two-thirds.[215] A solution of one-half teaspoon ordinary table salt or baking soda in one-half cup water may be used as a mouthwash. A half-and-half mixture of baking soda and salt has been found as effective as commercial dentifrice but some authorities recommend rotating plain salt, plain soda, and regular toothpaste on a three-day schedule.[168]

Periodic examinations by a dentist plus daily brushing and flossing are important, but "clean" teeth can decay when certain nutrients are insufficiently supplied.

Diet and Supplements

Most cavities are instigated by refined sugars and starches fermenting with saliva to form an enamel-eroding acid. Experts agree that frequency of ingestion rather than total amount of sweets consumed is responsible for the greatest percentage of tooth decay. Sweet or starchy foods that are part of a meal are less cavity-producing than between-meal snacks. Doctors at the National Institute of Dental Research found that cheese reduces bacteria-acid production. Citrus fruits also have an antibacterial action and the citric acid loosens plaque (see Mouth and Gum Problems). Food such as bananas and carrots cause bacteria to clump, making removal by brushing and flossing easier. Eating one-quarter of a raw apple after a meal has proven 30 percent more effective than brushing in removing food debris from the teeth.[215]

Strong, decay-resistant teeth have their beginnings before birth (see Pregnancy). Adequate vitamins and minerals are vital to tooth formation during early childhood. A varied diet including milk and natural foods should supply the essential nutrients but many authorities advocate supplements as well. (For children under 10, selenium tablets are not recommended as they may decrease the benefits of fluoride.[256]) Experimental studies involving supplementation with bone meal plus vitamins B and C from infancy have produced adults with no dental cavities whatsoever.[13, 261] Other tests have shown that older children and adults plagued with dental caries can limit new cavities and harden "soft" teeth with good oral hygiene, diet, vitamins, and minerals. Inert as teeth may seem, they require nutrients for continual renewal. A daily multi-vitamin-mineral tablet is suggested for all age groups, but, unless otherwise indicated, children should have only half the amounts of these daily supplements recommended for healthy decay-free teeth in adults.

> **Vitamin A**—10,000 to 25,000 units. Vitamin A is essential for the formation and preservation of sound teeth. A deficiency retards bone growth in infants, leads to orthodontic problems for children, and decay for adults.
>
> **Vitamin B-6**—50 milligrams. A year-long study of school children given lozenges containing B-6 showed a 40 to 50 percent reduction in their dental caries.[89, 261]
>
> **Bone Meal**—1,500 milligrams (six tablets or one teaspoon bone meal powder). Sweden has reported astounding success by using bone meal supplementation instead of water fluoridation. For infants under two, one-half teaspoon bone meal powder is stirred into the daily orange juice—one teaspoon for children and adults.[13, 261] Bone meal contains phosphorus as well as calcium, both of which are needed for tooth growth and renewal. If much meat or whole grain is included in the diet, magnesium-calcium supplements (dolomite) should be substituted for part of the bone meal to assure calcium-phosphorus absorption. Taking additional calcium for several days prior to tooth extraction is believed to lessen the danger of hemorrhage.[92]
>
> **Vitamin C**—1,000 to 10,000 milligrams. Vitamin C assists in calcium absorption to produce strong, thick tooth enamel. The *Journal of Preventive Medicine* (Spring, 1974) reported that children given 1,000 milligrams of vitamin C daily for each year of life up to age nine, and 10,000 milligrams

each day thereafter, recorded no cavities. Taking additional vitamin C, 10 milligrams B-1, and 75 to 100 milligrams zinc for several days before and after tooth extraction often decreases pain and accelerates healing.

Vitamin D (natural)—400 to 1,000 IU. Vitamin D is essential for utilization of the calcium needed for strong teeth. In addition, the acids in the mouth that attack tooth enamel are neutralized if saliva containing ample amounts of dissolved calcium can reach the area where the acids are being formed.

Vitamin E (see Caution, page 6)—100 to 400 IU. Required throughout life for stabilizing vitamin A and assuring healthy teeth, vitamin E deficiency during childhood can result in depigmentation and chalky-looking teeth. (A lack of pantothenic acid, one of the B vitamins, also contributes to depigmentation.)

Tissue Salts

For sharp, shooting pain: take three tablets of 6X Mag. Phos. each hour.
For deep-seated pain around the tooth: take tablets of 6X Silicea every hour.

Folk Remedies

Aloe Vera Gel—Rub aloe vera gel (available in health food stores) on the tooth and the gum surrounding it. Repeat every 15 minutes.

Alum—A mixture of equal amounts of powdered alum and salt applied to an aching tooth often brings quick relief.

Ammonia—Saturate a bit of cotton with ammonia and press over the cavity.

Ashes—Pack the sore tooth with damp ashes.

Bread Poultice—Soak toasted bread in alcohol to make a paste. Sprinkle with cayenne pepper, spread on gauze, then apply to the painful side of the face.

Cloves—Packing the cavity with cotton moistened with oil of cloves was the basic remedy for toothache. (Oil of cayenne or sassafras may be substituted.) Sucking on whole cloves or steeping them in hot water or honey, then chewing and holding them in the mouth next to the aching tooth is considered almost as effective.

Cold—a 10-minute cold footbath and/or an ice pack on the jaw often helps, as does a sliver of ice placed directly on the tooth.

Egg Yolk and Honey—Mix one teaspoon honey with one egg yolk, then apply as a compress on the jaw over the aching tooth.

Figs—Slice a fresh fig and squeeze the juice on the painful tooth.

Garlic—Keep a slice of fresh garlic in contact with the affected tooth for an hour and/or apply crushed garlic spread between pieces of gauze to the inside of both elbows and knees.

Heat—Hold hot compresses over the sore cheek while keeping the feet on a heating pad or hot water bottle for several hours.

Horseradish—Place grated horseradish on the gum by the aching tooth. Or, spread the horseradish between pieces of gauze and apply behind the ear on the painful side and to the bend of both arms and legs.

Mustard Seed—Chewing mustard seeds was believed to relieve toothache.

Onion—Bind half a roasted onion over the inside of the wrist opposite the aching tooth.

Salt Water—Rinse the mouth with warm salt water or epsom salts dissolved in hot water. Retain for several minutes and repeat at frequent intervals. This treatment was advised for toothache and also believed helpful following tooth extractions.

Vanilla—Place a few drops of vanilla on the painful tooth.

Vinegar—Warm a few tablespoons vinegar (with a sprinkling of cayenne pepper, if desired) and hold in the mouth to surround the throbbing tooth. Or, soak heavy brown paper in vinegar, sprinkle with grated ginger, and apply to the affected side of the face, leaving in place overnight.

Whiskey—A standard medication for temporarily deadening pain, whiskey was rubbed on the tooth, held in the mouth, or used as a gargle.

Case History

Eleven-year-old Adrianne A. was less than enthusiastic about spending two weeks of her summer vacation in a tent while her father "painted from nature" in the mountains. Being allowed to take her best friend along for company considerably improved her mental state, and the girls were having a great time until Adrianne felt the stabbing pain of a toothache. They were many miles from the nearest dentist. Adrianne's father proffered the bottle of whiskey he had brought along as a snake-bite remedy. Adrianne's mother read the pamphlet accompanying the tissue salts she had packed with the first-aid kit. Adrianne was doubtful of the results but let the tablets of 6-X Mag. Phos. dissolve under her tongue; winked at her friend as she swallowed a bit of the whiskey she was told to hold in her mouth; and felt no more pain until they returned to "civilization" and her dental carie was filled.

Nerve Massage

- Place the first two fingers of each hand against the hollow at the base of the skull. Massage firmly and slowly in a clockwise direction.
- Massage the hinge of the jawbone, and, if the aching tooth is in the lower jaw, rub the outer edge of the jawbone about 1½ inches from the bottom of the earlobe.
- If a front tooth on the left side is aching, massage the thumb and first finger of the left hand. If the painful tooth is on the back, left side, massage the last three fingers of the left hand. Massage the same fingers of the right hand for pain on the right side.

Nerve Pressure

Unless otherwise indicated, press each point for 10 seconds, release for 10 seconds, and repeat for a total of 30 seconds pressure.

- Press a point on the temple, 1½ inches in front of the top of the ear.
- Press inward and upward in the depression about 1 inch in front of the center of the ear.
- Using three fingers, push on the cheek an inch above the aching tooth, maintaining pressure for two or three minutes.
- Press the cheek 1 inch out from and even with the base of the nostril on the side with the toothache.

- Press the jaw ¾ inch below the base of the earlobe.
- Make a fist with the hand on the aching side. Press the highest part of the mound formed between thumb and index finger.
- On the aching side, press between the thumb and index finger—against the bone leading to the finger.
- For a toothache caused by neuralgia rather than a cavity: wrap the fingers with rubber bands—tightly enough to give firm pressure. Remove the moment the fingers start changing color, then repeat after a few minutes. Use the hand corresponding to the side with the aching tooth. For aching molars, wrap the middle and last two fingers. For the central part of the mouth, the thumb and first two fingers.

Sources (See Bibliography)

4, 6, 7, 8, 13, 19, 52, 53, 54, 62, 63, 67, 68, 78, 88, 89, 92, 142, 154, 156, 159, 168, 171, 173, 174, 189, 206, 214, 226, 227, 228, 229, 254, 256, 257, 260, 261, 269, 270, 281, 288, 310, 311, 325, 335, 345, 348, 349, 350.

ULCERS—PEPTIC, DUODENAL, AND GASTRIC

Despite the fact that ulcers are among civilization's most common maladies, terminology regarding them is confusing. As medically defined, peptic ulcers are sores on the lining of the stomach or the entrance to the upper intestine (duodenum). Although generally referred to as stomach ulcers, at least 90 percent of such ulcers are not in the stomach at all but are erosions of the duodenum.[174] Duodenal ulcers result from too much stomach acid either being produced or being allowed to reach this vulnerable area. Gastric ulcers are comparatively rare. Most gastric-ulcer sufferers generate normal amounts of digestive acids but retain food in the stomach for an extended period. This allows the acid more contact-time with the stomach lining—which has usually been weakened by gastritis (see Indigestion)—resulting in a portion of the stomach lining being "digested" to leave a raw sore.

All suspected ulcers should have medical diagnosis and attention. If allowed to progress unchecked, an ulcer can perforate (eat through the stomach wall), hemorrhage if it penetrates a blood vessel, or form a scar-tissue obstruction to block normal food movement into the intestines.

Once an almost exclusively masculine ailment, ulcers are becoming less discriminatory. In 1977, men outnumbered women 10 to one as victims of duodenal ulcers, with the gastric-ulcer ratio three to one. By 1980, there were only twice as many men as women afflicted with duodenal ulcers, and the gastric rate was even between the sexes.[18] No specific explanation has been found to account for this change, nor for the amazing predictability of attacks taking place in either spring or fall.

Ulcers occur when lining tissues fail in their protective role or when so much digestive acid is secreted linings are overwhelmed. Under laboratory conditions, ulcers have been formed by stress alone, by lack of practically any nutrient, or by combining stress with vitamin and mineral deficiencies. Heredity may play a role in the strength of the linings and the amount of acid secreted. Some people produce two to four times as much digestive acid as others. Chronic conditions such as diabetes, hypoglycemia, or lung disease may stimulate excess acid output. Aspirin, cortisone, and steroid medications can adversely affect stomach-lining cells.

Antacids have been the major ulcer treatment for decades but controlled studies indicate their value to be largely imaginary.[315] Tests have demonstrated that baking soda and commercial antacids provide temporary relief but speed stomach-emptying time to such a degree that ulcers, given longer exposure to corrosive stomach acids, are either made worse or caused to recur. Alkalis in various antacids can irritate ulcers. Some antacids contain aluminum, which has been related to memory loss and the instigation of Alzheimer's disease.

Milk of magnesia, magnesium carbonate, or magnesium trisilicate are believed the least harmful antacids because they act only in the stomach and intestines rather than being absorbed into the entire system, but they are laxatives to be used with discretion.[175] Antacids interfere with vitamin C absorption and can so disturb the body's metabolic balance that, as a counter-move, the stomach secretes twice as much acid at the next meal following a dose of antacid.[89] Appeasing an aggravated stomach with frequent offerings of protein-containing foods usually makes their use unnecessary.

The clinical development of ulcers is well-documented but causes as well as cures vary with individuals. Treatments are constantly being updated and the prognosis is encouraging—the increase of ulcer incidence is being matched by successful recoveries.

Diet and Supplements

Diet is the most controversial of all ulcer treatments. Traditional bland diets with milk and antacids taken every hour or so have generally been forsaken in the wake of numerous tests showing that ulcers heal as rapidly and recur no more frequently when a normal diet is followed. Some doctors feel the role of diet in ulcer treatment is of little importance and allow ulcer patients to eat whatever agrees with them, whenever they like. Other physicians advise a natural diet with plenty of fiber and few refined carbohydrates. (The British medical magazine, *Lancet* (October 2, 1982) published results of a study involving high-fiber vs bland-diet regimens for patients with recently healed ulcers. Ulcers reappeared in 80 percent of the bland-diet group but in only 45 percent of those on the high-fiber diet.) Fiber slows the passage of food and there is no danger of natural roughage puncturing tender ulcer-coverings since only acids can penetrate the stomach's protective lining.[305]

The "frequent feedings" rule is being questioned by some authorities, but it has been shown that both hunger and infrequent large meals tend to stimulate the over-secretion of digestive acids. Many duodenal ulcer victims have stomachs that empty too quickly, allowing acids to reach the duodenum before they have been completely neutralized by the reactions of digestion.

It is now believed that the time-honored "Sippy Diet" as well as other milk-and-cream diets may be too low in protein to promote healing, are deficient in vitamins and minerals, and may lead to atherosclerosis and heart disease. Milk has lost status as a remedy since it has been found to first neutralize then stimulate the secretion of stomach acids. Even if ineffective as a healing agent, milk does have a palliative effect on ulcer pain. Whole milk quiets an active stomach because its protein buffers stomach acids and the fat delays emptying time. When ulcers are painful, a fortified milk drink may be tolerated when other foods are not. Adelle Davis' recipe for fortified milk is given in her book, *Let's Get Well*[89], and simplified versions are listed in the Index. Blending one-fourth cup unsweetened protein powder with one quart milk (plus one-fourth cup malted-milk powder and/or an equal amount of brewer's yeast, if desired), then drinking one-half cup at least once each hour during the acute phase, is an even less complex method of supplying sufficient protein to neutralize stomach acids.

Carbohydrate foods require only about half the time needed by proteins for complete gastric processing. Sugar encourages the flow of digestive juices, and, when a sweet beverage or protein-free snack is taken on an empty stomach, there is little to neutralize those acids. The relationship between low blood sugar and ulcers is being examined since studies have shown 75 percent of peptic ulcer patients also have hypoglycemia[13]. Other tests show that an average of 40 percent of peptic ulcer cases stem from hypoglycemia.[171] The diet for Low Blood Sugar (which see) with its frequent, high-protein, small meals is ideal for those with ulcers. When protein foods are eaten at frequent intervals, stomach acids can usually be completely neutralized without ulcer irritation.

Including a little fat with each meal or snack slows stomach emptying to prevent long periods of exposure to digestive juices. Hydrogenated fats or deep-fried foods are not recommended but pan-frying is generally acceptable when butter or unsaturated oils are used and cooking temperatures kept low.

Eggs, either cooked or raw, are of great value in ulcer diets. Besides protein, fat, and other nutrients, they contain cystine. (A lack of this amino acid caused ulcers to develop in laboratory tests with animals.[89]) Early studies showed that raw egg white destroyed biotin, but later tests brought out the information that as many as three dozen raw egg whites could be eaten daily for a year without creating a biotin deficiency.[89]

Raw fruit and vegetable juices, including diluted citrus juices, often hasten rather than delay ulcer healing. (Raw papaya and raw pineapple are exceptions; they should not be used because they dissolve damaged tissue and could retard recovery.) Spicy foods, even hot chilies, curried, or vinegar-pickled items, do not adversely affect ulcers for some people. Nothing that can be swallowed at a meal is as irritating as the stomach's own digestive juices, but individual reactions are the best guide—anything that causes bloating or pain should be avoided.

Coffee (both regular and decaffeinated), tea, chocolate, and soft drinks containing caffeine have been found to stimulate acid production. Alcohol also stimulates the flow of gastric juices and has long been considered a stomach irritant forbidden for those with ulcers. However, tests at Cornell University Medical School showed no adverse stomach reaction even when 100-proof alcohol was administered.[89] Once past the acute stage, many ulcer victims have no problem with moderate use of these beverages as long as they are accompanied with protein-containing foods to neutralize the extra acid.

During ulcer attacks, protein from eggs, milk, and soy products may be more easily digested than meat, chicken, or fish. Pureeing fruits and vegetables may be helpful. Having foods and beverages at room or body temperature may also be beneficial as extremes of heat or cold can affect stomach reactions. Since digestion begins with the mouth's salivary glands, it is recommended that foods be thoroughly chewed, meals eaten slowly, and liquids sipped.

Vitamin and mineral therapy for ulcers has received little publicity, yet scientific studies and patient-practice by nutritionally oriented physicians have found it a most effective means of prevention and cure.

Vitamin A—10,000 to 75,000 units daily for a few weeks, then 10,000 to 25,000 units each day. Crucial for maintenance of stomach-lining tissues, extra vitamin A is needed by people who smoke or who live in highly polluted areas. Stress ulcers arising from severe burns or other injuries have been prevented by medically supervised administration of 10,000 to 400,000 units of water-soluble vitamin A.[260] When combined with vitamin E, vitamin A has a curative effect on existing ulcers. Carotene (a substance in carrots and other vegetables from which the body synthesizes vitamin A) has been found to prevent and help heal ulcers. Beta carotene is available in 10,000 or 25,000 IU capsules and is less inclined to create toxicity than other forms of vitamin A.

B Complex—One comprehensive tablet daily. The stress which either contributes to or is created by ulcers calls for B-vitamin supplementation. Deficiencies of B-2, folic acid, or pantothenic acid have been linked to ulcer formation. Many instances of complete cure have been recorded by ulcer victims taking 15 milligrams of B-2 daily for nine months.[4] Pantothenic acid decreases the secretion of stomach acid, and, when 50 to 100 milligrams are taken three times daily after meals, often brings rapid improvement. Taking 100 milligrams of B-6 each day plus large amounts of choline (present in lecithin or available as a separate supplement) has been credited with the swift healing of ulcers. (If choline is undersupplied, bile is continuously regurgitated from the intestines, irritating existing ulcers or causing new ones to form.[352]) Studies in Rumania have shown that additional amounts of B-12 neutralize the stress-ulcer-creating consequences of cortisone therapy.[261]

Bee Propolis—20 drops, or the equivalent in capsules, three times a day. Russian studies by F.D. Makarov (published in the Soviet-released book, *The Healing Art*) indicated that both duodenal and gastric ulcers responded favorably to this treatment.

Vitamin C—100 to 5,000 milligrams, preferably with bioflavonoids, in divided doses daily. The need for vitamin C is increased by stress. Ulcers can develop from its deficiency or refuse to heal when it is not amply supplied. Bioflavonoids improve vitamin C assimilation and strengthen newly formed tissue covering the ulcer. Taking vitamin C with milk or meals usually prevents stomach irritation, but it is available in buffered form or one-eighth teaspoon baking soda may be taken with each 500 milligrams of vitamin C to neutralize its acidity.

Vitamin E (see Caution, page 6)—100 to 1,200 IU daily. Vitamin E is essential for the assimilation of vitamin A. Laboratory tests have shown that stress ulcers can develop from a lack of vitamin E alone, that large amounts of this vitamin can lessen the formation of ulcers, preclude scar tissue in existing ulcers, at least partially dissolve old scars, and, when combined with vitamin A, prevent new ulcers from forming.

L-Glutamine—1,000 to 4,000 milligrams per day. This amino acid has been isolated from raw cabbage (see Folk Remedies, below) and has been beneficial for some ulcer sufferers.

Spirulina—1 to 3 tablets before each meal. Best known as a weight-reducing aid, spirulina has been found to contain potent anti-ulcerants which coat the stomach lining and inhibit pepsin secretion.

Tissue Salts—At the onset of an ulcer attack, take one each Kali. Phos. and Nat. Phos. in the 3X or 6X potency. Repeat at half-hourly intervals until relieved.

Zinc—90 milligrams taken three times a day with food. A high calcium intake increases the need for zinc. Controlled studies have shown this amount of zinc to triple the healing rate of ulcers without any side effects and, in many cases, effect a complete cure.[353]

Folk Remedies

Acidophilus Yogurt or Capsules—One-fourth cup plain yogurt eaten between meals, with or without the addition of two tablespoons brewer's yeast, or two acidophilus capsules with each meal. Long used for its stomach-soothing and ulcer-healing attributes, scientists have discovered acidophilus capable of destroying harmful stomach-acid-generating bacteria in the intestines.[89]

Alfalfa—One tablespoon dehydrated, ground alfalfa dissolved in a glass of water and taken once each day has brought immediate relief to many ulcer sufferers.[261] Alfalfa is also available in tablets, meal, or as seeds or leaves which can be steeped for a tea.

Almonds—Almond milk, made by whirring blanched almonds with water in an electric blender, is considered beneficial—possibly because it supplies high-quality protein that binds with stomach acids.

Aloe Vera Gel—Two tablespoons twice each day, mixed with juice for palatability, if desired. (The laxative action of aloe vera may necessitate a reduction in dosage after a few days.) Renowned for its healing properties for over 3,000 years, aloe vera gel is now available in health food stores and has been found to slow acid secretion, reduce inflammation, and promote regrowth of tissues lining the stomach.

Baker's Yeast—One cake (or one envelope dissolved in water or milk) each morning, noon, and night during acute attacks. Modern nutritionists fear this form of live yeast used for bread leavening will destroy helpful intestinal bacteria, but many successes with bleeding ulcers have been reported when as many as 22 yeast cakes were eaten each day.[37]

Cabbage or Potato Juice—One-half cup several times a day between meals. Scientific studies have shown both these raw vegetables to contain vitamin U which is necessary for maintenance of the protective stomach lining. This anti-ulcer factor is also present in raw milk but is destroyed by pasteurization or cooking. Both cabbage and potato juice must be made just before drinking to avoid rapid oxidation of their medicinal properties. Either juice may be diluted with water or mixed with fruit or vegetable juice to improve the flavor. When no juicer is available, nibbling on raw cabbage four or five times daily has been found helpful.

Goat's Milk—Drinking raw goat's milk in place of cow's milk is believed to help heal stomach ulcers. The milk may be more appetizing if a few drops of vanilla are added to each glass.

Herbal Teas—Drinking one to four cups catnip, comfrey, ginger, licorice root, or slippery elm tea each day is the herbalists' prescription for healing ulcers. The teas may be flavored with honey and lemon juice, if desired.

Honey—Eating a spoonful of honey several times a day was believed to speed ulcer healing. (Medical research has shown that a diet rich in honey decreases stomach acidity for those with gastric or duodenal ulcers.[106])

Okra—Cooked okra, either pureed or mashed and eaten with the cooking water, is thought to coat the stomach, neutralize stomach acid, and encourage healing. If preferred, it may be diluted with hot water or milk and sipped as a beverage.

Olive Oil—Taking a spoonful of olive oil three times each day was a favorite folk remedy for easing ulcers.

Potatoes—A diet of nothing but boiled, mashed potatoes for several days was advocated for acute ulcers by some folk therapists.

Nerve Massage

Several options are offered for relief of ulcer pain:

- Massage the soft pad at the base of each thumb. Then massage the webs between thumbs and index fingers.
- Massage the front or back of the wrists, whichever is tender.
- Massage the bottom of each foot, between the big-toe pad and the inner edge of the arch.

Nerve Pressure

Unless otherwise indicated, once or twice each day press each point for 10 seconds, release for 10 seconds, then repeat three times.

- Press above the nose where the eyebrows would meet, then press the top center of the nose where the bone ends and cartilage begins.
- Press down on the back of the tongue with a popsicle stick or the broad handle of a tablespoon.
- If the ulcer is causing pain and any of the fingers are tender, apply firm pressure on those fingers for from three to 15 minutes. Rubber bands may be wound around the fingers for even pressure, but should be removed the moment the fingers begin to change color.
- Press four points around the outer edge of the navel—upper left and right, lower left and right.

Smoking

Ulcer patients are often advised not to smoke because clinical tests have shown that nicotine in the blood increases the output of stomach acid while decreasing the buffering secretions that protect the duodenum. Other studies, however, have revealed that continuance of smoking does not alter ulcer-healing rates[353] and that the stress of attempting to stop smoking may be more harmful than helpful.[18] So, smoking, like diet selection, appears to be a matter of individual tolerance. Moderation, not smoking on an empty stomach, and the use of low-nicotine cigarettes is indicated for addicted smokers.

Stress

Any strong emotion—anger, anxiety, delight, sorrow, even remembered disappointments or frustrations—can trigger an outpouring of stomach acid. Dreaming of stressful situations has a similar effect, so midnight snacks may be well-advised. Every form of stress, mental or physical, increases the body's nutritional needs. Individuals whose diets have been deficient in protein or other nutrients are the ones most susceptible to ulcers. Taking 500 milligrams vitamin C plus 100 milligrams pantothenic acid with protein-reinforced milk or a high-protein snack such as a handful of peanuts or cheese crackers each hour during the onset of stress often helps prevent ulcer attacks.

Deliberate relaxation and auto-suggestion (see pages 9-10) may serve to relieve stomach-churning tension, especially when combined with intelligent analysis of immediate problems and selection of alternative solutions to avoid futile worrying. The old adage, "count to 10" was based on this premise even though it was advised for temper control. Physical exercise is another option. Literally walking briskly away from the pressures and irritants for a few minutes can be as effective as a tranquilizer.

Sources (See Bibliography)

1, 2, 3, 4, 7, 9, 13, 18, 23, 25, 34, 37, 52, 53, 54, 59, 63, 64, 68, 79, 80, 89, 104, 105, 106, 110, 126, 128, 142, 145, 152, 156, 165, 168, 171, 173, 174, 175, 180, 189, 215, 226, 227, 229, 232, 238, 250, 252, 260, 261, 269, 270, 288, 289, 297, 305, 309, 312, 315, 316, 321, 328, 333, 335, 337, 350, 352, 353, 354.

VARICOSE VEINS AND VARICOSE ULCERS

According to the world's first medical text, a 3,400-year-old Egyptian papyrus, bulging blue veins were a vexation long before Cleopatra's beauty-conscious era. Swollen veins most frequently occur in the legs because blood is pumped down the arteries by the heart and must be pulled back up, against gravity, through the veins. Visible varicose veins are evidence of the body bypassing invisible varicosities deep within the legs by utilizing smaller veins near the surface. (Varicose veins in the rectum are Hemorrhoids, which see.)

Although common (a 1972 U.S. Public Health Service survey showed well over one-third of the population afflicted with varicose veins), they are potentially dangerous. All obstructed blood vessels and varicose ulcers should receive medical attention. Reduced circulation in the legs can cause tissue to deteriorate so that any pressure can result in a slow-to-heal, open sore. (See Wounds and Cuts for additional healing remedies.) If ignored, the varicosities can lead to phlebitis (inflammation of the walls of the veins), or form clots which might break loose to instigate strokes or heart attacks.

Howard C. Baron's book, *Varicose Veins*[26], theorizes that hereditary weakness of the valves in the veins makes half the people in the world susceptible to varicose veins, and the remainder exempt. Other authorities attribute varicosities to constipation, high-heeled shoes that interfere with natural contraction of leg muscles, improper diet and lack of certain nutrients, insufficient exercise, obesity, occupations requiring long periods of sitting or standing, overly tight clothing, pregnancy (which causes increased pressure on leg veins), or vein damage from infection or injury. Natural correction of the cause offers more permanent relief than surgery—varicosities frequently reappear after being surgically removed.

Diet and Supplements

A diet high in body-firming proteins and bulky natural foods is recommended. Many nutritionally oriented doctors consider varicose veins the result of excessive consumption of refined carbohydrates. Stressing whole grains and regularly including small amounts of unprocessed bran has been found beneficial for both prevention and control of varicosities. One or two daily glasses of fresh fruit or vegetable juice— especially apple, beet, carrot, celery, citrus, parsley, or pineapple—may be useful. Antioxidants (see page 3) are considered helpful. A daily combination suggested for those with varicose veins is 2,000 to 3,000 milligrams vitamin C, 1,500 milligrams bioflavonoids (including 500 milligrams rutin), and 400 to 1,200 IU vitamin E (see Caution, page 6). Numerous studies have shown individual vitamins and minerals effective in preventing and treating varicose veins.

Vitamin A—10,000 to 25,000 units daily. Vitamin A assists varicose-ulcer healing, and is particularly important if cortisone has been prescribed.

B Complex—One comprehensive, high-potency tablet daily. Adequate B vitamins are necessary for maintenance of strong blood vessels and, when combined with vitamins C and E, help prevent blood clots. Improvement of phlebitis and clearing of blood clots within as little as 12 days has resulted from adding 50 to 100 milligrams pantothenic acid to this combination.[88] Persistent varicose ulcers have healed in three months when 5 milligrams of folic acid was taken three times each day.[260] (Folic acid not only speeds healing but widens blood vessels to create auxiliary routes for blood transmission around clogged arteries.)

Vitamin C and Bioflavonoids—500 to 5,000 milligrams vitamin C plus 300 to 1,000 milligrams bioflavonoids taken at intervals throughout the day. Bioflavonoids aid vitamin C absorption and intensify its effect. Both strengthen tissues to avoid capillary rupture. Vitamin C also enhances the beneficial action of vitamin E.

Calcium—500 to 1,000 milligrams daily. Besides its function in maintaining bones and teeth, calcium is essential for the strength of soft tissues—which can weaken to allow varicosities.

Vitamin E (see Caution, page 6)—400 to 1,600 IU daily. Alpha tocopherol opens collateral circulation in the legs to take pressure off the varicosities, enables congested tissues to better utilize oxygen, and eliminates internal blood clots while interfering only slightly (or not at all) with the clotting of blood to seal wounds. When taken each morning and night, vitamin E dilates even the smallest capillaries to improve circulation and open new channels of blood supply. If there is pain in the varicosities immediately after beginning vitamin E therapy, it is believed a positive symptom of improved circulation. However, starting with 100 IU daily and working up to larger amounts may be more comfortable.

Vitamin E may or may not improve the appearance of existing varicose veins, but has been found to reduce swelling and aching, and halt the natural tendency of varicosed veins to worsen. Vitamin E ointment (or oil squeezed from capsules) relieves skin irritation when applied locally. Used with oral supplements, topical applications promote the healing of varicose ulcers.

Zinc—50 to 100 milligrams daily. Zinc deficiency may be at least partially responsible for leg ulcers. Clinical studies have shown this dosage to triple the speed of varicose ulcer healing.[78]

Elastic or Support Stockings

Rather than inhibiting circulation as tight garters or girdles do, elastic stockings reduce both pain and swelling of varicosities by forcing the blood into deeper veins in the legs.

Exercise and Leg Elevation

Walking, swimming, running, or bicycling encourages contraction of leg muscles and stimulates blood flow in the veins. The indoor exercise of lying on the back with legs in the air and pretending to pedal a bicycle for 30 seconds at a time is excellent therapy. Exercising the calf muscles massages the veins to prevent blood pooling in the legs. Alternating activity with resting with the legs elevated allows the veins to drain by gravity and is especially effective during early stages of varicosity.

Standing still or sitting with the legs crossed should be avoided. When standing for prolonged periods, shift body weight from one foot to the other, and, if possible, elevate one foot a few inches on any support available—block, bar rail, or cabinet shelf under the kitchen sink. To compensate for lengthy sitting, at least once each hour flex the leg muscles and take 10 deep breaths, forcing out all old air before inhaling. Relaxing in a reclining chair or on a slant board, or elevating the foot of the bed a few inches, assists the return of blood from the legs.

Folk Remedies

Aloe Vera—For itching varicosities: apply split aloe vera leaves or aloe vera gel from a health food store.

Apple Cider Vinegar—Each morning and night, drink a glass of water mixed with two teaspoons of the vinegar. Then apply full-strength apple cider vinegar to the varicosed veins.

Apples—A poultice of rotten apples was an old remedy for varicose ulcers.

Cabbage—Bind bruised cabbage leaves over ulcerated varicose veins.

Herbs—Drinking a daily cup of marjoram, sassafras, or white oak bark tea was considered helpful for varicose veins. Foot and leg baths or poultices of camomile, comfrey, elder, juniper berry, slippery elm, or white oak bark tea were used to relieve pain and itching. A compress made from a handful of mixed comfrey root, camomile, and sage, simmered for 15 minutes in a little water and wrapped in cloth, was also believed beneficial.

Hot and Cold Water—Alternating hot-and-cold foot or leg baths for 30 minutes twice each day is an effective treatment for eczema or ulcers resulting from varicosed veins. Beginning with two minutes hot and 30 seconds cold, then gradually increasing the cold-bath time to two minutes is recommended. When baths are not feasible, apply moist hot-and-cold towels alternately for 30 minutes, four times a day.

Marigold Flowers—Adding a few chopped, fresh marigold flowers to a daily salad was believed to nourish the veins.

Onions—Applying a poultice of minced brown onions was folk-therapy for slow-healing varicose ulcers.

Violet Leaves and Flowers—Place one handful crushed, fresh violet leaves and flowers in the foot-bath water, or use as a compress over distended veins.

Nerve Massage

Massage the pad under the little toe on the right foot. Then, massage both feet from just above the heel pad to the center of the arch.

Nerve Pressure

Press each point for 10 seconds, release for an equal length of time, and repeat for a total of 30 seconds pressure.

- Press the hinge of both jawbones, 1 inch in front of the ears.
- Press the breast muscle 2 inches toward the center of the chest from the right armpit.
- Press the outer aspects of each side of the pubic bone, 4 inches below the hipbones.

Stress

Some authorities believe emotional upsets involving suppressed anger cause excessive amounts of blood to surge into the leg because of a primitive urge to kick out when things go wrong. Kicking a pillow was Adelle Davis'[89] solution. Practicing relaxation techniques (pages 9-10) may also help release tension in the veins.

Sources (See Bibliography)

4, 9, 12, 13, 19, 25, 26, 34, 52, 53, 62, 64, 78, 80, 88, 89, 98, 142, 154, 168, 171, 173, 174, 181, 189, 190, 229, 241, 243, 252, 254, 256, 260, 261, 269, 274, 284, 288, 299, 301, 302, 303, 304, 305, 312, 315, 316.

VISION PROBLEMS (See Also Cataracts, Conjunctivitis, and Glaucoma)

Eyes are affected by emotions and environmental conditions as well as the nourishment with which they are supplied. Wearing protective goggles while working with high-speed electric tools or lawn mowers guards against eye injuries from flying particles of wood, metal, or stone. Many vision problems can be prevented, halted, or reversed by natural means, but regular examinations are wise, and any injury or continuing abnormality should have medical attention.

Twenty-five hundred years ago Hippocrates recommended raw liver to his patients with dimming vision. During the intervening ages, folk practitioners have used foods and herbs to treat visual disturbances. Sipping a mixture of two teaspoons each apple cider vinegar and raw honey in a glass of water with every meal is a folk remedy credited with preserving good eyesight well past old age. Today, nutritionally oriented ophthalmologists suggest vitamin and mineral supplementation in addition to corrective lenses.

Visual purple, a substance formed in the eyes from vitamin A, is essential for both day and night sight. It is used up, much in the manner of camera film, by nerve impulses relaying images to the brain and must be replenished from stored vitamin A while the eyes are closed. Persons who do close work or are exposed to bright light much of the time require exceptionally large amounts of this vitamin.

Every nutrient plays a role in eye health. Three or four months of nutritious diet with a multi-vitamin-mineral formula plus 25,000 to 50,000 units vitamin A and 50 to 100 milligrams zinc daily may retard or regress deterioration to make new glasses unnecessary.

A few seconds of daily nerve massage or nerve pressure have also proven successful in alleviating general vision problems.

- Starting at the outer corner of the eye and searching for tender spots, gently massage the curved bone above and surrounding the eye.
- Hook the index fingers under the jawbone just beneath each ear and pull forward for 10 seconds. Release for 10 seconds and repeat three times.
- Squeeze and massage the first two fingers and the webs between them on both hands. If only one eye is affected, massage the fingers on that side only.
- Press above the center of the foot where the ankle joins the bone of the leg. Release for 10 seconds, then repeat for a total of 30 seconds pressure on the side affected.
- Massage the pads beneath the second and third toes with two fingers while using the thumb to massage the top of the foot where the second and third toes begin. Repeat with the other foot if both eyes are involved.

Blurred and Dimmed Vision

Illness or nutritional deficiencies can reduce visual acuity. Fluctuations in blood-sugar levels can result in fuzzy or double vision which normalizes with proper sugar control (see Diabetes and Low Blood Sugar). Since the eyes are nourished by the body's blood supply, circulatory problems or High Blood Pressure (which see) may be responsible. Taking three tablespoons of lecithin granules daily has rectified some cases of dimming vision related to high cholesterol levels. Medical evaluation is indicated if the condition persists as it might be symptomatic of the increased ocular pressure of glaucoma.

Amblyopia (dim vision without organic reason), sometimes called tobacco blindness and attributed to smoking and alcohol consumption, has been corrected by massive amounts of vitamins B-1, B-12, and C. Vitamins A, B-2, and the balance of the B complex are needed for clear sight. Vitamin C helps maintain normal vision. Vitamin E protects both vitamin A and the retina of the eye. Even mild deficiencies of any of these vitamins can result in general dimming of sight. Suggested daily supplements:

Vitamin A—10,000 to 30,000 units
B Complex—One comprehensive tablet each morning and evening
B-2—5 to 250 milligrams
Vitamin C with Bioflavonoids—1,000 to 4,000 milligrams in divided doses
Vitamin E (see Caution, page 6)—100 to 400 IU each morning and evening

The supplements for dim vision usually improve blurred vision as well, but, in some cases, 50 to 200 milligrams B-6 plus 100 to 300 milligrams pantothenic acid are needed for correction. Taking four tablets of the tissue salt Calc. Fluor. four times a day in the 6X potency has been reported helpful. An equal dosage of Nat. Phos. is suggested for blurring that comes and goes.

Lack of exposure to natural outdoor light can cause the retina to become insensitive and vision to dim. Marilyn Rosanes-Berret[283] recommends stimulating the retina by sitting in direct sun with closed eyes (without glasses) and slowly turning the head from side to side. The time should gradually be increased from two minutes to 10 minutes—several short periods are believed better than one or two long ones. On cloudy days, an unshielded 150-watt light bulb can be substituted for sunlight.

Massaging the pads at the base of the second and third fingers on both hands a few seconds each day has improved dim vision for some individuals. Others have benefited from applying 30 seconds pressure, at 10 second intervals, to two points in the middle of the forehead above the inside corner of each eye.

Eye Strain

When eye strain persists despite an optometrist's assurance of correctly fitted lenses, natural remedies may resolve the problem. Supplements of vitamins A, E, and the entire B complex often help relieve eye strain. Visual fatigue has shown improvement within 24 hours after additional B-2 was taken.[189] Vitamin A frequently does away with the itching that accompanies eye strain. Calcium is important for controlling excessive watering and blinking.

Folk practitioners advised putting one drop of castor oil in each eye or bathing the eyes with strained camomile, fennel, or lemon grass tea. Other eye-washes used to invigorate tired eyes: one tablespoon Witch Hazel, one teaspoon honey or baking soda, or one-half teaspoon salt, each stirred in one cup water; or a half-and-half mixture of lukewarm milk and water. (Excessive eye-bathing can dilute tears and reduce their protective antibacterial action.[241]) Compresses of cooked mashed beets, grated raw potato, or moist slippery elm or pekoe tea leaves placed over closed eyes were other options.

Tension is another possible cause of eye strain. The relaxation techniques described on pages 9-10 plus these external remedies may provide relief.

- With the eyes closed, relax, and take 10 deep breaths. Then rotate the head around the shoulders three times each to the right and to the left.
- Cup the palms over the closed eyes for five minutes. When this is done several times each day, it is believed to keep eye muscles relaxed.

Nerve massage and nerve pressure offer alternative methods for alleviating eye strain.

- Use the thumbs to push up on the bone just under the beginning of each eyebrow above the nose. Press for 10 seconds, release for an equal length of time, and repeat for a total of three pressures.
- Firmly press the tips of the index and middle fingers on each hand for a few minutes daily.
- Tightly squeeze the knuckles of the first two fingers on both hands, applying pressure to upper and lower surfaces as well as sides, for five minutes at a time once each day. Rubber bands may be wound around the fingers for even pressure but should be removed the moment the fingers begin to turn blue.
- Massage the entire big toe, then rotate it—first left, then right—until it feels loose. If both eyes are affected, treat both big toes; otherwise, left toe for left eye, right toe for right eye.
- Massage the bottom of each foot, midway between the heel pad and the ball of the foot.

Farsightedness

Formerly regarded as an inescapable adjunct of aging, farsightedness has been treated with corrective lenses and witticisms regarding arms growing shorter. Many cases, however, have improved with vitamin supplementation and the remedies for blurred and dimmed vision (see above). Taking brewer's yeast, increasing the amount of protein in the diet, and eating one-fourth to one-half cup sunflower seeds daily has also been of help.

Floaters and Spots

A common complaint among adults, "floaters" are specks of opaque tissue floating in the transparent substance of the eyeball between lens and retina. They are considered harmless and usually become less noticeable with time. In some instances, floaters have disappeared after two months of daily supplementation with 50 milligrams of B-2. If these floaters are large enough to interfere with vision, an ophthalmologist may remove them surgically—or may prescribe high doses of vitamin D, calcium, choline, inositol, and the amino acid, methionine.

Case History

Jennifer N. had holes in her eyes. At least that was what she called the clear, blank spots that sometimes floated through her field of vision. The spots were beautiful—jaggedy-edged "holes," each surrounded with a little halo of light— but Jennifer seldom had time to admire their attractive qualities; the spots were a nuisance. She was a receptionist-secretary, the "holes" usually appeared just when she was busiest, and she couldn't "see through" them to read the copy from which she was typing. Thinking that glasses might solve the problem, she had her eyes checked. Jennifer didn't need glasses, was relieved by the doctor's explanation of her "floaters" (see paragraph above), and opted for postponing surgical removal until they became more serious. Then a fortuitous bit of serendipity occurred. Jennifer's new roommate so convincingly described the virtues of the vitamin supplements she unpacked onto a kitchen shelf that Jennifer decided to try some of them herself. After a month of supplementing her diet with a daily multiple-vitamin-mineral, 1,000 milligrams of vitamin C, a B-complex tablet, and a potent calcium-plus-A-and-D caplet, Jennifer came to a surprising realization. She no longer had "holes" in her eyes! How much of which vitamin did away with her floaters Jennifer will never know, because she is not about to discontinue her vitamin supplementation. Besides enjoying her newfound sense of well-being, Jennifer does not want to risk a recurrence of the "holes" in her eyes.

Dark spots in front of the eyes frequently respond to B-complex therapy but may be due to a lack of protein and require additional supplements of vitamins B-2, B-6, or C. Halos around bright lights or objects (if not associated with migraine headaches) may disappear with the same treatment. Light spots in the field of vision often vanish when 2,000 milligrams of vitamin C is taken each hour for 16 hours.[3] Although this amount of vitamin C is not toxic, the dosage may need to be reduced if diarrhea occurs.

Nearsightedness (Myopia)

Diet can be especially important in arresting or improving myopic conditions. Controlled hospital tests showed that enriching children's diets with additional protein halted the development of myopia and, in many cases, bettered vision.[261] In 1981, *Documenta Ophthalmologica* (Vol. 28) cited deficiencies of calcium and chromium, and an over-abundance of sugar as possible causes of myopia. Doctors have known for some time that diabetics with high blood sugar levels are prone to nearsightedness. They now are attributing much of the increased incidence of myopia to the extensive use of refined carbohydrates.[354] Carbonated beverages are suspect as contributing factors in nearsightedness. In addition to the sugar they contain, it appears that the carbonic acid can waterlog tissues in the eye, causing swelling and distortion that can result in myopia.[280]

The *American Journal of Ophthalmology* (May, 1950) stated that nearsightedness might be due to lack of vitamin A and calcium. (Folk medicine advises taking two teaspoons of apple cider vinegar in a glass of water with each meal to assist calcium absorption.) Vitamin D is necessary for the metabolization of calcium (which affects the strength of eye muscles). The addition of vitamin D alone has improved vision for nearsighted children and adults. The natural vitamin D from fish-liver oils is less toxic than the synthetic, irradiated form (ergosterol). Taking large amounts of vitamin C helps detoxify any excess from either form. Suggested daily supplements for myopic adults are:

Vitamin A—25,000 units
Vitamin C—500 to 1,000 milligrams with each meal
Calcium—800 to 2,000 milligrams
Chromium—100 to 250 micrograms (essential for carbohydrate metabolism)
Vitamin D (natural)—1,000 to 2,500 IU

Exposing the closed eyes to direct sunlight for a few minutes each day has helped myopia as well as dim vision. Daily eye exercises, such as those developed by William Horatio Bates during the 1920's and detailed in *Do You Really Need Eyeglasses?*[283] have been credited with regressing myopia.

Night Blindness

Adjustment to bright light is rapid but average eyes require about 10 minutes to adapt from bright to dim light. The efficiency of vitamin A as a specific for night blindness was well-publicized during World War II when carrots were added to the diets of airplane pilots. Diminished ability to see in dim light is an early-warning-sign of vitamin A deficiency which, if not corrected, can lead to blindness. Adequate, complete protein is essential for the body's assimilation of vitamin A. When night blindness is a problem, vegetarians in particular may be well-advised to analyze their protein intake. Continued exposure to sunlight can destroy the visual purple produced by the body from vitamin A. Extra supplements before a day at the beach or behind the wheel of a car may prevent temporary night blindness.

Other nutrients also are involved in night sight. A lack of vitamin B-2 may contribute to night blindness and the addition of zinc supplements has corrected some chronic cases. Studies conducted by the U.S. Department of Health, Education, and Welfare in 1974 showed that the carbon monoxide and nicotine in cigarette smoke reduces oxygen supply to the eyes and their ability to adapt to darkness. Vitamins B-15, C, and E are believed to help compensate for this reaction. Daily supplements suggested for adult night blindness:

Vitamin A—25,000 units
Vitamin B-2—10 to 100 milligrams, in two divided doses
Vitamin C with Bioflavonoids—1,000 to 3,000 milligrams in divided doses
Vitamin E (see Caution, page 6)—100 to 400 IU
Zinc—30 to 150 milligrams, in two divided doses

Sources (See Bibliography)

3, 4, 9, 24, 34, 38, 44, 52, 53, 61, 63, 64, 71, 72, 78, 88, 89, 98, 110, 128, 154, 156, 168, 171, 173, 176, 180, 189, 190, 192, 211, 226, 228, 229, 230, 236, 241, 244, 252, 254, 256, 261, 272, 276, 280, 283, 297, 311, 318, 333, 345, 353, 354.

WARTS AND MOLES

Most warts and moles are harmless happenstances but any bleeding, crusting, or sudden increase in size warrants medical attention. Common warts (verucca vulgaris) can occur on any part of the body and sometimes disappear by themselves if left alone. Believed caused by a virus (possibly related to herpes) that can be destroyed by the body's own antibodies, wart development may have a psychological factor since mental suggestion has effected cures. A plantar wart (verruca plantaris) on the bottom of the foot is often contagious and may be contracted or spread by walking barefoot in shower rooms or public areas. Forced by the weight of the body to grow up into the foot, a plantar wart may have a hard surface like a corn but has blood vessels and nerve endings, as all warts do. Relieving pressure on a plantar wart by padding the foot eases discomfort and speeds recovery. Attempting to remove warts by scraping or bathroom surgery could be dangerous. There are various medical and surgical methods of wart removal but none guarantee against recurrence.

Dietary Supplements

Many orthomolecular physicians favor stimulating the body's immune mechanism with vitamins A, C, and E to produce antibodies which will attack the wart virus. Both common and plantar warts have responded to these daily amounts for adults:

Vitamin A—30,000 to 100,000 units for four weeks, then reduced to 25,000 units. Most brown spots and flat moles are impervious to treatment, but dry, raised moles frequently flake away when oral supplements are accompanied by topical applications of natural vitamin A several times daily.

Vitamin C—1,000 to 10,000 milligrams in divided doses. Applying a paste of powdered vitamin C and water to warts each night for several months is said to remove even a plantar wart without leaving a crater.

Vitamin E (see Caution, page 6)—200 to 1,200 IU taken internally plus external applications of vitamin E from a pierced capsule twice each day. The favorite modern folk-remedy for warts, another option is to saturate the gauze portion of an adhesive bandage with vitamin E, cover the wart for 24 hours, then replace with a freshly saturated bandage.

Some warts have vanished after a few weeks of vitamin therapy, others have lingered for months. Adding 60 milligrams of zinc daily and/or taking three tablets of the 3X tissue salts Kali. Mur., Nat. Mur., and Silicea in alternate doses at four-hour intervals may hasten their disappearance. Plantar warts have reportedly been cured by taking 40,000 units of vitamin A daily plus three tablets of 6X Silicea three times during the day.

Case History

When Laura G. noticed the mole on her back she knew exactly what to do about it. Two years earlier she had had one in almost the same place, and, by following a friend's suggestion for treating it with vitamin A, had gotten rid of it in a month. For the next four weeks Laura dutifully rubbed her mole with vitamin

A each morning and evening, and added 25,000 units of carotene to her daily supplements. Nothing happened. This mole did not even begin to flake away as the first one had. Discouraged, Laura asked her friend for further advice, and was given a new clipping about warts and moles. According to this article, some warts and moles may look alike, but respond to different remedies. Feeling challenged by her stubborn mole-wart, Laura decided to try treating it with vitamin E before resorting to having it surgically removed. She covered it with vitamin E-saturated gauze and adhesive tape each morning. In addition to an extra 200 IUs of vitamin E, she took a 30-milligram zinc tablet every day and dissolved tissue-salt-pellets of Kali. Mur., Nat. Mur., and Silicea under her tongue every morning, noon, and night. Laura's efforts were rewarded. This mole must have been a wart because it did not flake away in tiny fragments; it simply vanished during her shower one morning!

Folk Remedies

Folk medicine wart-cures include practically everything, including talking them to death, and apparently are successful in direct proportion to patient faith in the treatment. When performed on a self-help basis, "wart charming" consists of simply telling the wart each day that it is no longer wanted and visualizing the affected area as being smooth and wart-free. An old English custom was to cut an apple in two, rub each half over the wart, tie the apple together, and bury it near a cemetery.

Aloe Vera Gel—Pat aloe gel over warts or moles three or four times each day or cover them with cotton saturated with the gel. Common warts often vanish in a few weeks but plantar warts may take six months.

Asparagus—Eat one-fourth cup cooked, pureed asparagus twice each day until the warts disappear.

Bacon—Secure a piece of bacon or salt pork over the wart each night.

Bandaging—Covering the wart with an air-tight bandage is a slow but apparently effective cure.

Carrots—Apply freshly grated raw carrot (mixed with olive oil, vitamin E, or table salt, if desired) several times during the day and bandage in place at night.

Castor Oil—There were several options for using this standard folk remedy. The wart or mole could be rubbed with the oil 20 times each night and morning, or gauze saturated with warm castor oil could be applied three times a day. For faster, possibly irritating results, a paste of baking soda and castor oil was to be rubbed on the wart for at least three successive evenings. Alternate applications of castor oil and cranberry have caused some moles to fade away.

Chile Pepper—According to Carolyn Niethammer's book, *American Indian Food and Lore* (Macmillan, 1974), Southwestern Indians bandaged slices of raw chile pepper over warts to drive them away.

Cod Liver Oil—Rubbing warts with cod liver oil every morning and evening has produced results in a few weeks.

Dandelion or Milkweed—Rub the milk from the cut end of dandelion or milkweed stems on the wart two or three times a day.

Figs or Papaya—Securing crushed, fresh figs or unripe papaya pulp against the warts is a Hindu remedy said to be effective within three months.

Garlic—Applying sliced raw garlic twice a day and eating garlic (or taking three garlic perles) daily is credited with curing warts in a month. A quicker, but painful, option was to apply a paste of garlic powder, cayenne pepper, and oil, then cover with an airtight bandage. The wart was to be lightly scraped each day before applying a fresh dressing.

Lemon—Squeeze a few drops of fresh lemon juice on the wart each morning and night. If desired, chopped raw onion may be placed over the wart for 10 minutes following the application of lemon juice. Other options are to soak the warts for 30 minutes each night in a mixture of lemon juice and warm water; or to steep fresh lemon rind in vinegar for 24 hours, then apply the inner side to the wart for three hours—repeating daily with a fresh lemon.

Liver—Taking three desiccated liver tablets three times each day is believed to build immunity to warts and cause existing ones to disappear after six months.

Marigold—The *Farmer's Almanack* for 1798 recommended applying crushed fresh marigold flowers to warts twice each day.

Peas—On the first day of a new moon, rub each wart with a different raw pea, wrap the peas in cloth, and throw them over the left shoulder. If a nine-pea pod can be obtained, rubbing it over the wart and throwing it away while chanting, "Wart, wart; fly away, fly away" is considered an infallible cure.

Potato or Radish—Rub the wart with sliced raw radish or white potato several times each day for two weeks. Chanting, "Go 'way" three times and burying the vegetable slices is said to improve the cure's effectiveness.

Raw Meat—Rub the wart with a piece of raw meat once or twice each day.

Soda and Vinegar—Keep the warts moist with a solution of baking soda and vinegar for 10 minutes three or four times a day. Cooperative warts can be expected to vanish within a few weeks.

Sources (See Bibliography)

13, 19, 28, 52, 53, 62, 68, 78, 84, 88, 89, 142, 152, 168, 174, 181, 201, 214, 226, 229, 251, 254, 260, 261, 277, 288, 305, 310, 311, 315, 316, 318, 325, 335, 345.

WORMS—TRICHINOSIS AND INTESTINAL WORMS

Body-inhabiting worms sound like part of a science-fiction scenario too horrendous to consider, but they are alive and residing—even in these twentieth-century, sanitary United States. Ringworm is a fungus infection rather than a worm, but the remainder of these revolting creatures persist in using humans as hosts. Modern medicine has progressed beyond folk cures, so professional help is advisable whenever worms are suspected. Natural preventives and remedies, however, can often augment orthodox treatment to avoid worm invasion or speed their departure.

Trichinosis—Caused by a roundworm, *trichinella spiralis,* it usually appears after eating raw or inadequately cooked pork, ham, sausage, or other pork products containing embryo parasites in dormant form. (Bear meat, also, has been found to contain trichina.) The best treatment is prevention. Pork should be well-cooked—to at least 170 degrees. Using a meat thermometer for oven roasts and cutting pork into serving-size portions for ease in turning during microwave cooking are precautionary measures.

The incubation period from the time inhabited pork is eaten until the onset of symptoms is from seven to 14 days. If trichinosis is suspected within two or three days, thoroughly cleansing stomach and bowels with purgatives, laxatives, and enemas may be helpful. Ingested larvae are liberated in the stomach and intestines where, in about three days, they reach adulthood. Trichinosis is not contagious, the worms do not lay eggs that pass out of the body. They produce great numbers of young worms that burrow into tissues, are transported by the blood, and finally become encysted in muscles where they may lie dormant for as long as 20 years. Embryo production continues for approximately six weeks. During this period there may be fever, chills, swollen eyelids, abdominal and muscular pain. Blood studies or a bit of muscle tissue (a biopsy) can confirm trichinosis at this stage. Standard treatment consists of bed rest, nutritious diet, ample fluids, hot baths, and painkillers. During the 1800's, taking one tablespoon oral glycerine or 100-proof alcohol each hour for eight hours on an empty stomach was believed to absorb fluid from the minute animal bodies, causing them to dry up and die.[142] (This should not be attempted without medical approval.) Once the parasites are encysted in muscles they no longer create obvious symptoms but may be responsible for some cases of neuritis.

Intestinal worms most often found in North America are pinworms, roundworms, hookworms, and tapeworms. Due to better control of water supplies and sewage, human infestation by these parasites is becoming less common. They appear in children more frequently than in adults and are more prevalent in tropical climates. The majority of worms that molest people are harbored in the intestines and transmitted through contamination of food, soil, or water by human feces. Neither children nor adults should go barefoot in suspected areas. Washing the hands before handling or eating food and after going to the toilet are routine measures of personal hygiene that help avoid fecal-borne worm infestation.

These parasitic creatures secure food from the contents of the intestine in which they live, or from the victim's blood. They rarely overwhelm their host but can create a variety of unpleasant symptoms and cause gradual weakening. Professional diagnosis is recommended as specific medications (vermifuges or anthelmintics) are required for each type of worm.

Hookworm—An ancient ailment known throughout the world, hookworm is still prevalent in some southern states. The source of infection is fecal contamination of soil. Occasionally larvae are introduced into the body through contaminated food or water but more commonly penetrate the skin, usually through the feet. Shoes should be worn in suspect areas—the pleasurable squish of mud between the toes creates an ideal opportunity for invaders. Inflammation and intense itching, called "ground itch" is the first symptom of their presence.

When larvae enter the body through the skin they tunnel into a blood vessel and are carried to the lungs, where they may produce a lung inflammation sometimes mistaken for pneumonia. They then travel up the bronchial tubes to the throat, are swallowed, and finally reach the intestines where they grow into adult hookworms fastened to the lining of the bowel. It takes about six weeks for larvae to become egg-laying adults after penetrating the skin. If acquired by mouth, their progress is much more rapid.

An adult hookworm, ¼ to ½ inch long, "hooks" itself to an intestinal wall and feeds from the host's blood, taking up to ½ cc. each day. Hookworms excrete a toxic substance that may burst small blood vessels to which they are attached, then prevent the released blood from coagulating. The 15,000 eggs laid daily by each female are excreted in bowel movements where their presence makes positive diagnosis possible. Hookworm infestation is rarely fatal but, if not corrected, anemia caused by blood loss can make the victim an invalid, retard children's growth, and create heart problems. "Strongyloides," a different and less common worm, produces similar effects and can be evicted by the same means. Without treatment, about 90 percent of the worms will be eliminated within a year or two; complete eradication can take up to seven years.[288]

Pinworms (oxyuriasis)—Also called seatworms or threadworms, these are the most common parasitic nematodes—frequently infesting children in temperate climates. The tiny, white, threadlike worms can be carried into the mouth on contaminated fingers or toys or may enter the body through contact of hands or bare feet with polluted soil. (Filariasis, a rare threadworm, is insect borne.) The worms are from ⅛ to ½ inch long and as many as 5,000 at one time may inhabit the lower bowel. They do not burrow into tissues, but occasionally migrate to the appendix or vagina. The female worm lays thousands of eggs at once in the tender skin at the anal orifice, causing intense itching. A worm that cannot find its way back to the bowel may occasionally be found on bed linen or underwear.

Scrupulous personal hygiene is necessary to prevent anything that touches the anus from conveying pinworm eggs and larvae to the mouth. Antiseptic, soothing ointments may ease itching, but, if pinworms are discovered, it is advisable for all household members to be treated. Even family pets can become infested and disperse the infection if they defecate in sandboxes or other areas where children play.

Roundworms (ascariasis)—Large, white worms that infest the intestinal tract; females may grow to 15 inches, but an average roundworm is 6 inches in length and the thickness of an ordinary lead pencil. Roundworms are exceedingly prolific—one female can lay 200,000 eggs a day. These eggs are excreted in the feces, then develop on the moist soil of unsanitary regions. They return to human intestines by ingestion of unwashed root vegetables, or from touching contaminated objects and placing soiled fingers in the mouth.

The roundworm's normal habitat is the small intestine where it maintains position by pushing against opposite sides of the walls. A few roundworms may not produce any symptoms or may be mistaken for allergy. A large number may cause intestinal obstruction or appear to be a tumor. They may wander through the body plugging up the Eustachian tube from throat to ear, the common bile duct, or appendix, and have even been responsible for hemorrhagic pneumonia. Effective prescriptive medications for their expulsion can be prescribed after diagnosis has been made from eggs or worms found in the stools.

Tapeworm—There are four kinds of these nightmarish creatures: beef *(taenia saginata),* fish *(diphyllobothrium latum),* pork *(taenia solium),* dwarf *(hymenolepis nana).* Tapeworms are long, flat worms consisting of a head followed by a ribbon-like string of segments. The head has little hooks or sucking disks which attach to the bowel lining. Each worm is supplied with male and female reproductive organs and each segment is usually capable of producing both eggs and additional segments.

The dwarf tapeworm, seldom over ½ inch long, is common among children in the southern United States. It enters the mouth from environmental contamination by human or animal feces. Other tapeworms are acquired by eating raw or insufficiently cooked meats containing embryos. Salting or smoking does not destroy larvae, but thorough cooking does. Beef tapeworms may grow to a length of 30 feet but have no hooklets so are dislodged with comparative ease when appropriate medication is taken. Fish tapeworms are rare in America but infest fresh-water fish in many parts of the world. Pork tapeworm larvae are usually in the neck, tongue, and shoulders of infected swine but human infestation is uncommon in this country.

Tapeworms may produce abdominal distress and appendicitis-like symptoms, ravenous appetite and false hunger pains despite weight loss, bowel obstruction, diarrhea, anemia, general weakness, and nervousness. Diagnosis is made from microscopic examination of stools.

Whipworm (trichuriasis)—Found primarily in the Gulf Coast region, whipworms are 1½ to 2 inches long, live chiefly in human intestines, and are evicted by the same means as hookworms or tapeworms. They enter through the mouth as eggs from fecal contamination of soil. Whipworms produce large numbers of eggs—as many as 1,000 worms have been found in one person.[312] They may retard growth or cause appendicitis symptoms in children; induce diarrhea, nausea, and anemia in adults. The worms are usually detected by being passed in the stools.

Diet and Supplements

Although infestation by intestinal parasites is relatively common, there are no official studies showing the efffect of dietary improvement on their hosts. However, laboratory tests have shown that animals with deficiencies of protein, vitamins A, B-1, B-2, biotin, folic acid, or other nutrients were infested with many types of worms, including trichina. If the worms were destroyed by medication but the diets not improved, the animals died from intestinal infection. When these same parasites were implanted in animals on optimum diets, infestations did not occur.[89] Research does indicate that humans with adequate diets have greater resistance to intruders in their systems and that, when any type of parasite invades, the diet should be unusually nutritious.

Normal stomach acids can often destroy many parasites picked up from infested foods. Reinforcing these acids with betaine HCL tablets or apple cider vinegar may be advisable, particularly when in areas subject to worm infestation. Yogurt, acidophilus milk, and acidophilus capsules encourage growth of beneficial bacteria in the intestines to fend off invaders. Since pinworms and many other parasites thrive on sugar, reducing the amount of refined carbohydrates and soft drinks is recommended.[254] Taking additional vitamin A may help prevent secondary infections. Folklore advises drinking carrot juice and eating generous amounts of apples, cherries, peaches, rhubarb, rutabagas, and water chestnuts to help dislodge worms.

Folk Remedies

Potent vermifuges favored by folk practitioners are no longer available. Pink hydrastin, santonin, extract of spigelia, and worm-seed are as difficult to come by as the metal flakes from a blacksmith's anvil. Some of the kitchen-medicines, however, have borne the test of time and many are still being used, either as the sole treatment or to augment medical prescriptions.

Berries—Fresh black raspberries, strawberries, or huckleberries, eaten with each meal for three consecutive days, was a worm-remedy for children.

Birch Bark or Elm Bark—One-eighth teaspoon dried, powdered birch bark taken before breakfast was believed to get rid of worms. If necessary, a second dose could be taken in two weeks. Solid pieces of elm bark were soaked in water, bits of the bark chewed during the day and the liquid sipped. The elm bark treatment was used for tapeworms or hookworms because the thick mucilage from the bark was thought to loosen the worm's grasp. One or two tablespoons of turpentine and castor oil were to be taken to speed the worm's passage. This bark treatment was to be continued for several days after any worm portions were seen in the evacuations.

Coconut—Fresh coconut, including the milk, is a general vermifuge in India where it is considered particularly effective against tapeworms.

Garlic—Employed by ancient Babylonians, Chinese, Greeks, Romans, and Hindus, garlic is the original natural remedy for worms. Garlic-oil capsules are believed as effective as fresh garlic and may be used as alternatives to eating minced garlic or squeezing it into tomato juice with a garlic press. For children who refused to swallow garlic, an old method of medication was to place peeled garlic cloves in their shoes. As the child walked, the garlic was crushed, the worm-killing oil absorbed by the skin, then carried by the blood to the intestines. For pinworms, several large garlic bulbs were chopped and simmered in two cups of water until the liquid was reduced to one cup. A few tablespoons of the infusion were injected into the rectum on three successive nights.

Case History

Allison D. had been at their summer cabin for less than a week when little Allie displayed symptoms of pinworms. Not wanting to make the long trip back to the city for medical diagnosis and treatment, Allison decided to take the advice of a neighboring camper and try garlic as a remedy. As she attempted to grate a clove of garlic so she could conceal it in her daughter's vegetables, the garlic clove slipped out of her fingers and landed close to Allie. The toddler plopped the garlic in her mouth, chewed it up, and swallowed it with obvious enjoyment. Surprised but relieved at the ease of "administering the medication," Allison gave Allie a lot of garlic—either by itself or mashed and spread on buttered bread—during the following days. No one wanted to get too close to Allie because of her "garlic breath," but the natural remedy was successful. When they returned to the city, Allie's pediatrician could detect no traces of pinworms.

Herbs—Teas made from chaparral, parsley, or sage were thought to expel worms when taken before breakfast and several times during the day. Dried sage was mixed with honey or molasses and taken in frequent doses of one teaspoon each. Drinking strong spearmint tea and injecting a small amount in the bowel every night for one week was another option. Tea made from peach tree leaves and flowers was given to children with round or pinworms.

Milk and Honey—Drinking warm milk sweetened with honey was believed to "turn" worms, especially if a little alum was added to the mixture.

Onions—There are several options for utilizing the worm-destroying capabilities credited to onions. Chop one large onion into a glass of water and let stand overnight. Strain, then drink the liquid before breakfast. Or, layer minced onions with sugar, let stand at least eight hours, then take the liquid in teaspoonful doses. Or, cook onions in milk and take one teaspoonful each night and morning.

Papaya Seeds—Chewing and swallowing one tablespoon fresh or dried papaya seeds on an empty stomach was thought to expel worms. The dosage should be repeated several times.

Pineapple Juice—Fresh pineapple juice is used as an anthelmintic in India and South America. Its protein-digesting enzymes are believed to digest and destroy intestinal parasites.

Pomegranate—Both the dried rinds and the root bark have been employed in the treatment of tapeworms since ancient times. (The rinds are easier to acquire and are considered more effective.) Two heaping teaspoons of dried, finely ground pomegranate rind are to be simmered with two cups water in a porcelain or glass utensil for 30 minutes. After fasting for 12 to 24 hours, one-fourth cup of the strained liquid should be taken each hour for six hours. For best results, a laxative should follow the last dose. The treatment is to be continued for two more days, stopped for three days, then repeated for three days.

Pumpkin Seeds—A standard folk remedy for tapeworms, pumpkin (or winter squash or large, ripe cucumber) seeds may be used either fresh or dried, eaten plain or taken in "emulsions." The outer hulls of pumpkin or squash seeds should be removed by soaking in hot water, then 4 ounces of the seeds taken in three divided doses an hour apart on an empty stomach. (Children should have 1 ounce of the dried seeds.) If desired, the seeds can be ground or pulverized, mixed with half their amount of sugar, and stirred in one pint of warm water.

Another option is to make a syrup from brown sugar or honey and ground seeds, then flavor with cinnamon. A laxative should be taken one hour after the last dose of pumpkin seeds. If necessary, the treatment can be repeated for four or five days.

Salt—Drinking strong salt water and heavily salting all food for a week or two has been known to evict pinworms. Eating garlic at the same time is recommended.

Sulphur and Lard—Combining sulphur powder (available in pharmacies) with lard and smearing over the rectal (plus vaginal, for girls) area often hastens the demise of pinworms.

Tobacco—When fresh tobacco leaves are available, take a strong laxative, then pound the tobacco leaves with honey and lay them on the abdomen.

Sources (See Bibliography)

13, 19, 27, 52, 59, 69, 73, 81, 89, 98, 142, 152, 156, 176, 184, 226, 227, 254, 261, 288, 297, 312, 315, 318.

WOUNDS—ABRASIONS, CUTS, LACERATIONS, PUNCTURES
(See Also Bedsores, Burns, and Varicose Ulcers)

Current medical advice is to cleanse all wounds with cold water and, if possible, wash surrounding areas with soap and water to avoid contamination of the injury. An abrasion (outer layer of skin scraped away) seldom bleeds profusely but benefits from chilling before bandaging. Cuts, lacerations (torn or jagged-edged wounds that may have crushed tissue), and puncture wounds from nails or other pointed objects usually bleed freely. A small amount of bleeding brings healing cells to the site but excessive bleeding should be stopped by applying pressure with sterile gauze or clean cloth. (An ice cube wrapped in the cloth slows blood flow.) Adults can lose as much as a pint of blood without serious effect. "Pressure points" and tourniquets went out of vogue after World War II. A tourniquet (which, if improperly applied, can cause loss of a limb) should be used only in cases of arterial bleeding that can be controlled no other way.

The value of antiseptics is being questioned since those strong enough to kill germs could also destroy human cells responsible for preventing infection and healing wounds. After the wound is dry, its edges should be pressed together and secured with a gauze-centered adhesive bandage. Longer cuts may require strips of adhesive tape trimmed into dumbbell or butterfly shapes—with the narrow centers across the incision. To lessen pain: injured hands or feet can be soaked in ice water for 10 minutes before bandaging, other wounds covered with ice in a plastic bag after the tape is applied. A moderately tight bandage, an ice pack, or elevating the injured part above heart level helps stop blood seepage. Extensive wounds, especially on the face, or those caused by rusty metal or an object recently in contact with unclean substances that might cause tetanus, should have immediate medical attention.

Case History

Five-year-old Bret and his friend Tom were having a great time playing under the sprinkler. When Tom's mother reminded them that Bret was to have gone home at 5, and it was now 5:10, Bret grabbed his towel in one hand, his shoes in the other, ran down the alley, and rushed into his kitchen—leaving a trail of bloody footprints. Bret admitted that he had stepped on something sharp, but did not feel any pain until his mother cleansed the cut and pulled out a thin piece of glass. She filled a pan with ice cubes and water, told Bret to soak his foot until the pain went away, then applied a bandage, and considered the accident to be merely another vicissitude of a small boy's existence. The next morning, however, there was a red spot on Bret's instep, and, fearing blood poisoning, she took him to the doctor. After examining the cut and extracting another piece of curved glass, the doctor gave Bret a tetanus shot and suggested a continual soaking of the foot in a warm solution of epsom salts. Apparently Bret had stepped on a broken light bulb and any attempt to surgically remove the remaining fragment might result in permanent damage to his foot. Bret's father brought home a miniature lounge chair so Bret could soak his foot in comfort while he watched TV. Bret's mother supplied cookies and soft drinks to the children who came to play board games with the invalid. During the nights, they took turns in replenishing the epsom-salts pack under the heating pad wrapped around Bret's foot. Gradually the red spot on his instep diminished; after a seemingly endless month, an inch-long sliver of glass emerged from the cut, and the combination of professional care plus a home remedy was a complete success.

Diet and Supplements

Any sudden injury creates a stress situation within the body, withdraws nutritional reserves, and causes tremendous amounts of protein to break down. After a severe wound, the diet should be exceptionally high in protein, with at least 1,000 additional daily calories obtained to allow this protein to be used for forming new tissue rather than for caloric needs. When much blood has been lost, milk, buttermilk, yogurt, eggnogs, and juices are recommended in preference to tea or coffee as they help rebuild both blood and tissue. Milk and egg yolks also contain amino acids required by newly formed tissue. All nutrients aid in forming new cells for healing. Supplementary vitamins and minerals can accelerate recuperation.

   Vitamin A—25,000 to 100,000 units daily for a week or two. Vitamin A helps prevent infection and assists vitamin C in forming new tissue. For those who have been taking cortisone (which depletes the body's store of vitamin A and hinders healing), vitamin A supplementation is particularly important.

   B Complex—One comprehensive, high-potency tablet once or twice daily. Besides combating the stress of injury, B vitamins such as B-2, B-6, and folic acid are needed for rapid healing. Taking up to 1,600 milligrams pantothenic acid daily for one or two weeks following severe injuries helps avoid adrenal exhaustion.

   Vitamin C—500 to 1,000 milligrams each hour or two for a few days, then gradually reduced. The amount of vitamin C varies with severity of the injury and individual tolerance. Wound healing requires formation of connective tissue which, although made of protein, cannot be synthesized in the body without vitamin C. Hundreds of studies have shown that resistance to infection, speed of recovery, and strength of new tissue is dependent upon the amount of vitamin C obtained. Taking 1,000 to 3,000 milligrams of bioflavonoids each day increases absorption and efficiency of vitamin C as well as helping strengthen new tissues.

Calcium—Restorative tissue depends on calcium as well as vitamin C and protein. If the equivalent of at least one quart of milk is not obtained daily, calcium supplements may encourage healing.

Vitamin E (see page 6)—200 to 800 IU daily, taken internally, plus vitamin E oil rubbed on the wound each day. Vitamin E protects cells from harm when blood vessels have been cut, promotes formation of new tissue, and prevents contraction so permanent scars do not form.

Tissue Salts

- To mitigate bleeding and shock, take one each 6X Ferr. Phos. and Kali. Phos. at 10-minute intervals until bleeding subsides. A dressing saturated with a solution of three tablets each of these two tissue salts dissolved in one-half cup warm water is often helpful and can be renewed through the bandage without removing it.

- If the injury is swollen, take three or four doses of 6X Kali. Mur.
- If the wound is festering, take three daily doses of 6X Calc. Sulph. and Silicea.

Zinc—150 milligrams in three divided doses daily for a week or two, then gradually reduced. Zinc helps mobilize stored vitamin A and build proteins needed for forming new skin and tissue.

Folk Remedies

Aloe Vera—Cover the injury with aloe vera gel or with a dethorned section of a split leaf secured with a bandage.

Case History

In the dusky twilight Olivia J. tripped over the curb in front of her daughter's home. Feeling more embarrassment than pain, she scrambled to her feet and walked into the house with blood dripping through her torn stocking from knee to ankle. Olivia's daughter feared the wound warranted a trip to the hospital emergency room, but her mother insisted that a bandage would be sufficient until she saw her doctor for her regular appointment the following day. After cleansing and disinfecting the wound, and an ineffectual search for gauze or a bandage large enough to cover the bleeding shin, they decided to use a dethorned leaf of the aloe vera plant in the kitchen window. The throbbing discomfort Olivia was beginning to feel was relieved by the cooling aloe gel, and when her medical appointment had to be postponed for two days, she simply taped on fresh leaves from the supply her daughter had given her. The doctor was startled at the sight of the aloe leaf taped to Olivia's leg. Apologetically, she explained about the accident and the excuse for using aloe; then she asked the doctor what medication she *should* apply to speed healing and prevent scarring. He removed the aloe leaf, carefully examined the extensive wound, and just as carefully retaped the long green leaf. With a twinkle in his eye, the doctor stated in his most professional manner, "Your wound is healing beautifully, nothing I could suggest would be any more effective. My recommendation is that you continue with the present treatment."

Alum—Binding wounds with cloth squeezed out of a weak alum-and-water solution was believed to hasten healing.

Apple Cider Vinegar—For slow-healing wounds, folk practitioners advised stirring two teaspoons apple cider vinegar in a half or whole glass of water six times a day, sponging one spoonful over the injury and drinking the remainder. To subdue inflamed wounds, the vinegar was poured into warm milk to make curds which were applied externally at frequent intervals.

Bacon—Covering cuts with moldy bacon was an old-fashioned remedy also used as a specific for drawing infection from puncture wounds. (Scientists have found that bacon mold is a relative of penicillin.[310])

Baking Soda—Washing an open wound with a solution of two tablespoons soda and one teaspoon apple cider vinegar stirred in one cup warm water was the conservative treatment. Hardier individuals doused the area with cold soda water and sprinkled black pepper over the wound.

Bread—Soak bread or breadcrumbs in boiling beer, milk, or water for five minutes. Spread over the wound after draining any excess liquid.

Butter—Rub unsalted butter or Vaseline with minced fresh catnip or parsley leaves. Sugar may be included, if desired. Smooth over skinned knees or similar injuries.

Cabbage—Place bruised raw cabbage leaves, boiled cabbage, or fresh cabbage juice over the wound and secure with a bandage. Replace every four hours. Juliette de Bairacli Levy reported in *Health Quarterly Plus Two* (Vol. 2, No. 1, 1977) that Gypsies in Israel tied whole cabbage leaves over wounds to draw out impurities. The leaves were replaced when they darkened but were removed at night.

Carrots—Possibly because of their high vitamin-A content, carrots have long been a favorite wound-healing remedy. Minced raw carrots were applied to fresh wounds. Cooked carrots, mashed with a little oil to prevent hardening, (or made into a paste with flour and unsalted butter) were used to cover injuries. Open or infected wounds were bathed with liquid from carrots cooked in milk, then poulticed with the mashed vegetable. A salve for all kinds of wounds was made by simmering carrot juice until it was the consistency of thick syrup.

Comfrey Tea—Drinking strong comfrey tea and/or applying tea-saturated cloths or a poultice of moist tea leaves was the herbalists' remedy. (Comfrey contains allantoin, a cell-proliferating substance that speeds wound healing.[215])

Cottage Cheese—To promote healing of minor cuts or scratches, cover with cottage cheese.

Cucumber—European folk healers apply ripe cucumber juice to small, open wounds.

Eggs—For minor cuts, apply the moist surface of the inside coating (skin) of a raw or boiled egg. For more serious wounds, beat one cup each apple cider vinegar and turpentine into one beaten egg and sponge over the injury.

Flour—To stanch the flow of blood, cover cuts with a handful of flour, or a paste of flour, salt, and vinegar.

Garlic—An ancient medication for controlling infection and healing wounds, minced raw garlic, applied externally, was used with success during World War I. Pressed garlic or garlic juice mixed with raw honey or water is also effective. Eating garlic (or taking garlic capsules) often augments external treatment.

Geranium Leaves—For abrasions, bind crushed, fresh geranium leaves over the raw skin.

Honey—A remedy for wounds since earliest recorded times, the bacteria-fighting capabilities of raw honey are now medically recognized. (Hospitals have used it with dry bandages for awkwardly placed wounds.[86]) Honey does not stick to the skin and the dressings do not adhere to the wounds. Folk practitioners have combined bee pollen with honey, or prepared an ointment by mixing equal parts of honey and flour with a little water, to accelerate healing. When raw honey is not available, black molasses or granulated sugar can be substituted. All these substances draw moisture from infected wounds and surrounding tissues to help destroy inflammation-producing bacteria.

Jojoba Oil—Now available in pharmacies or health food stores, jojoba has a long history as a wound healer. As recorded by Carolyn Niethammer in *American Indian Food and Folklore* (Macmillan, 1974), a Jesuit priest wrote in 1763 that southern California's Cahuilla Indians placed jojoba fruit in arrow wounds and spread jojoba oil on cuts to prevent swelling and speed healing.

Lemon—Squeezing juice from a fresh lemon over a wound was believed to disinfect and help heal it.

Oatmeal—Stir boiling water into dry oatmeal to make a thick paste. Spread between pieces of gauze and cover the wound.

Onions—A kitchen-medicine favorite, raw or cooked onions were minced, grated, sliced, or mashed, then applied directly to wounds. Poultices were made from chopped, roasted onions mixed with diced salt pork or bacon, or by blending boiled onions with bread crumbs and warm milk. For minor wounds, a salve of mashed onions, honey, and apple cider vinegar was used.

Papaya—Applying slices of fresh papaya to stem the flow of blood from cuts or to clear infected wounds is a treatment adopted from African folk healers by modern health professionals.

Peach Tree Leaves—To ease painful wounds, steep a handful of fresh peach tree leaves in one cup boiling water for 10 minutes. Mash the leaves and apply as hot as can be borne.

Potato—Grated raw potato, applied either hot or cold, was used to prevent infection and hasten recovery.

Pumpkin Seeds—Pulverized dried, unsalted, shelled pumpkin seeds have been used as successful healing agents.

Salt—Binding salt over open cuts is a centuries-old remedy.

Slippery Elm Tea—For an updated version of an American Indian treatment for wounds, stir dry slippery elm tea with hot water to make a paste. Spread between pieces of gauze and apply to the injury. Renew several times with freshly prepared poultices.

Spider Webs—Placing spider webs across an open cut is said to stop bleeding; even cobwebs have been used with the spider webs to stanch blood flow from massive lacerations.[121] Some folk practitioners recommend cleansing wounds with turpentine before applying the webs.

Tobacco—In the days of roll-your-own cigarettes, wet tobacco or a dampened cigarette paper was used to halt bleeding from a cut.

Turnip—For slow-healing, open wounds, apply scraped or grated raw turnip every four hours, night and day, until healing has obviously commenced.

Turpentine or Kerosene—Both were standard remedies for cleansing wounds and relieving their pain. To halt bleeding or prevent infection, brown sugar mixed with turpentine or kerosene was bound over the wound. Sponging the area with turpentine makes skin sufficiently transparent for imbedded slivers to be seen and removed.

Sources (See Bibliography)

3, 4, 5, 7, 8, 24, 27, 28, 62, 68, 69, 73, 78, 81, 86, 88, 89, 91, 98, 111, 121, 142, 152, 156, 165, 174, 190, 215, 226, 227, 228, 229, 241, 252, 256, 260, 276, 293, 297, 301, 305, 310, 315, 318, 324, 330, 333, 335, 345, 350.

BIBLIOGRAPHY

1   Aagaard, Orlena, *Tasty Cooking for Ulcer Diets,* Crown, 1969

2   Abrahamson, E.M. and Pezet, A.W., *Body, Mind and Sugar,* Pyramid, 1971

3   Adams, Rex, *Miracle Medicine Foods,* Parker, 1977

4   Adams, Ruth and Murray, Frank, *Complete Home Guide to Vitamins,* Larchmont, 1978 edition

5   _____*Health Foods,* Larchmont, 1975

6   _____*Improving Your Health with Vitamin A,* Larchmont, 1978

7   _____*Improving Your Health with Vitamin C,* Larchmont, 1978

8   _____*Improving Your Health with Calcium and Phosphorus,* Larchmont, 1978

9   _____*Is Low Blood Sugar Making You a Nutritional Cripple?,* Larchmont, 1975

10   Aero, Rita, *The Complete Book of Longevity,* Putnam, 1980

11   Aihara, Herman, *Acid and Alkaline,* George Ohsawa Macrobiotic Found., 1980 edition

12   Airola, Paavo, *Health Secrets from Europe,* Parker, 1970

13   _____*How to Get Well,* Health Plus, 1974

14   _____*Sex and Nutrition,* Health Plus, 1970

15   _____*Stop Hair Loss,* Health Plus, 1965

16   Albright, Peter and Elizabeth, *Body, Mind and Spirit,* Stephen Greene, 1980

17   Alexander, Dale, *Arthritis and Common Sense,* Simon and Schuster, 1954

18   Allen, Oliver E. and editors, *Secrets of Good Digestion,* Time-Life, 1982

19   Anderson, Clifford R., *Modern Ways to Health,* Southern Publishers Assn., 1962

20   Anderson, James W., *Diabetes: A Practical New Guide to Healthy Living,* Arco, 1981

21   Andron, Michael, *Reflex Balance: A Foot and Hand Book for Health,* New York, 1980

22   Ashmead, DeWayne (editor), *Chelated Mineral Nutrition in Plants, Animals and Man,* Charles C. Thomas, 1982

23   Atkins, Robert C., *Dr. Atkins' Diet Revolution,* Bantam Books, 1973

24   _____*Dr. Atkins' Nutrition Breakthrough,* Perigord, 1981

25   Bailey, Herbert, *Vitamin E, Your Key to a Healthy Heart,* ARC Books, 1971 ed.

26   Baron, Howard C. with Gorin, Edward, *Varicose Veins,* William Morrow, 1979

27   Beeton, Isabella, *Book of Household Management,* S.O. Beeton, London, 1861

28   Benham, Jack and Sarah, *Rocky Mountain Receipts and Remedies,* Reporter Printing, 1966

29   Bennet, Hal Zina, *Cold Comfort,* Clarkson N. Potter, 1979

30   _____*The Doctor Within,* Clarkson N. Potter, 1981

31   Bennet, Iva and Simon, Martha, *The Prudent Diet,* David White, 1973

32   Benson, Herbert with Klipper, Miriam Z., *The Relaxation Response,* William Morrow, 1975

33   Bergeron, Victor, *Trader Vic's Bartender's Guide,* Doubleday, 1972 edition

34   Bergson, Anika and Tuchak, Vladimir, *Zone Therapy,* Pinnacle Books, 1974

35   Berkley, George, *Arthritis Without Aspirin,* Prentice-Hall, 1982

36   Bernhardt, Roger and Martin, David, *Self-Mastery Through Self-Hypnosis,* Bobbs-Merrill, 1977

37   Bieler, Henry G., *Food Is Your Best Medicine,* Random House, 1965

38   Biermann, June and Toohey, Barbara, *The Diabetic's Book,* Houghton Mifflin, 1981

39   Blaine, Tom R., *Goodby Allergies,* Citadel, 1968

40   Blanc, Albert D.G., *So You Have Asthma!,* Charles C. Thomas, 1966

41   Bland, Jeffery, *Your Health Under Siege,* Stephen Greene, 1981

42   Blauer, Stephen, *Rejuvenation,* Hippocrates Health Institute, 1980

43   Boericke, William and Dewey, Willis, *The 12 Tissue Remedies of Schuessler,* Harjeet

44   Bogert, L. Jean, *Nutrition and Physical Fitness,* W.B. Saunders, 1960, 7th ed.

45   Bootzin, Richard R., *Behavorial Self-Management,* Brunner/Mazel, 1977

46   Boyd, Nathaniel Welsher, III, *Stay Out of the Hospital,* Dorrance, 1976

47   Brady, William, *An Eighty-Year-Old Doctor's Secrets of Positive Health,* Prentice-Hall, 1961

48   Brennan, R.O. with Mulligan, William C., *Nutrigenetics, New Concepts for Relieving Hypoglycemia,* Signet, 1977

49   Brennan, Richard O. with Hosier, Helen Kooiman, *Coronary? Cancer? God's Answer: Prevent it,* Harvest House, 1979

50   Brewer, Gail Sforza and Brewer, Tom, *What Every Pregnant Woman Should Know: The Truth About Diets and Drugs in Pregnancy,* Random House, 1977

51   Bricklin, Mark, *The Natural Healing Cookbook,* Rodale, 1981

52   _____*The Practical Encyclopedia of Natural Healing,* Rodale, 1976

53   _____*Rodale's Encyclopedia of Natural Home Remedies,* Rodale, 1982

54   Brody, Jane, *Jane Brody's Nutrition Book,* Bantam Books, 1982

55   Bronfen, Nan, *Nutrition for a Better Life,* Capra, 1980

56   Butler, Pamela E., *Talking to Yourself,* Stein & Day, 1981

57   Buxbaum, Robert and Micheli, Lyle J., *Sports for Life*, Beacon, 1979

58   Cameron, Ewan and Pauling, Linus, *Cancer and Vitamin C*, Warner Books, 1981

59   Cameron, Myra, *The GNC Gourmet Vitamin Cookbook*, Keats, 1980

60   Carey, G.W., *The Biochemic System of Medicine*, Biochemic Publications

61   Carey, Geo. W., *The 12 Cell Salts of the Zodiac*, Health Research

62   Carroll, David, *The Complete Book of Natural Medicines*, Summit, 1980

63   Carter, Mildred, *Hand Reflexology: Key to Perfect Health*, Parker, 1975

64   _____*Helping Yourself with Foot Reflexology*, Parker, 1969

65   Cayce, Hugh Lynn, editor, *Edgar Cayce on Diet and Health*, Coronet Comm., 1969

66   Challem, Jack Joseph, *Vitamin C Updated*, Keats, 1982

67   Chan, Pedro, *Finger Acupressure*, Ballantine, 1974

68   Chapman, Esther, *How to Use the 12 Tissue Salts*, Pyramid, 1971

69   Chase, A.W., *Dr. Chase's Recipes, Information for Everybody*, Ann Arbor, 1866

70   Cheraskin, E. and Ringsdorf, W.M., *New Hope for Incurable Diseases*, Exposition Press, 1971

71   Cheraskin, E; Ringsdorf, W.M. and Brecher, Arline, *Psychodietics*, Stein & Day, 1974

72   Cheraskin, E; Ringsdorf, W.M. and Sisley, Emily L., *The Vitamin C Connection*, Harper Row, 1983

73   Child, Mrs., *The American Frugal Housewife*, Carter, Hendee & Co., 1835

74   Cilentro, Lady, *You Don't Have to Live With: Chronic Ill Health*, Whitcombe & Tombs, Australia, 1977

75   Clark, Linda, *Get Well Naturally*, Arco, 1968

76   _____*Handbook of Natural Remedies for Common Ailments*, Devin-Adair, 1976

77   _____*How to Improve Your Health*, Keats, 1979

78   _____*Know Your Nutrition*, Keats, 1981 edition

79   Cleave, T.L., *Peptic Ulcer, Causation, Prevention and Arrest*, John Wright & Sons, 1962

80   _____*The Saccharine Disease*, Keats, 1978

81   Coleman, Lester D., *All Your Medical Questions Answered*, Good Housekeeping Books, 1977

82   Collins, R. Douglas, *What Every Patient Should Know About His Health and His Doctor*, Exposition Press, 1973

83   Consumer Reports editors, *The Medicine Show*, Pantheon Books, 1980 edition

84   Cooley, Donald G., *After-40 Health and Medical Guide*, Meredith Corp., 1980

85   Coon, Nelson, *Using Plants for Healing*, Rodale, 1979 revised edition

86   Crane, Eva, *A Book of Honey*, Charles Scribner's Sons, 1980

87   Davis, Adelle, *Let's Cook It Right*, Harcourt Brace, 1974 edition

88   _____*Let's Eat Right to Keep Fit,* Signet, 1970 edition

89   _____*Let's Get Well,* Signet, 1972 edition

90   _____*Let's Have Healthy Children,* Harcourt, Brace & World, 1959

91   _____*Let's Stay Healthy,* Harcourt Brace Jovanovich, 1981

92   _____*You Can Get Well,* The Original Health Book People, 1975

93   Davis, Francyne, *The Low Blood Sugar Cookbook,* Grosset & Dunlap, 1973

94   Dawson, Adele, *Health, Happiness and the Pursuit of Herbs,* Stephen Greene, 1980

95   Degan, Charles, *Age Without Fear,* Exposition Press, 1972

96   Denenberg, Herb, *Smart Shopper's Guide,* Chilton, 1978

97   de Spain, June, *Little Cyanide Cookbook,* American Media, 1976

98   Dick, William B., *Dick's Encyclopedia of Practical Receipts and Processes, or How They Did It in the 1870s,* Funk & Wagnalls reprint

99   Di Cyan, Erwin, *Vitamins in Your Life,* Simon & Schuster, 1972

100   Dong, Collin H. and Banks, Jane, *New Hope for the Arthritic,* Thomas Y. Crowell, 1975

101   Donsbach, Kurt W., *Menopause,* International Institute of Natural Health Sciences, 1977

102   _____*Stress,* International Institute of Natural Health Sciences, 1981

103   Dowd, Mary T. and Dent, Alberta, *Elements of Foods and Nutrition,* John Wiley & Sons, 1937

104   Dreyfack, Raymond, *The Complete Book of Walking,* Writer's House, 1979

105   Dufty, William, *Sugar Blues,* Warner Books, 1976

106   Ehrlich, David with Wolf, George, *The Bowel Book,* Schocken Books, 1981

107   Ehrmantraut, Harry C., *Headaches: The Drugless Way to Lasting Relief,* Autumn Press, 1977

108   Eichenlaub, John E., *A Minnesota Doctor's Home Remedies for Common and Uncommon Ailments,* Prentice-Hall, 1980

109   Ellis, John M. and Presley, James, *Vitamin B-6: The Doctor's Report,* Harper & Row, 1973

110   Elwood, Catharyn, *Feel Like a Million,* Devin-Adair, 1956

111   Emery, Carla, *Old-Fashioned Recipe Book,* Bantam Books, 1977

112   Eshleman, Ruthe and Winston, Mary, *American Heart Association Cookbook,* David McKay, 1979, third edition

113   Esko, Wendy, *Introducing Macrobiotic Cooking,* Japan Publications, 1978

114   Faelton, Sharon and editors of *Prevention Magazine, The Complete Book of Minerals for Health,* Rodale, 1981

115   _____*Vitamins for Better Health,* Rodale, 1982

116   Farb, Stanley M., *The Ear, Nose, and Throat Book: A Doctor's Guide to Better Health,* Appleton-Century Crofts, 1980

117   Feingold, Ben, *Why Your Child Is Hyperactive,* Random House, 1975

118   Finneson, Bernard E. and Freese, Arthur S., *Dr. Finneson on Low Back Pain,* Putnam's Sons, 1975

119   Fishbein, Morris, editor, *Modern Family Health Guide*, Doubleday, 1967 edition

120   Fisher, Arthur and Time-Life editors, *The Healthy Heart*, Time-Life, 1981

121   Fisher, M.F.K., *A Cordiall Water*, North Point Press, 1981 edition

122   Flaxman, Ruth, *Home Remedies for Common Ailments*, Putnam's Sons, 1982

123   Frazier, Claude A. and Brown F.K., *Insects and Allergy and What to Do About Them*, University of Oklahoma Press, 1980

124   Fredericks, Carlton, *Arthritis, Don't Learn to Live with It*, Grosset & Dunlap, 1981

125   _____*Eat Well, Get Well, Stay Well*, Grosset & Dunlap, 1980

126   _____*Psycho-Nutrition*, Grosset & Dunlap, 1976

127   _____*Winning the Fight Against Breast Cancer: The Nutritional Approach*, Grosset & Dunlap, 1977

128   Fredericks, Carlton and Bailey, Herbert, *Food Facts and Fallacies*, Arco, 1965

129   Fredericks, Carlton and Goodman, Herman, *Low Blood Sugar and You*, Constellation International, 1969

130   Freese, Arthur S., *The End of Senility*, Arbor House, 1978

131   Friedman, Sandor; Steinheber, Francis; and Lass, Abraham, *The Doctor's Guide to Growing Older*, New American Library, 1980

132   Fries, James, *Vitality and Aging*, W.H. Freeman, 1981

133   Galton, Lawrence, *The Disguised Disease: Anemia*, Crown, 1975

134   _____*The Silent Disease: Hypertension*, Crown, 1973

135   Garten, M.O., *The Health Secrets of a Naturopathic Doctor*, Parker, 1967

136   Gelb, Barbara Levine, *The Dictionary of Food*, Ballantine, 1979

137   Gerras, Charles, editor, *Feasting on Raw Foods*, Rodale, 1980

138   Gibbons, Euell, *Feast on a Diabetic Diet*, McKay, 1969

139   Gilmore, C.P. and Time-Life editors, *Exercising for Fitness*, Time-Life, 1981

140   Goldbeck, Nikki & David, *The Supermarket Handbook*, Signet, 1976

141   Goldberg, Phillip and Kaufman, Daniel, *Natural Sleep, How to Get Your Share*, Rodale, 1978

142   Goodenough, Josephus, *Dr. Goodenough's Home Cures and Herbal Remedies of 1904*, Crown, 1982 edition

143   Green, Bernard and Schwarz, Ted, *Goodbye Blues*, McGraw-Hill, 1981

144   Guerra, Luis, *The Bio-Diet*, Crown, 1982

145   *Guide to Consumer Product Information*, Bristol-Meyers, 1978

146   Haggard, Howard D., *Devils, Drugs and Doctors*, Harper & Brothers, 1929

147   Hales, Dianne, *The Complete Book of Sleep*, Addison Wesley, 1981

148   Hall, Dorothy, *The Herb Tea Book*, Keats, 1980

149   Hamilton, Richard, *The Herpes Book*, St. Martin's Press, 1980

150   *Handbook for Home Growing and History of the Ornamental and Exotic Aloe Vera Plant*, Nurserymen's Exchange, 1977

151   Harris, Ben Charles, *The Compleat Herbal*, Larchmont, 1972

152   _____*Kitchen Medicines*, Weathervane Books, 1968 edition

153   Harris, M. Coleman and Shure, Norman, *All About Allergy*, Prentice-Hall, 1969

154   Hauser, Gayelord, *Treasury of Secrets*, Farrar, Straus & Co., 1963 edition

155   Healthful Living Today editors, *Natural Foods and Your Health Food Store, What's in It for You?*, Keats, 1974

156   Heimlich, Henry J. with Galton, Lawrence, *Home Guide to Emergency Situations*, Simon & Schuster, 1980

157   *Heinz Handbook of Nutrition*, McGraw-Hill, 1959

158   Herter, George Leonard and Berthe E., *Bull Cook and Authentic Historical Recipes and Practices, Volume 11*, Herter's Inc., 1973 edition

159   _____*Bull Cook and Authentic Historical Recipes and Practices, Volume III*, Herter's Inc., 1974

160   Herter, Geroge L. and Berthe E., *George the Housewife*, Herter's Inc., 1973 ed.

161   Hess, John L. and Karen, *The Taste of America*, Penguin Books, 1977

162   Hess, Mary Abbott and Hunt, Anne Elise, *Pickles and Ice Cream*, McGraw-Hill, 1982

163   Hewitt, Edward R., *Lecithin and Health*, Health Publishing Co., 1977 edition

164   _____*The Years Between 75 and 90*, Health Publishing Co., 1957

165   Hill, Ann (editor), *Visual Encyclopedia of Unconventional Medicine*, Crown, 1979

166   Hill, Howard E., *Introduction to Lecithin*, Pyramid, 1972

167   Hills, Hilda Cherry, *Good Food to Fight Migraine*, Keats, 1978

168   Hirschhorn, Howard H., *Pain-Free Living: How to Prevent and Eliminate Pain All Over the Body*, Parker, 1977

169   Hoehn, Gustave, *Acne Can Be Cured*, Arco, 1977

170   Hoffer, Abram and Walker, Morton, *Nutrients to Age Without Senility*, Keats, 1980

171   _____*Orthomolecular Nutrition, New Lifestyle for Super Good Health*, Keats, 1978

172   Hoffman, Joyce and editors of *Prevention Magazine, Here's to Your Good Health*, Rodale, 1980

173   Houston, F.M., *The Healing Benefits of Acupressure*, Keats, 1974 edition

174   Hurdle, J. Frank, *A Country Doctor's Common Sense Health Manual*, Parker, 1975

175   _____*Low Blood Sugar, A Doctor's Guide to Its Effective Control*, Parker, 1969

176   Hutchinson, E., *Ladies' Indispensable Assistant*, New York, 1852

177   Huxley, Alyson and Back, Philippa, *The Two-in-One Herb Book*, Keats, 1982

178   Jacobson, E., *Progressive Relaxation*, University of Chicago Press, 1938

179   James, Claudia V., *That Old Green Magic*, Amitra Books, Canada, 1952

180   Jarvis, D.C., *Arthritis and Folk Medicine*, Fawcett, 1960

181 _____*Folk Medicine,* Holt, Rinehart & Winston, 1958

182 Jencks, Beata, *Your Body: Biofeedback at Its Best,* Nelson Hall, 1977

183 Jennings, Isobel, *Vitamins in Endocrine Metabolism,* Charles C. Thomas, 1970

184 Kadans, Joseph M., *Encyclopedia of Fruits, Vegetables, Nuts and Seeds for Healthful Living,* Parker, 1973

185 Kamen, Betty and Si, *Total Nutrition During Pregnancy,* Appleton-Century-Crofts, 1981

186 Keim, Hugo A., *How to Care for Your Back,* Prentice-Hall, 1981

187 Kelley, Wm. Donald, *One Answer to Cancer,* Kelley Foundation, 1974 edition

188 Kirban, Salem, *The Getting Back to Nature Diet,* Keats, 1978

189 Kirschmann, John D. (director, Nutrition Search), *Nutrition Almanac,* McGraw-Hill, 1977, plus 1979, revised edition

190 Kloss, Jethro, *Back to Eden,* Woodbridge Press, 1975 edition

191 Kordel, Lelord, *Natural Folk Remedies,* Putnam's Sons, 1974

192 Kraskin, Robert, *You Can Improve Your Vision,* Doubleday, 1968

193 Krause, Marie V. and Hunscher, Martha A., *Food, Nutrition and Diet Therapy,* W.B. Saunders Co., 1972, fifth edition

194 Kugler, Hans J., *Dr. Kugler's 7 Keys to a Longer Life,* Stein & Day, 1978

195 _____*Slowing Down the Aging Process,* Pyramid, 1973

196 Kugler, Matthew J., *Fever: Its Biology, Evolution and Function,* Princeton University Press, 1979

197 Kulvinkas, Victoras, *Love Your Body,* Omangod Press, 1974

198 Kunin, Richard, *Mega-Nutrition,* McGraw-Hill, 1980

199 Kyser, Franklin A., *Therapeutics in Internal Medicine,* Thomas Nelson & Sons, 1950

200 Lamb, Lawrence E., *Metabolics,* Harper & Row, 1974

201 Lang, George, *Lang's Compendium of Culinary Nonsense and Trivia,* Clarkson N. Potter, Crown, 1980

202 Lansky, Vicki, *The Taming of the C.A.N.D.Y. Monster,* Meadowbrook Press, 1978

203 Lappe, Frances Moore, *Diet for a Small Planet,* Ballantine, 1971

204 Law, Donald, *A Guide to Alternative Medicine,* Doubleday Dolphin, 1976

205 Lee, William, *Bee Pollen: Nature's Energizer,* Keats, 1983

206 Lehner, Ernst and Johanna, *Folklore and Odysseys of Food and Medicinal Plants,* Tudor, 1962

207 Lenz, Frederick P., *Total Relaxation,* Bobbs-Merrill, 1980

208 Leonard, Jon N.; Hofer, J.L. and Pritikin, N., *Live Longer Now,* Charter Communications, 1974

209 Lewis, David, *How to Be a Gifted Parent,* W.W. Norton, 1979

210 Light, Marilyn, *Hypoglycemia: One of Man's Most Widespread and Misdiagnosed Diseases,* Keats, 1983

211 Lowenfeld, Claire and Back, Philippa, *Herbs, Health and Cookery,* Gramercy, 1965

212 Lowenkopf, Anne, N., *Osteopuncture,* Medical Arts Press, 1976

213   Lubowe, Irwin I., *A Teenage Guide to Healthy Skin and Hair*, E.P. Dutton, 1979
214   Lucas, Richard, *The Magic of Herbs in Daily Living*, Parker, 1972
215   _____*Nature's Medicines*, Parker, 1966
216   Mackarness, Richard, *Living Safely in a Polluted World*, Stein & Day, 1980
217   Maltz, Maxwell, *Psycho-Cybernetics*, Prentice-Hall, 1960
218   Margo, *Growing New Hair*, Autumn Press, 1980
219   Margolius, Sidney, *Health Foods, Facts and Fakes*, Walker &Co., 1973
220   Maroon, Joseph C., *What You Can Do About Cancer*, Doubleday, 1969
221   Marshall, John L. with Barbash, Heather, *The Sports Doctor's Fitness Book for Women*, Delacorte Press, 1981
222   Marshall, Mel, *Real Living with Real Foods*, Fawcett, 1974
223   McGuire, Thomas L., *The Tooth Trip*, Random House/Bookworks, 1972
224   McLeish, John A.G., *The Ulyssean Adult*, McGraw-Hill, 1976
225   Mendelsohn, Robert S., *Confessions of a Medical Heretic*, Contemporary, 1979
226   Meyer, Clarence, *American Folk Medicine*, New American Library, 1973
227   _____*Vegetarian Medicines*, Meyerbooks, 1980
228   Mindell, Earl, *Earl Mindell's Quick and Easy Guide to Better Health*, Keats, 1982
229   _____*Earl Mindell's Vitamin Bible*, Warner Books, 1979
230   Mirsky, Stanley and Heilman, Joan Rattner, *Diabetes: Controlling it the Easy Way*, Random House, 1981
231   Montagu, Ashley, *Life Before Birth*, New American Library, 1964
232   Morales, Betty Lee, *Aloe Vera—The Miracle Plant*, Health in Mind & Body, 1977
233   Morrison, Lester M., *The Low-Fat Way to Health and Longer Life*, Prentice-Hall, 1958
234   Murphy, Wendy, *Coping with the Common Cold*, Time-Life, 1981
235   _____*Dealing with Headaches*, Time-Life, 1982
236   _____*Touch, Taste, Smell, Sight and Hearing*, Time-Life, 1982
237   Mylander, Maureen, *Great American Stomach Book*, Ticknor & Fields, 1982
238   Newbold, H.L., *Mega-Nutrients for Your Nerves*, Berkley, 1978
239   Newby, Hayes A., *Audiology*, Appleton-Century Crofts, 1972, third edition
240   Noble, Elizabeth, *Having Twins*, Houghton Mifflin, 1980
241   Norfolk, Donald, *The Habits of Health*, St. Martin's Press, 1976
242   Notelovitz, Morris, *Stand Tall: The Informed Woman's Guide to Preventing Osteoporosis*, Triad, 1982
243   Null, Gary and Steve, *Complete Handbook of Nutrition*, Dell, 1972
244   Ott, John, *Health and Light*, Simon & Schuster, 1976
245   Outerbridge, David E., *Hangover Handbook*, Harmony Books, 1981
246   Padus, Emrika, *Woman's Encyclopedia of Health and Natural Healing*, Rodale, 1981
247   Page, Robin, *Cures and Remedies the Country Way*, Summit Books, 1978
248   Passwater, Richard A., *Cancer and Its Nutritional Therapies*, Keats, 1978

249   _____*Selenium as Food and Medicine*, Keats, 1980

250   _____*Super-Nutrition*, Simon & Schuster Pocket Books, 1975

251   Pauling, Linus, *Vitamin C, the Common Cold and the Flu*, W.H. Freeman, 1970

252   Pearson, Durk and Shaw, Sandy, *Life Extension*, Warner Books, 1983

253   Pelletier, Kenneth R., *Holistic Medicine: From Stress to Optimum Health*, Delecorte/Seymour, 1979

254   Pelstring, Linda and Hauck, Jo Ann, *Food to Improve Your Health*, Walker & Co., 1974

255   Pfeiffer, Carl C., *Mental and Elemental Nutrients*, Keats, 1975

256   _____*Zinc and Other Micro-Nutrients*, Keats, 1978

257   Pfeiffer, Carl and Banks, Jane, *Total Nutrition*, Simon & Schuster, 1980

258   Philpott, William H. and Kalita, Dwight K., *Brain Allergies*, Keats, 1980

259   Plaut, Martin E., *The Doctor's Guide to You and Your Colon*, Harper & Row, 1982

260   *Prevention Magazine* Staff, *The Complete Book of Vitamins*, Rodale, 1977

261   _____*The Encyclopedia of Common Diseases*, Rodale, 1976

262   _____*No More Headaches*, Rodale, 1982

263   _____*Rub Your Headache Away*, Rodale, 1979

264   Price, Joseph M., *Coronaries, Cholesterol, Chlorine*, Pyramid, 1971

265   Price, Weston, *Nutrition and Physical Degeneration*, Price-Pottenger, 1977

266   Pritikin, Nathan and McGrady, Patrick, Jr., *The Pritikin Program*, Grosset & Dunlap, 1978

267   Rapaport, Howard and Linde, Shirley M., *The Complete Allergy Guide*, Simon & Schuster, 1970

268   Rapp, Doris, *Allergies and Your Family*, Sterling Publishing, 1981

269   Reader's Digest, *Eat Better, Live Better*, Reader's Digest Association, 1982

270   _____*Our Human Body*, Reader's Digest Association, 1962

271   Regnier, Edme, *The Administration of Large Doses of Ascorbic Acid in the Prevention and Treatment of the Common Cold*, Review of Allergy, 1968

272   Reilly, Harold H., and Brod, Ruth Hagy, *The Edgar Cayce Handbook for Health Through Drugless Therapy*, Macmillan, 1975

273   Reuben, David, *Everything You Always Wanted to Know About Nutrition*, Simon & Schuster, 1978

274   _____*The Save Your Life Diet*, Ballantine, 1975

275   Revell, Dorothy, *Hypoglycemia Control Cookery*, Berkley, 1973

276   Riker, Tom and Robert, Richard, *Directory of Natural and Health Foods*, Paragon, 1979

277   Rinzler, Carol Ann, *The Dictionary of Medical Folklore*, Ballantine, 1980

278   Rivlin, Richard, *Riboflavin*, Plenum Press, 1975

279   Roberts, Sam E., *Exhaustion: Causes and Treatment*, Rodale Press, 1967

280   Rodale, J.I., *If You Must Smoke*, Pyramid, 1968

281   Rodale, J.I. and staff of Prevention Magazine, *Bone Meal for Good Teeth*, Rodale, 1972

282   _____*Complete Book of Minerals for Health*, Rodale, 1972

283 Rosanes-Berret, Marilyn, *Do You Really Need Eyeglasses?*, Hart, 1974

284 Rose, Jeanne, *Herbs and Things*, Grosset & Dunlap, 1972

285 Rose, Louisa, *The Menopause Book*, Hawthorn/E.P. Dutton, 1977

286 Rubin, Herman H., *Your Life Is in Your Glands*, Auburn Press, 1948

287 Schauss, Alexander, *Diet, Crime and Delinquency*, Parker House, 1980

288 Schifferes, Justus J., *Family Medical Encyclopedia*, Little, Brown, 1959

289 Schneider, L.L., with Stone, Robert B., *Old Fashioned Health Remedies That Work Best*, Parker, 1977

290 Schulman, Brian and Smoller, Bruce, *Pain Control*, Doubleday, 1982

291 Schultz, William, *Shiatsu*, Bell Publishing, 1976

292 Schwartz, Alice Kuhn and Aaron, Norma S., *Somniquest*, Harmony Books, 1979

293 Scott, Cyril, *Cider Vinegar, Nature's Great Health-Promoter*, Athene, England, 1982, revised edition

294 Seaman, Barbara, *Women and the Crisis in Sex Hormones*, Rawson, 1977

295 Seegmiller, J.P., *Gout*, Grune & Stratton, 1967

296 Segerberg, Osborn, Jr., *Living to Be 100*, Charles Scribner's Sons, 1982

297 Sehnert, Keith W. with Eisenberg, Howard, *How to Be Your Own Doctor (Sometimes)*, Grosset & Dunlap, 1981 edition

298 Shames, Richard and Sterin, Chuck, *Healing with Mind Power*, Rodale, 1978

299 Shute, Evan V., *Common Questions on Vitamin E and Their Answers*, Keats, 1979 ed.

300 Shute, Wilfrid E., *Health Preserver*, Rodale, 1977

301 ———*Vitamin E Book*, Keats, 1978 edition

302 ———*Vitamin E for Ailing and Healthy Hearts*, Pyramid, 1969

303 Siegal, Sanford, *Dr. Siegal's Natural Fiber Permanent Weight-Loss Diet*, Dell, 1975

304 Slaughter, Frank G., *Science and Surgery*, Perma Books, 1956

305 Smith, Lendon, *Feed Your Kids Right*, Dell, 1979

306 ———*Improving Your Child's Behavior Chemistry*, Simon & Schuster Pocket Books, 1977

307 Spock, Benjamin, *Baby and Child Care*, Simon & Schuster, 1976

308 Stern, Jess, *Edgar Cayce, the Sleeping Prophet*, Doubleday, 1967

309 Stone, Irwin, *The Healing Factor: Vitamin C Against Disease*, Grosset & Dunlap, 1972

310 Stoppard, Miriam, *Healthcare*, Weidenfeld & Nicolson, London, 1980

311 Svensson, Jon-Erik, *Folk Remedies, Receipts and Advice*, Berkley, 1977

312 Swartout, Hubert O., *Modern Medical Counselor*, Review & Herald, 1943

313 Talbot, Richard, *How to Succeed with Your Own Body*, Mr. Health, Inc., 1973

314 Tanner, Ogden, *The Prudent Use of Medicines*, Time-Life, 1981

315 Taylor, Robert B., *Dr. Taylor's Self-Help Medical Guide*, Arlington House, 1977

316 ———*Feeling Alive After 65*, Arlington House, 1973

317 Tenenbaum, Frances, *Over 55 Is not Illegal*, Houghton Mifflin, 1979
318 Thomas, Mai, *Grannies' Remedies*, Gramercy, 1965
319 Thompson, William A.R., *Herbs That Heal*, Charles Scribner's Sons, 1976
320 Tilden, J.H., *The Pocket Dietitian*, Brock-Haffner Press, 1918
321 Time-Life editors, *Wholesome Diet*, Time-Life, 1981
322 Tobe, John, *Cataract, Glaucoma and Other Eye Disorders*, Provoker Press, 1971
323 Turin, Alan C., *No More Headaches*, Houghton Mifflin, 1981
324 Tyree, Marion Cabell (editor), *Housekeeping in Old Virginia*, John P. Morton, 1879
325 Van Fleet, James K., *Extraordinary Healing Secrets from a Doctor's Private Files*, Parker, 1977
326 Vaughan, Clark, *Addictive Drinking*, Viking, 1982
327 Vaughan, Warren, T., *Practice of Allergy*, C.V. Mosby, 1939
328 _____*The Story of Allergy*, Blue Ribbon Books, 1940
329 Verdesca, Arthur S., *Live, Work and Be Healthy*, Van Nostrand Reinhold, 1980
330 Wade, Carlson, *Bee Pollen and Your Health*, Keats, 1978
331 _____*Carlson Wade's Lecithin Book*, Keats, 1980
332 _____*Catalytic Hormones*, Parker, 1982
333 _____*Health Secrets from the Orient*, Parker, 1973
334 _____*Helping Yourself with New Enzyme Catalyst Health Secrets*, Parker, 1981
335 _____*Natural Folk Remedies*, Globe, 1979
336 Walford, Roy L., *Maximum Life Span*, W.W. Norton, 1983
337 Walker, Norman W., *Pure and Simple Natural Weight Control*, O'Sullivan Woodside, 1981
338 Warner, Rebecca; Wolfe, Sidney M.; and Rich, Rebecca, *Off Diabetes Pills*, Public Citizen's Health Research Group, 1978
339 Watt, Bernice K. and Merrill, Annabel L., *Composition of Foods: Raw, Processed*, (Handbook #8) U.S. Dept. of Agriculture, 1975
340 Weg, Ruth B., *Nutrition and the Later Years*, University of Southern California Press, 1978
341 Welk, Lawrence, *You're Never Too Young*, Prentice-Hall, 1981
342 Weller, Charles, *New Way to Live with Diabetes*, Doubleday, 1966
343 Wentzler, Rich, *The Vitamin Book*, Gramercy, 1980 edition
344 White, Ellen G., *Healthful Living*, Medical Missionary Board, 1898
345 Wigginton, Eliot (editor), *The Foxfire Book*, Doubleday Anchor Books, 1972
346 Wigmore, Ann, *Be Your Own Doctor*, Hemisphere Press, revised seventh printing
347 Williams, Roger J., *Alcoholism, the Nutritional Approach*, University of Texas Press, 1951
348 _____*Nutrition Against Disease*, Pitman, 1971

349 _____*Nutrition in a Nutshell,* Doubleday, 1962

350 Williams, Roger J. and Kalita, Dwight K., *Physician's Handbook on Ortho-Molecular Medicine,* Keats, 1977

351 Wilson, Fisher and Fuqua, *Principles of Nutrition,* John Wiley & Sons, 1975 ed.

352 Wordsworth, Jill, *Diet Revolution,* St. Martin's Press, 1977

353 Wright, Jonathan V., *Dr. Wright's Book of Nutritional Therapy,* Rodale, 1979

354 Yudkin, John, *Sweet and Dangerous,* Bantam Books, 1973

INDEX